501 BEST

HIGH-INTENSITY

EXERCISES

General Disclaimer

The contents of this book are intended to provide useful information to the general public. All materials, including texts, graphics, and images, are for informational purposes only and are not a substitute for medical diagnosis, advice, or treatment for specific medical conditions. All readers should seek expert medical care and consult their own physicians before commencing any exercise program or for any general or specific health issues. The author and publishers do not recommend or endorse specific treatments, procedures, advice, or other information found in this book and specifically disclaim all responsibility for any and all liability, loss, or risk, personal or otherwise, which is incurred as a consequence, directly or indirectly, of the use or application of any of the material in this publication.

MOSELEY ROAD INC.
International Rights and Packaging
22 Knollwood Avenue
Elmsford, NY 10523
www.moseleyroad.com

President Sean Moore
Project editorial and art director Lisa Purcell
Production director Adam Moore

Photography Naila Ruechel
www.nailaruechel.com

With thanks to CROSSFIT VALKYRIE
www.crossfitvalkyrie.com

Printed in China

ISBN 9781626691421

19 18 17 16 15 1 2 3 4 5

501 BEST HIGH-INTENSITY EXERCISES

THE ULTIMATE RESOURCE FOR CRAFTING HEART-POUNDING WORKOUTS

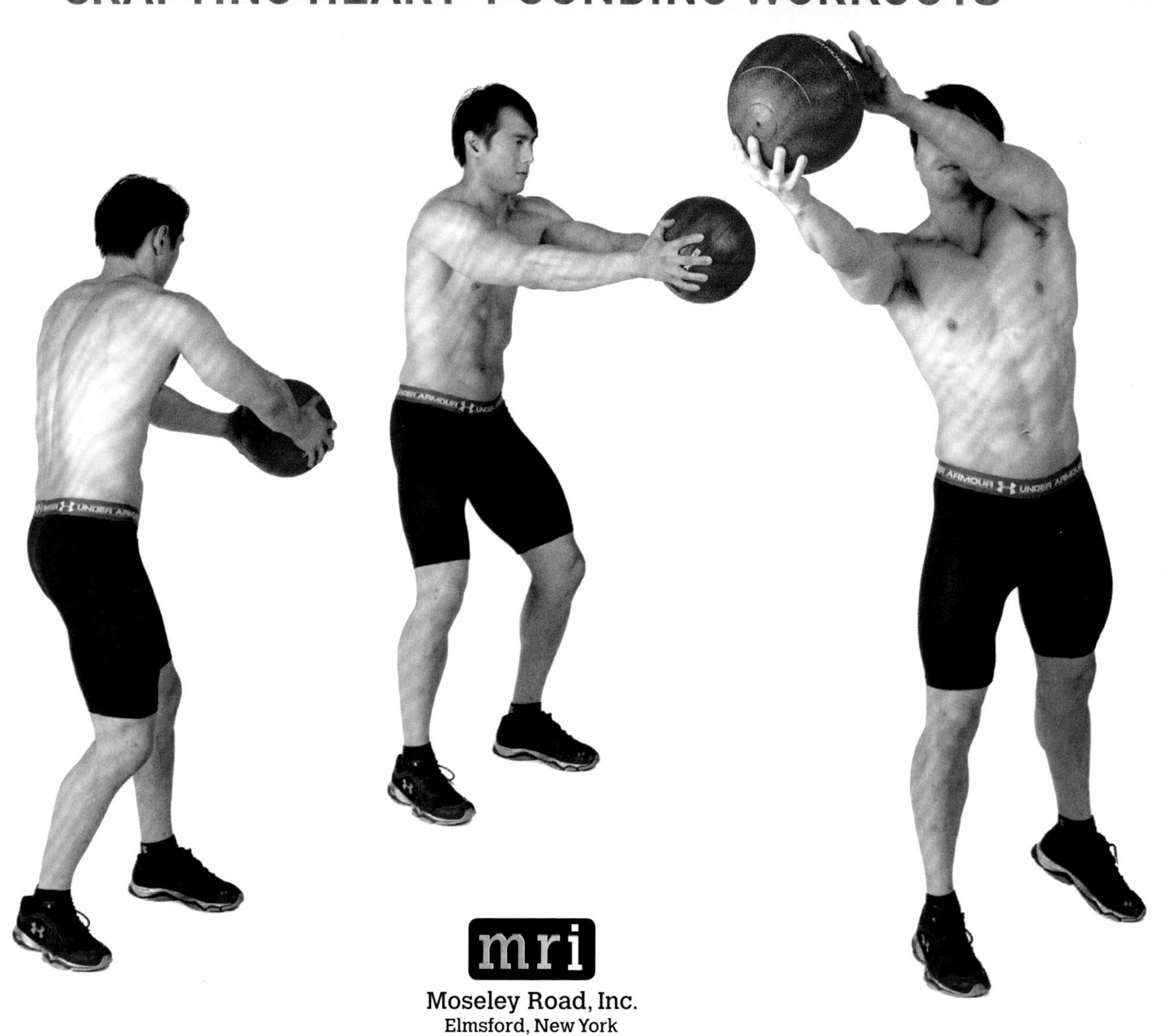

mri

Moseley Road, Inc.

Elmsford, New York

CONTENTS

CONTENTS

INTRODUCTION

UP YOUR FITNESS LEVEL WITH A HIGH-INTENSITY WORKOUT PROGRAM

Gym-goers these days are increasingly turning to high-intensity regimens, whether they are signing up for tried-and-true aerobic and spin classes or checking out fitness boot camps, functional training programs, group dance classes, battle rope regimens, suspension training, cardio boxing workouts, and scores of other demanding disciplines. You can incorporate aspects of all of these—and more—to craft your own high-intensity plan—a plan that will allow you to reap the greatest benefits for your hard work.

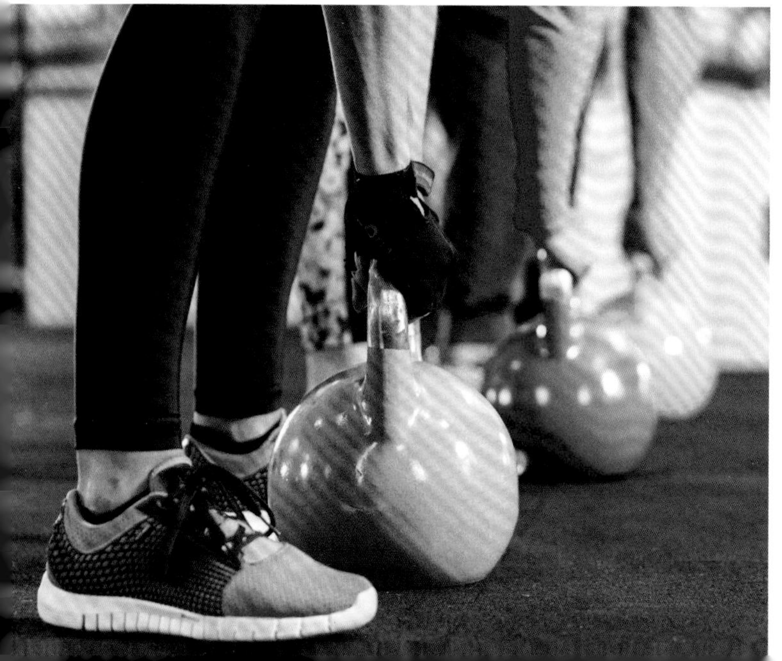

WHAT IS A HIGH-INTENSITY WORKOUT PROGRAM?

High-intensity workout programs feature multiple components: classic cardio training, such as running and cardio machine work; functional fitness moves, like Mountain Climbers and Squats that use everyday movement patterns; and exercises like the Push-Up (and its scores of variations) that help you build power and strength. In these pages you will find 501 of the best exercises to help you attain these benefits. You can incorporate them into a workout routine like HIIT, add them to a strength training regimen, or weave them into your cardio program. You can take the list to the gym, or you can perform most of them right at home or in your backyard.

CRAFTING YOUR OWN HIGH-INTENSITY WORKOUT

There are probably just as many ways to put a workout program together as there are exercises to incorporate into them. Still, there are a few guidelines to help you figure out how to achieve your individual fitness goals.

You can start by trying out a sampling of some of the featured exercises. Say that you want to work on lower-body toning—look for exercises like the many Squat and Lunge variations. Want to burn fat? Try one of the jumps or some of the ones labeled "plyo" or "plyometric," which are moves designed to incinerate calories and get your rate going. There are plenty, like the Burpees, which have multiple benefits, combining hard-core strength training with high-energy cardio. These exercises also work well in interval training or high-intensity interval (HIIT) regimens. This popular form of exercise combines two of the most effective fat-burning methods: a high-intensity component (like Mountain Climbers) and lower-intensity components (like Barbell Rows).

The high-intensity component means that, in a quick burst, you push your body to the absolute maximum in order to achieve muscle fatigue and maximum oxygen (keep in mind that the harder you work your muscles, the more oxygen they will require). Working your body at its near-maximum levels trigger what is known as the afterburn effect—in other words your body continues to consume oxygen and burn calories up to 48 hours after your workout. Of course, even elite athletes can only work at maximum levels for short bursts, so you need to incorporate intervals of lower-intensity activity. For example, you would first perform a 5-minute warm-up like jumping rope, then follow that with an eight-rep set of a strength exercise like Barbell Rows, and then follow that with a burst of fast Mountain Climbers for a minute. You would then repeat the entire routine for a 45-minute session. You vary this type of training by alternating one of he many strength moves found in this book with any one of its cardio or plyometric moves or with cardio machine work.

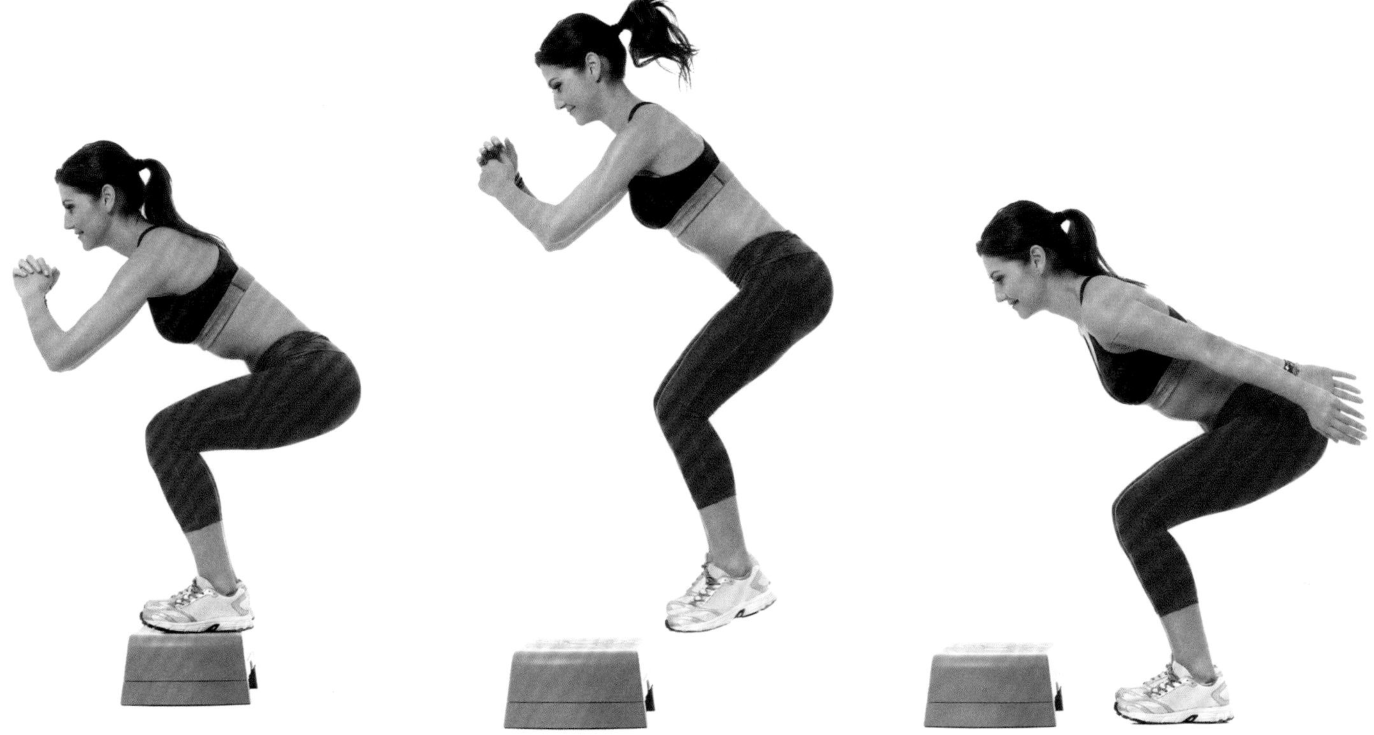

ADD IN SOME CLASSIC CARDIO

Along with the exercises featured in the following pages, a well-rounded high-intensity fitness program can include classic cardio work—those rows and rows of machines that fill just about every gym and health club these days. Here is a breakdown of a few of the most common.

Treadmill The mainstay of both commercial gyms and home fitness rooms, a treadmill allows you to get in your daily run or walk no matter what the weather. Jogging at a moderate pace for a half hour will burn about 350/half hour. You can use it to walk, jog, or run on an even surface or you can adjust the incline for a rigorous uphill workout. They help you lose weight, tone muscle, relieve stress, and improve your cardiovascular health.

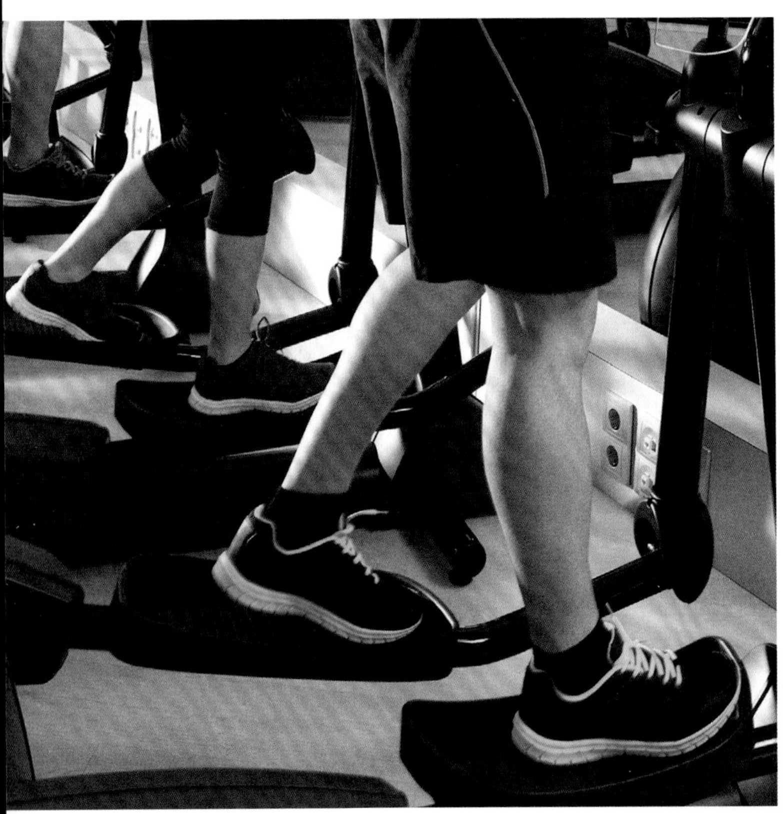

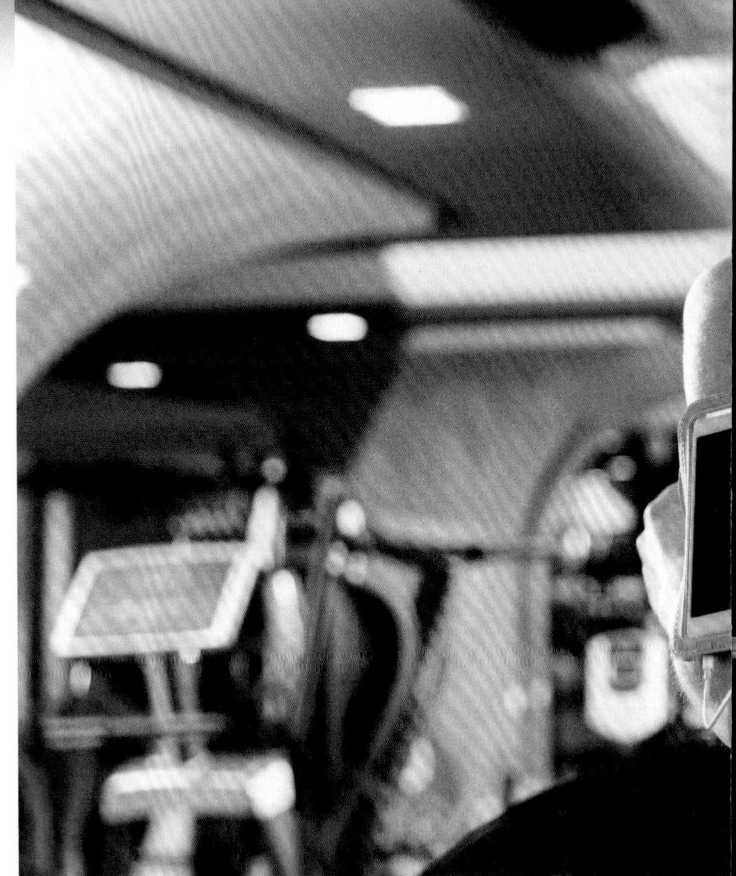

Stationary Bike This old-school piece of equipment offers high value. Working at a moderate pace, you can burn up to 650 calories per hour and improve heart and lung health, tone and strengthen muscles, and improve balance and coordination. It is also a low-impact form of exercise. You can find various versions at the gym—the standard upright, spin models, and recumbent styles that give you back support.

Elliptical Trainer No longer the new kid on the block, the elliptical trainer has become one of the most popular of the cardio machines, the go-to piece of equipment if you want an effective cardio workout with little stress on the joints. Spending a half hour on an elliptical will burn through 350 calories. It can help with blood pressure, improve heart and lung health, and build stronger bones.

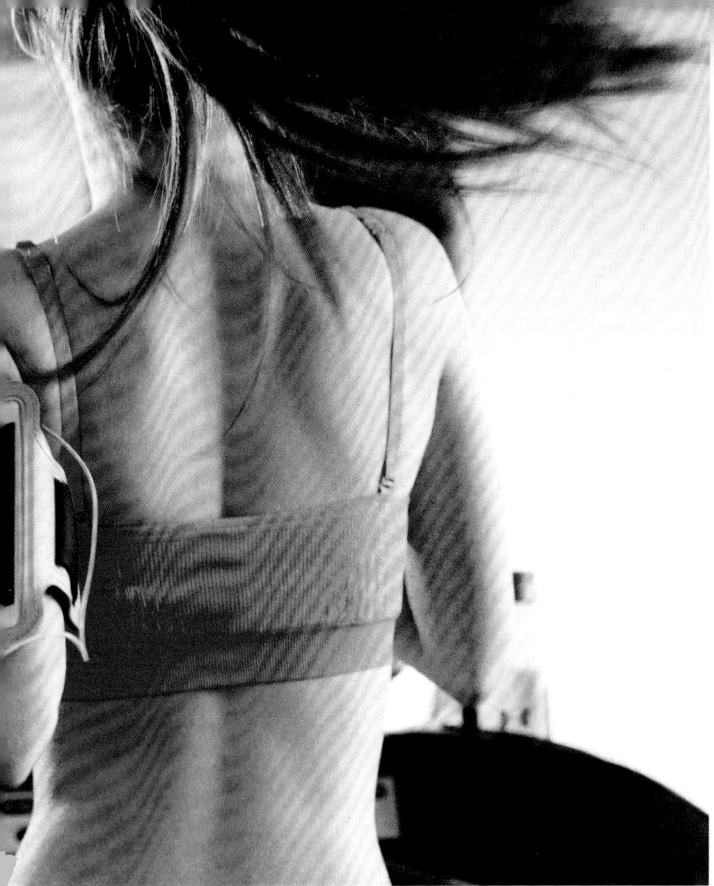

GET TO WORK!

Taken all together, combining a program of exercises and cardio will give you a high-intensity workout. This kind of program will help you to build lean muscle, burn fat, improve heart health, and increase oxygen utilization, while you also improve your balance, posture, coordination, agility, endurance, flexibility, and power. The work may be hard, the sweat copious, but who wouldn't want these benefits?

Rowing Machine Rowing machines are one of the cardio favorites of HIIT and functional training devotees, combining the best of a cardiovascular workout with powerful strength and endurance training. Rowing at a moderate pace for a half hour will burn about 200 calories and improves heart and lung health, tones and strengthens muscles, helps you drop the pounds, and reduces stress.

Stair Climber Also known as the stair machine, stair stepper, tread-climber or step machine, this star of the 1980s gym has proved its value over the years, becoming a favorite with gym-goers looking for a high-intensity workout. It offers efficient cardio, increases strength and body tone in your entire lower body, improves your balance, and engages your core muscles with every step. Working on a climber with burn about 180 in a half hour.

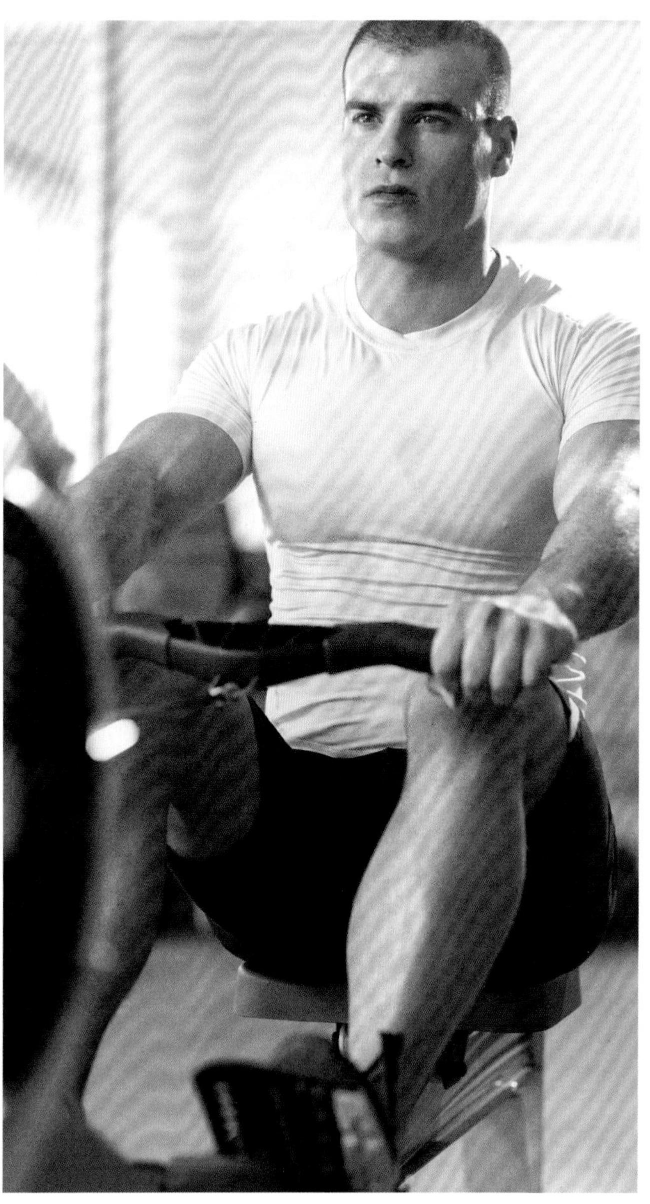

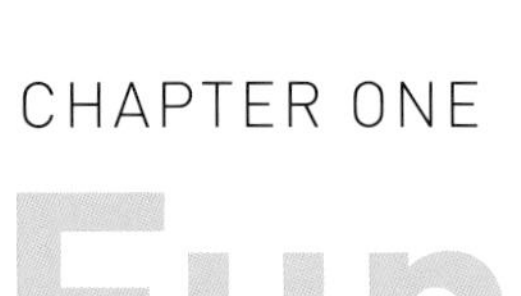

CHAPTER ONE

Functional Moves

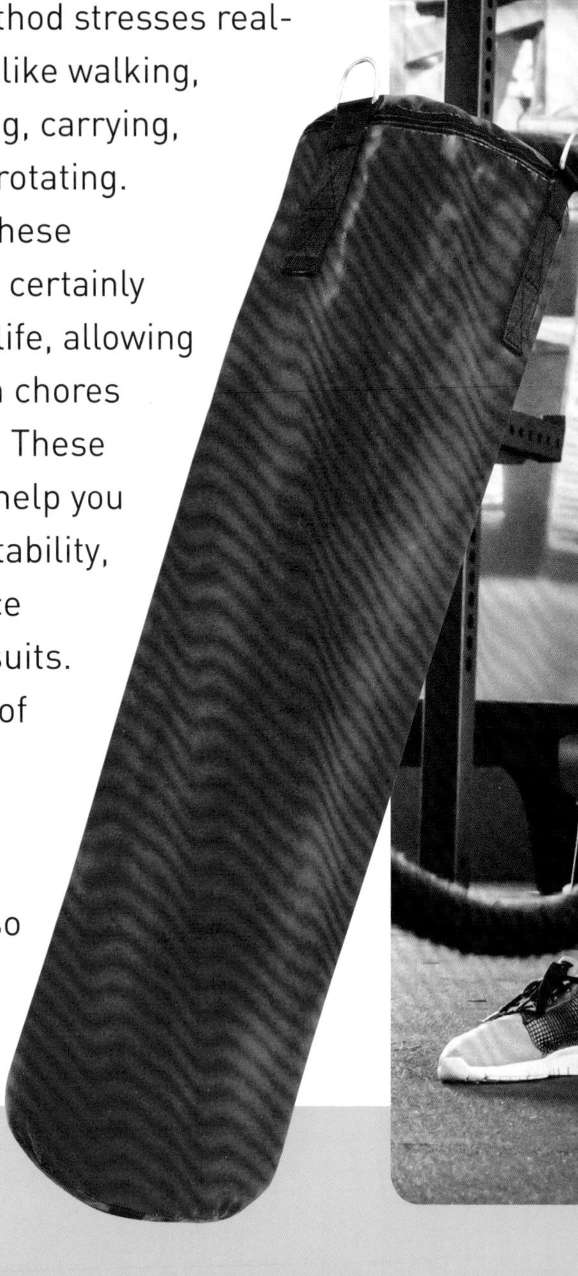

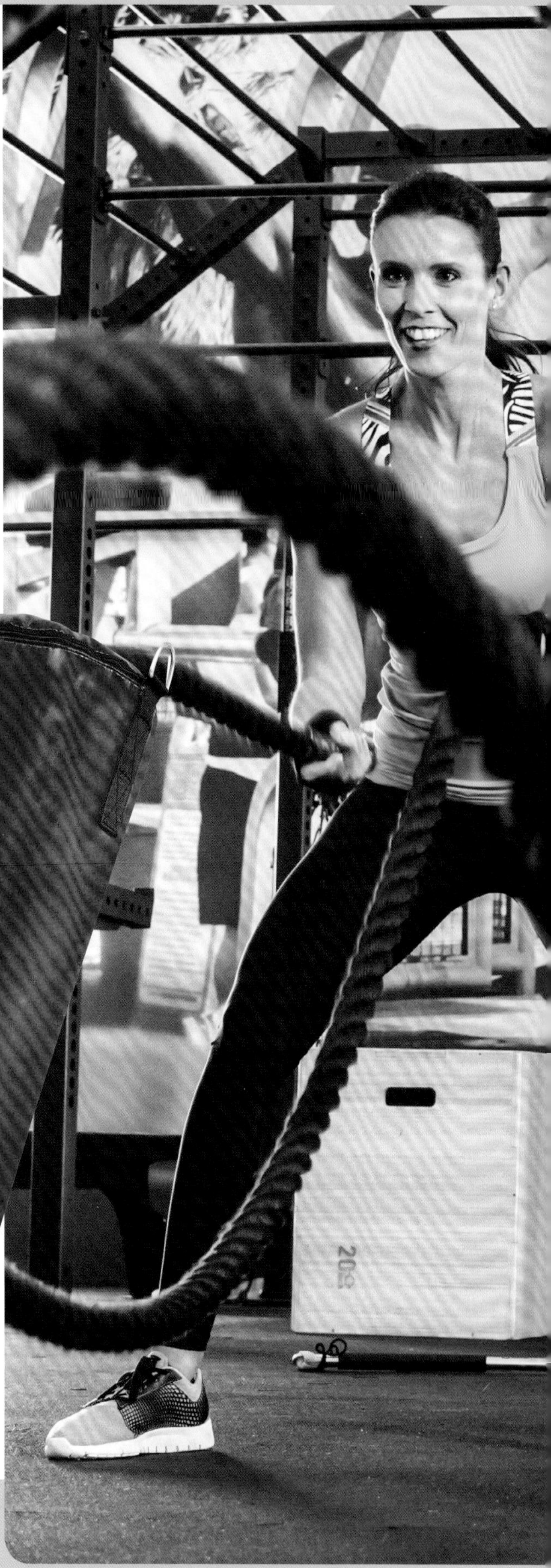

In recent years, functional training has become an entrenched part of the fitness scene. This training method stresses real-life movement patterns like walking, running, pushing, pulling, carrying, hinging, squatting, and rotating. Building proficiency in these movement patterns can certainly enhance your everyday life, allowing you to perform common chores and activities with ease. These kinds of exercises also help you to attain the strength, stability, flexibility, and endurance needed for athletic pursuits. Revving up these kinds of exercises during high-intensity functional training boosts their aerobic benefits and also increases your power and builds muscles.

Functional Moves

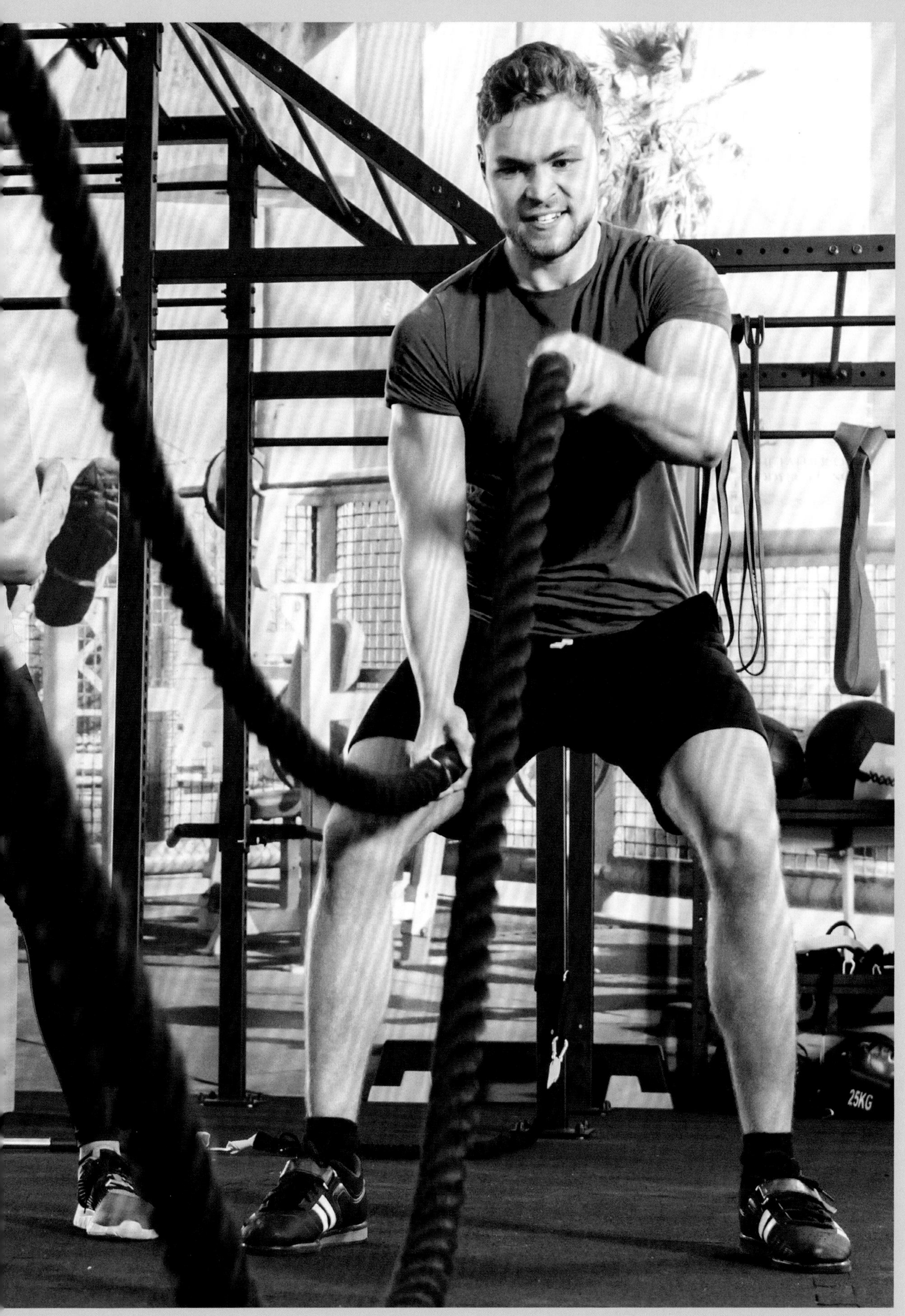

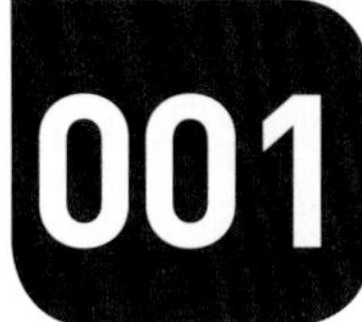

Basic Squat

Often called the "king of all exercises," the squat—and its many variations—is a hard-working exercise that fits into just about any workout regimen, from concentrated bodybuilding to high-intensity boot camp training. It is a compound movement that mimics natural, everyday movement patterns, working multiple joints and just about all your muscles, especially the thighs and glutes. Regularly performing squats can help you develop a strong core, increase lower body-strength and size, and promote joint health. Squats can also test your mental toughness; just try performing 20 well-executed reps. The movement may look simple, but pay close attention to your form: a poorly done squat can be hard on your hips, knees, and ankles.

- Stand with your legs and feet parallel and shoulder-width apart, and your knees bent very slightly. Tuck your pelvis slightly forward, lift your chest, and press your shoulders down and back.
- Extend your arms in front of your body for stability, keeping them even with your shoulders. With your feet planted firmly on the floor, curl your toes slightly upward.
- Draw in your abdominal muscles and bend into a squat. Keep your heels planted on the floor and your chest as upright as possible, resisting the urge to bend too far forward. Exhale, and return to the original position. Repeat for the desired repetitions.

FIND YOUR FORM

There is much debate about just how low you should squat. A general rule of thumb is that you should only go as low as you can while still maintaining a neutral, straight spine.

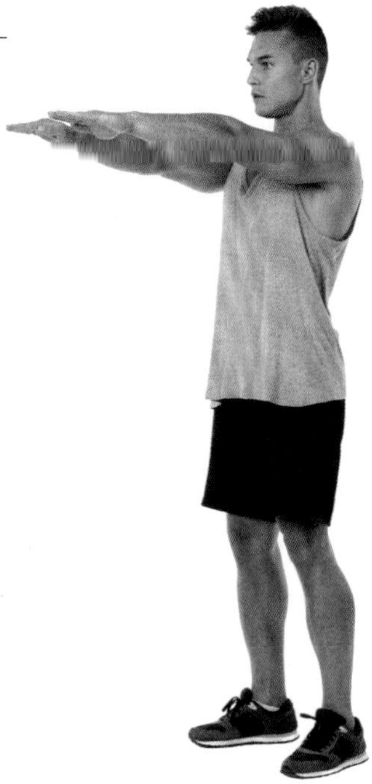

MUSCLE ANNOTATION KEY
Black bold = primary
Black = deep primary
Gray bold = secondary
Gray = deep secondary

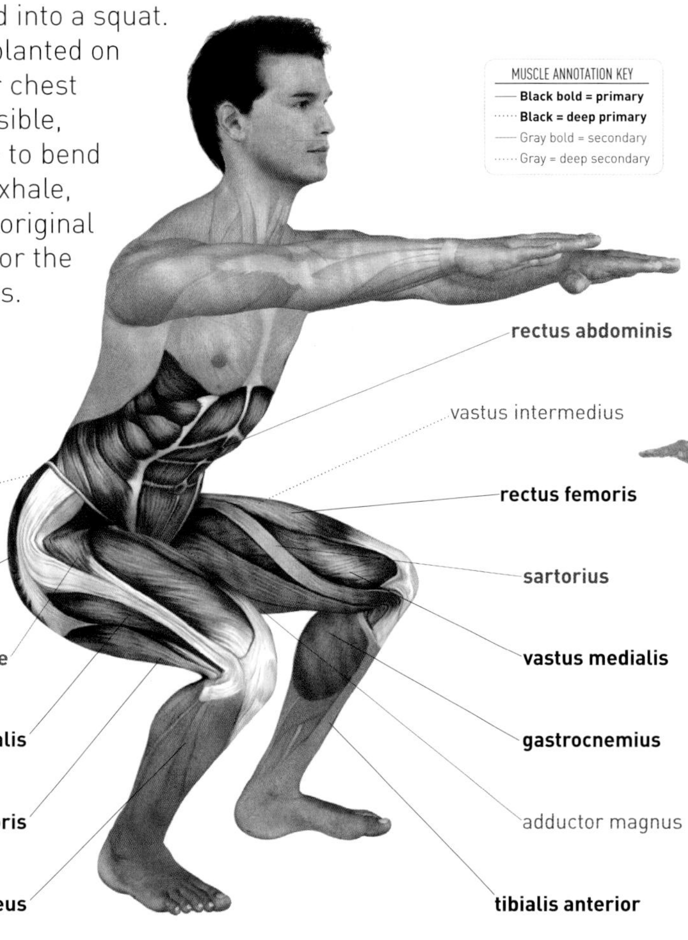

rectus abdominis
vastus intermedius
gluteus medius
rectus femoris
gluteus maximus
sartorius
tensor fasciae latae
vastus medialis
vastus lateralis
gastrocnemius
biceps femoris
adductor magnus
soleus
tibialis anterior

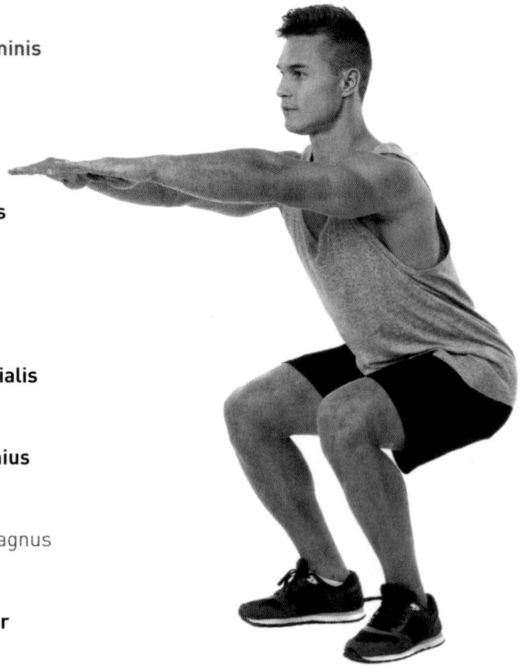

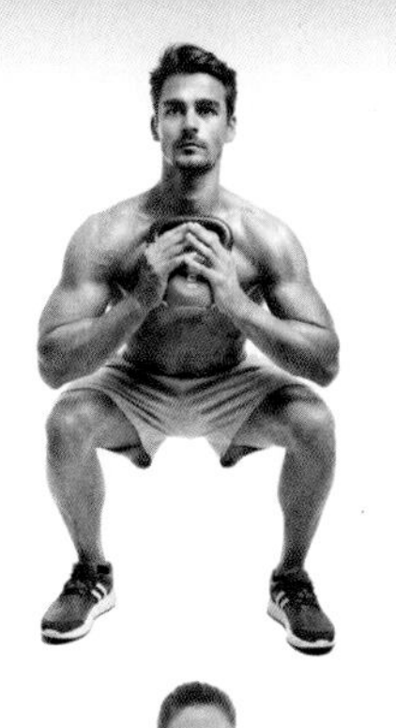

002 Goblet Squat

Hold a dumbbell or kettlebell vertically next to your chest, with both hands cupping the dumbbell head or kettlebell handle, as if it were a heavy goblet. Keeping your abs braced, push your hips back, and bend your knees to lower your body until your thighs are parallel to the floor. Pause, and then press upward back to the starting position, and repeat.

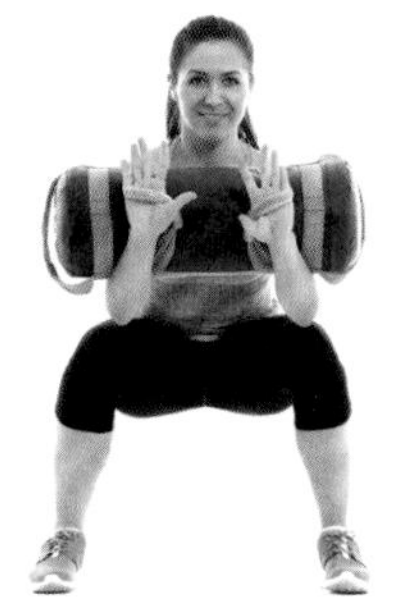

003 Sandbag Squat

Stand with your feet shoulder-width apart holding a sandbag across your upper chest. Push your hips back, and bend your knees to lower your body until your thighs are parallel to the floor. Drive your heels into the floor to push yourself explosively back up.

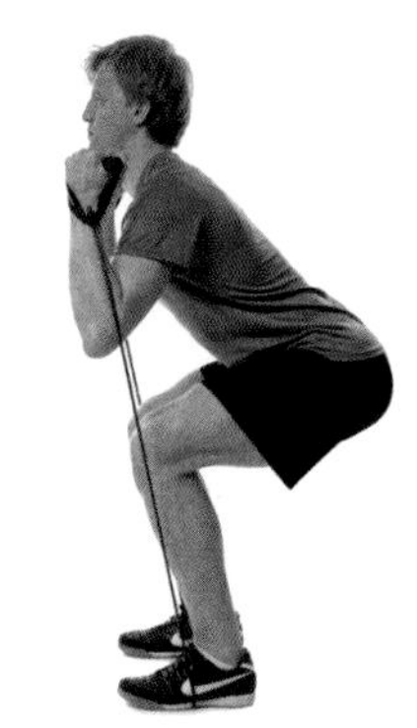

004 Resistance Band Squat

Secure a resistance under both feet. Stand with feet shoulder-width apart, and then with an end in each hand, bring your hands to shoulder level. Keeping your knees aligned with your toes, bend your knees, and lower your body. Keeping your back straight, raise yourself back to starting position, and repeat.

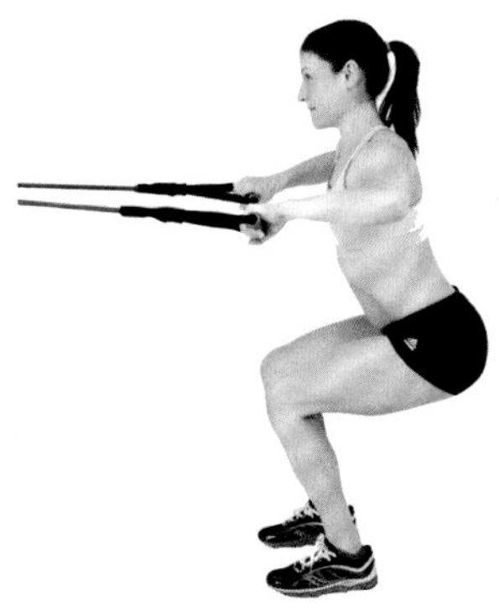

005 Squat and Row

Stand upright, holding both ends of a resistance band. Plant your feet hip-width apart, making sure your back is neither arched nor slumped. In a smooth movement, begin to bend your knees. At the same time, bend your elbows as you pull both ends of the band in toward your body. Keeping the rest of your body stable and your abdominals engaged, use both hands to pull the band even further toward your body. Smoothly return to starting position.

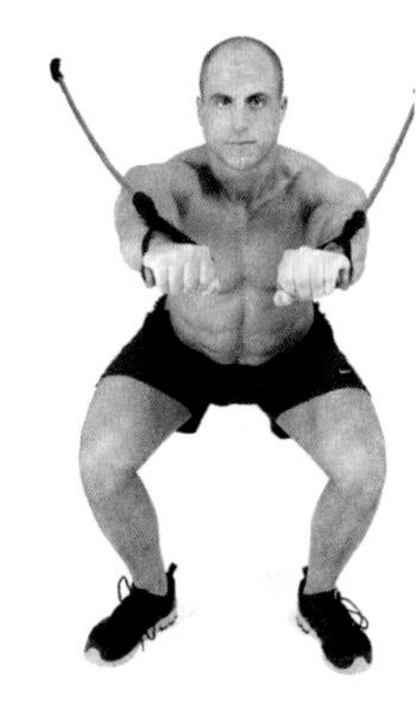

006 Press and Squat

Loop a resistance band around a weight machine. Stand facing away from the machine, your feet planted hip-distance apart or slightly wider, and grasp one handle in each hand. Bend your elbows, feeling resistance from the band as you raise both handles to shoulder height. Bend your knees into a squat position. Simultaneously straighten both arms in front of you, feeling resistance as you press. Gradually straighten your knees and release the handles, returning your arms to starting position.

THE BOSU BALANCE TRAINER

Invented by David Weck, a BOSU is an inflated rubber hemisphere attached to a rigid platform. You can use it with the dome side up or down. When facing up, the dome provides unstable surface while the device remains stable. Facing down, it becomes highly unstable. Either side works to add functional balance challenges for athletic drills, aerobic activities, and other exercises.

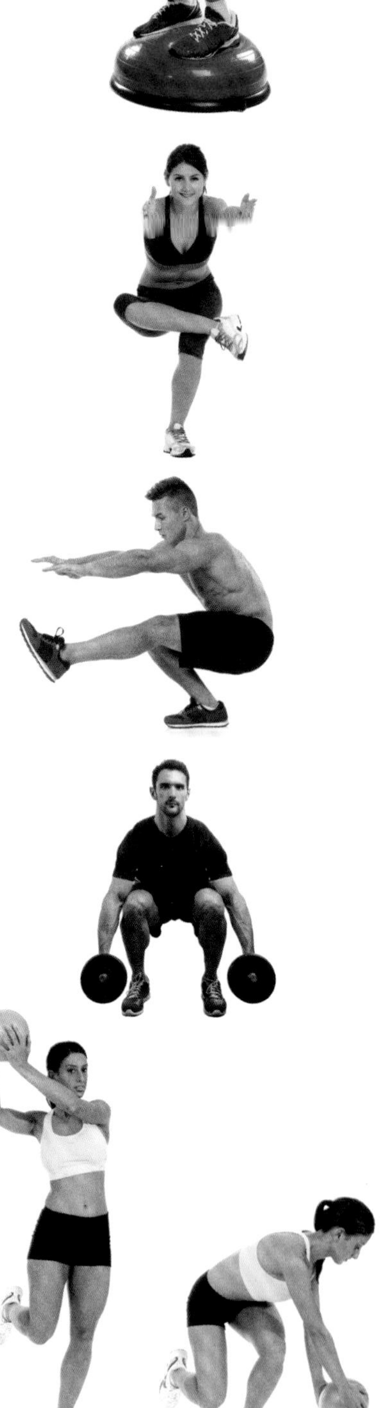

007 BOSU Squat

Up the level of difficulty by performing a Basic Squat (#001) on the dome side of a BOSU ball.

008 Single-Leg Squat

Stand holding your arms straight out in front of your body at shoulder level. Raise your right leg, and cross it over your left so that your right ankle rests just above your left knee. Push your hips back, and lower your body as far as you can. Hold for a count of one, and then push your body back to the starting position.

009 Pistol Squat

Stand holding your arms straight out in front of your body at shoulder level. Raise your right leg off the floor, and hold it there. Push your hips back, and lower your body as far as you can. Hold for a count of one, and then push your body back to the starting position.

010 Dumbbell Squat

Grasp a dumbbell in each hand, and stand with your legs and feet parallel and shoulder-width apart. Keeping your knees aligned with your toes, bend your knees, and lower your body into a squat position. Keeping your back straight, raise yourself back to starting position, and repeat.

011 Power Squat

Stand straight, holding a weighted ball in front of your torso. Shift your weight to your left foot, and bend your right knee, lifting your right foot toward your buttocks. Bend your elbows, and draw the ball toward the outside of your right ear. Bend at your hips and knee, and lower your torso to the left, bringing the ball toward your right ankle. Press into your left leg and straighten your knee and torso, returning to the starting position, and repeat.

012 Barbell Squat

The Barbell Squat is the most commonly performed of the weighted squats. Also known as High Bar Back Squat or Olympic Squat, you hold the bar right at the base of your neck across the top of your trapezius muscles. There are many variations of a this kind of squat—it all depends on how and where you hold the barbell. In a Low Bar Barbell Squat, for example, the bar sits lower on your back, and in front versions, you hold it in front of your chest. No matter which version, the Barbell Squat is a key exercise for training your lower body. As with any exercise, form is essential, and safety is crucial—this kind of weight movement calls for a high level of mobility at the hips, spine, and shoulders.

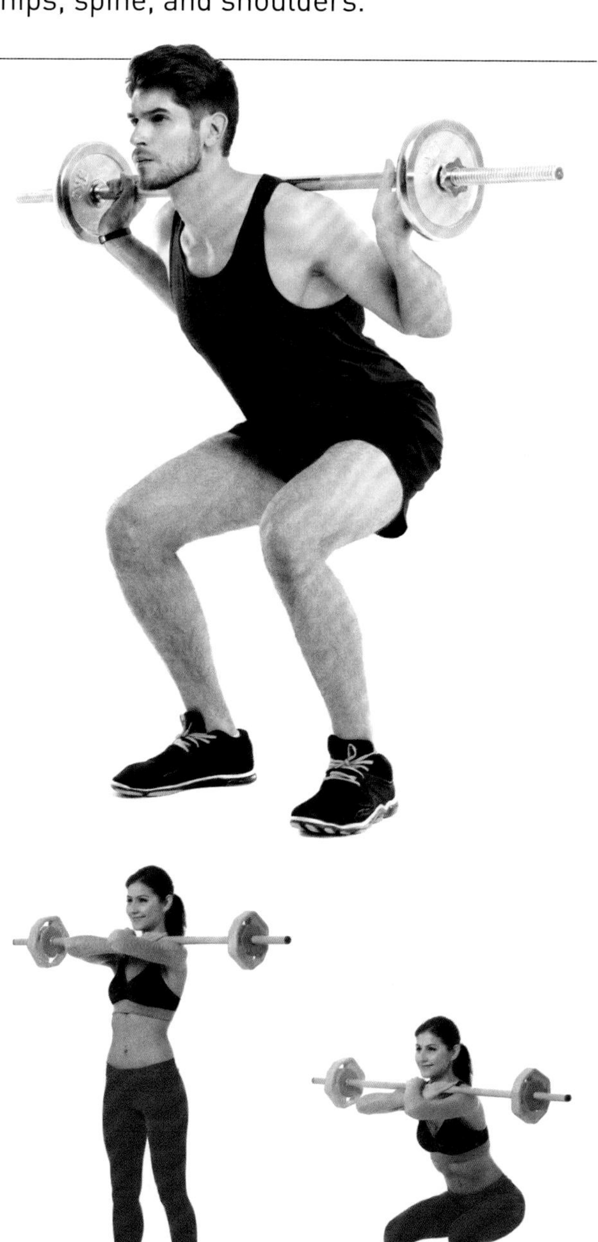

- Set up the barbell on a squat rack so that it is at the same height as your upper chest. Position your body under the bar, with your knees bent so that the bar is resting high on the back of your shoulders.
- Grip the bar with your hands comfortably wider than your shoulders. Slowly straighten your legs to push upwards, lifting the barbell from the rack and take one step forward.
- Standing with your legs shoulder-width apart, bend your knees forward and allow your hips to bend back as if your were sitting down until your thighs are parallel to the floor.
- Hold for a count of one, and then push up through your heels while straightening your hips and knees, until you have returned to the starting position.
- Repeat for the desired repetitions.

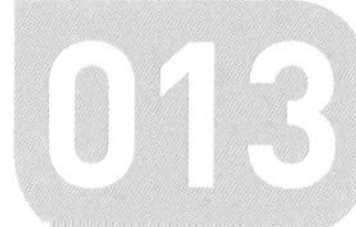

013 Front Barbell Squat

Stand upright, and take a barbell from a rack (or have a spotter help you), letting it rest along your upper chest Position your feet shoulder-width apart with your toes pointed slightly outward. Move your shoulders back and your chest out so your back is flat and your torso erect. Cross your forearms in front of your chest so that your upper arms are parallel to the floor and each hand is grasping the bar near the opposite shoulder. Perform a Basic Squat (#001), and then push up through your heels while straightening your hips and knees, to return to the starting position.

014 Suspended Squat

Face the anchor point of a suspension system, and grasp the foot cradles with both hands. Lower your hips down and back. Push up to return. Repeat for the desired repetitions.

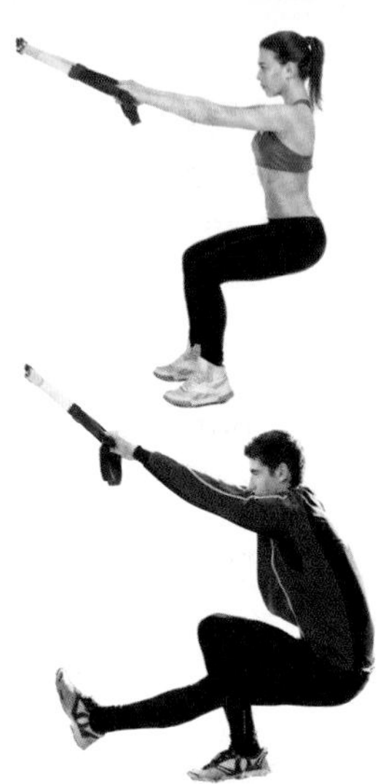

015 Suspended Single-Leg Squat

Face the anchor point, and grasp the foot cradles with both hands. Stand on one leg, and lower your hips down and back. Push up to return. Repeat for the desired repetitions, and then switch sides.

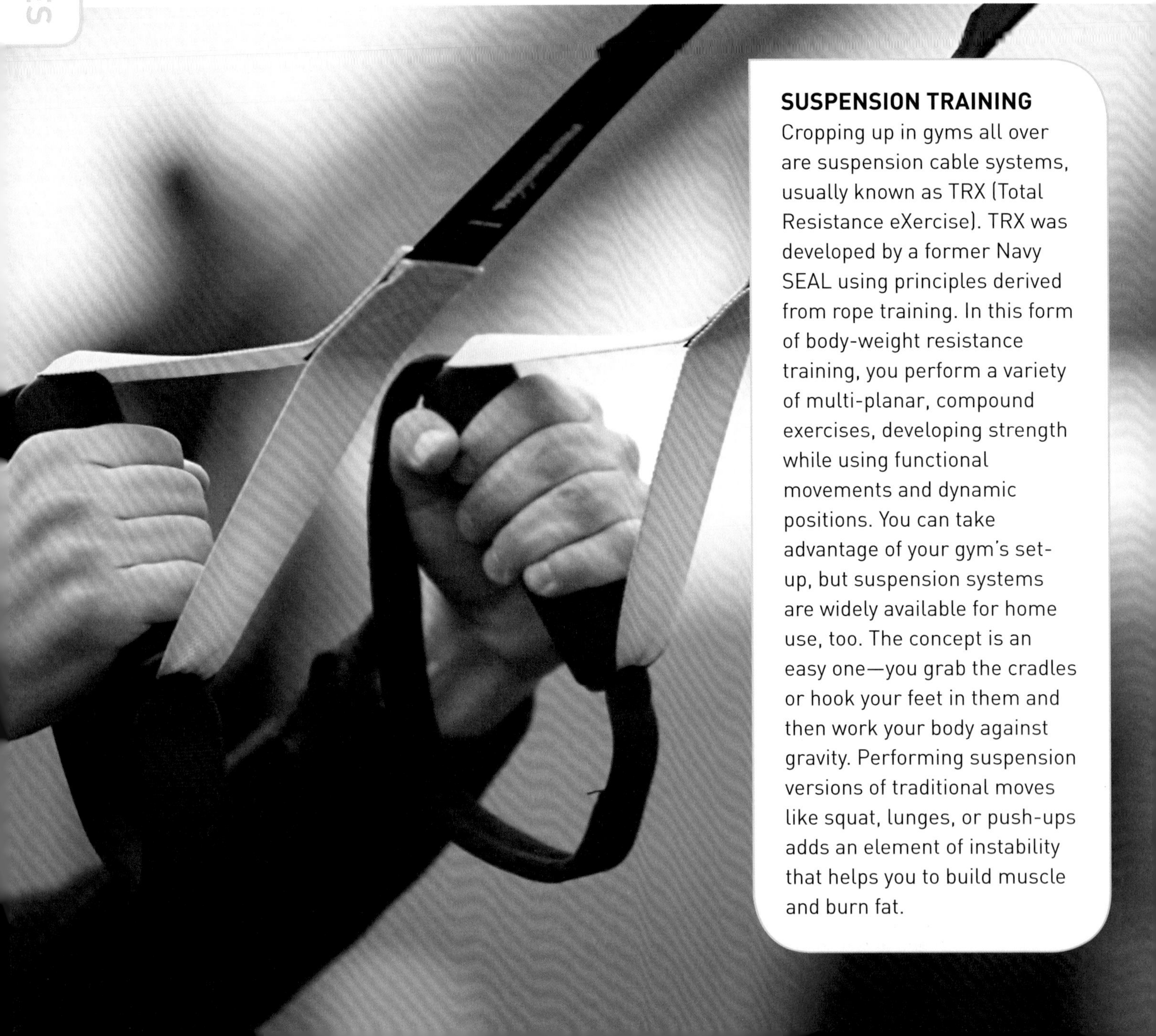

SUSPENSION TRAINING

Cropping up in gyms all over are suspension cable systems, usually known as TRX (Total Resistance eXercise). TRX was developed by a former Navy SEAL using principles derived from rope training. In this form of body-weight resistance training, you perform a variety of multi-planar, compound exercises, developing strength while using functional movements and dynamic positions. You can take advantage of your gym's set-up, but suspension systems are widely available for home use, too. The concept is an easy one—you grab the cradles or hook your feet in them and then work your body against gravity. Performing suspension versions of traditional moves like squat, lunges, or push-ups adds an element of instability that helps you to build muscle and burn fat.

016 Medicine Ball Squat

Grasping a weighted medicine ball in both hands, stand with your legs and feet parallel and shoulder-width apart. Keeping your knees aligned with your toes, bend your knees, and lower your body into a squat position. Keeping your back straight, raise yourself back to starting position, and repeat.

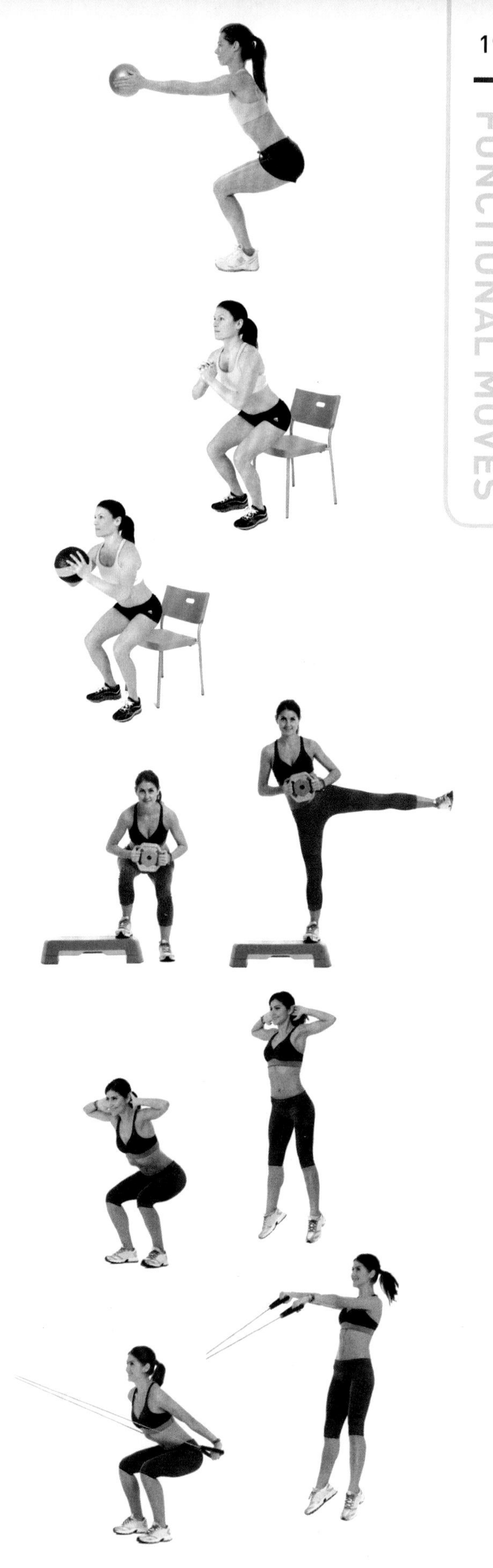

017 Chair Squat

Stand upright in front of a chair. Clasp your hands in front of your chest. Slowly lower into a squat position. Continue lowering until you are resting on the chair. With control, rise back up to the starting position, and repeat.

018 Medicine Ball Chair Squat

Perform as you would the Chair Squat (#017), but challenge yourself by holding a medicine ball in both hands at chest height in front of you throughout the exercise.

019 Box Squat with Side Leg Lift

Stand with right foot on a step grasping a disc weight or medicine ball at waist level. Keeping your knees aligned with your toes, bend your knees, and lower your body into a squat position. Keeping your back straight, raise yourself, shifting all your weight to your right foot as you lift your left leg straight out to the side. Return to the starting position, repeat for the desired repetitions, and then perform on the other leg.

020 Jump Squat

Place your fingers on the back of your head and pull your elbows back so that they're in line with your body. Dip your knees into a squat in preparation to leap, and then explosively jump as high as you can. When you land, immediately squat down, and jump again.

021 Resistance Band Jump Squat

Stand upright, holding both ends of a resistance band in your hands. Your feet should be planted hip-width apart, your back neither arched nor slumped. Pull your arms back as you dip your knees into a squat in preparation to leap, and then explosively jump as high as you can. When you land, immediately squat down, and jump again.

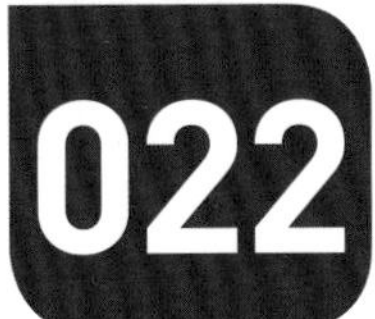

Sumo Squat

Like any squat, the Sumo Squat is a terrific lower-body exercise that tones your thighs, butt, and calves. Its execution is similar to a Basic Squat, but your stance is wider and your toes sharply angled away from the midline of your body. This kind of squat—which gets its name from the stance of a Japanese sumo wrestler—adds an inner-thigh focus to your workout. There are many variations, including weighted ones.

- Stand with your feet planted beyond shoulder width and your toes turned out. Bend your knees very slightly and tuck your pelvis slightly forward, lift your chest, and press your shoulders downward and back.
- Place your hands on your thighs.
- Squat down until your thighs are parallel to the floor, keeping your weight on your heels.
- Push off with your heels at the bottom of the squat, squeezing your glutes and inner thighs to rise back to the starting position.

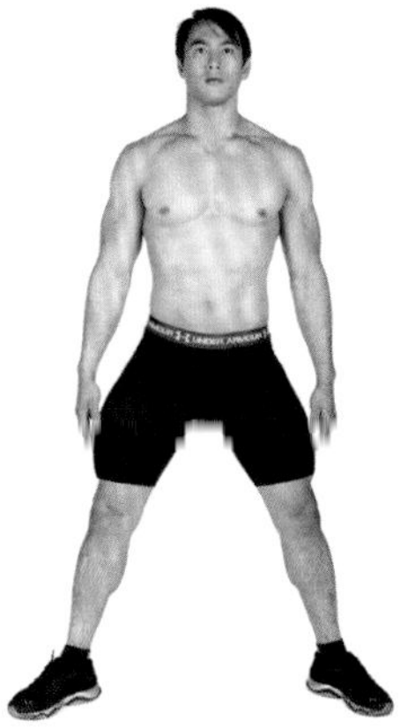

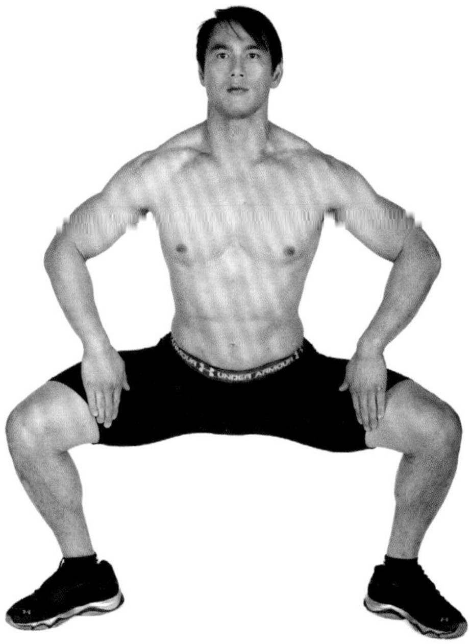

FIND YOUR FORM

Imagine that you are balancing a book on top of your head. This will help you keep your chest elevated and the weight of your upper body over your hips.

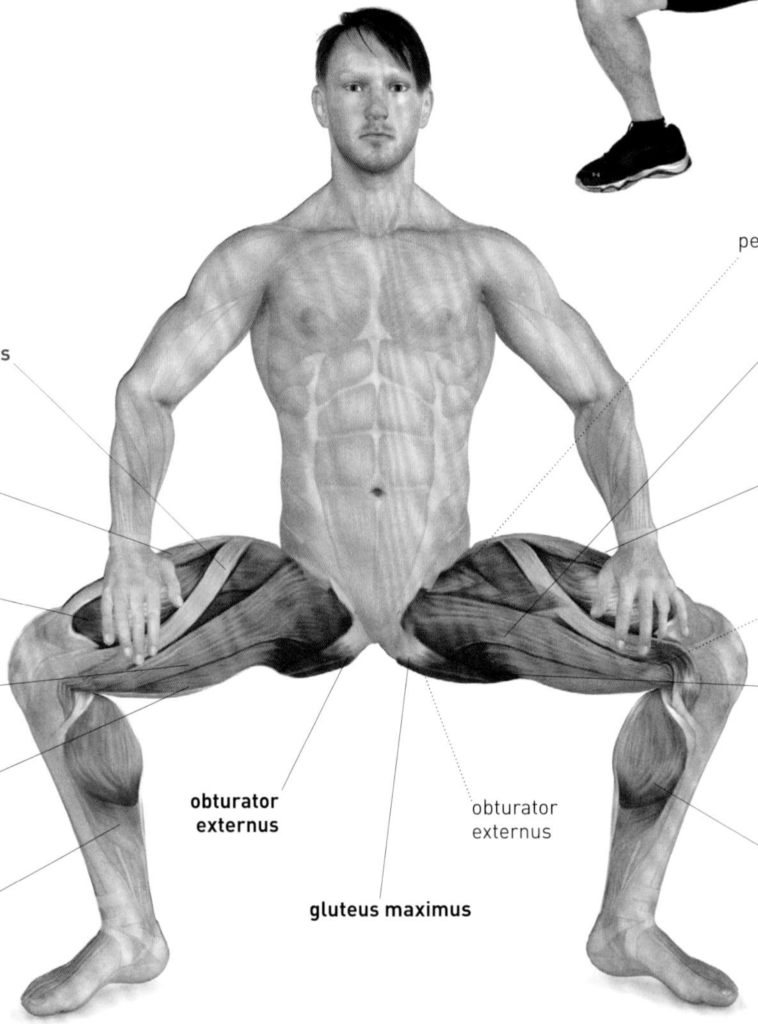

pectineus
sartorius
adductor brevis
rectus femoris
vastus lateralis
vastus medialis
gracilis
adductor longus
adductor magnus
biceps femoris
obturator externus
obturator externus
soleus
gluteus maximus
gastrocnemius

MUSCLE ANNOTATION KEY
— **Black bold = primary**
····· Black = deep primary
— Gray bold = secondary
····· Gray = deep secondary

023

Chair Plié

Stand with your feet in a wide stance, with toes turned out and a chair in front of you. Keeping your knees aligned with your toes, bend your knees, and lower your body into a squat position. Keeping your back straight, raise yourself back to starting position, and repeat.

024

Side-Leaning Sumo Squat

Begin at the bottom position of a Sumo Squat (#022), with your knees bent and thighs parallel to the floor. Drop your right forearm onto your right thigh, just above the kneecap. Bring your left arm and hand straight up and reach over to the right side. Hold this position as you stretch. Round your left arm down so that both forearms are on your thighs, and bring your head back to the center. Push off with your heels at the bottom of the squat, squeezing your glutes and inner thighs to rise back to the starting position. Switch sides, and repeat, alternating right and left reaches.

025

Toe-Touch Sumo Squat

Perform as you would a Sumo Squat (#022), and then bend forward to toe your toes. Return to standing position, and repeat.

026

Toe-Touch Sumo Squat with Reach

Perform as you would a Toe-Touch Sumo Squat (#025), and then at the bottom of the move, rotate your torso to extend one arm toward the ceiling. Return to the toe-touch position, and then extend the opposite arm. Return to standing position, and continue, alternating toe touches and arm reaches.

027

Medicine Ball Sumo Squat with Overhead Lift

Stand holding a medicine ball at chest height. Perform as you would a Sumo Squat (#022), extending your arms straight downward. As you return to standing position, lift the ball straight up toward the ceiling. Continue lowering and raising the ball as you alternate squatting and standing.

028

Weighted Sumo Squat

Stand holding a weight such as a disc weight, kettlebell, dumbbell, or medicine ball, and perform as you would a Sumo Squat (#022).

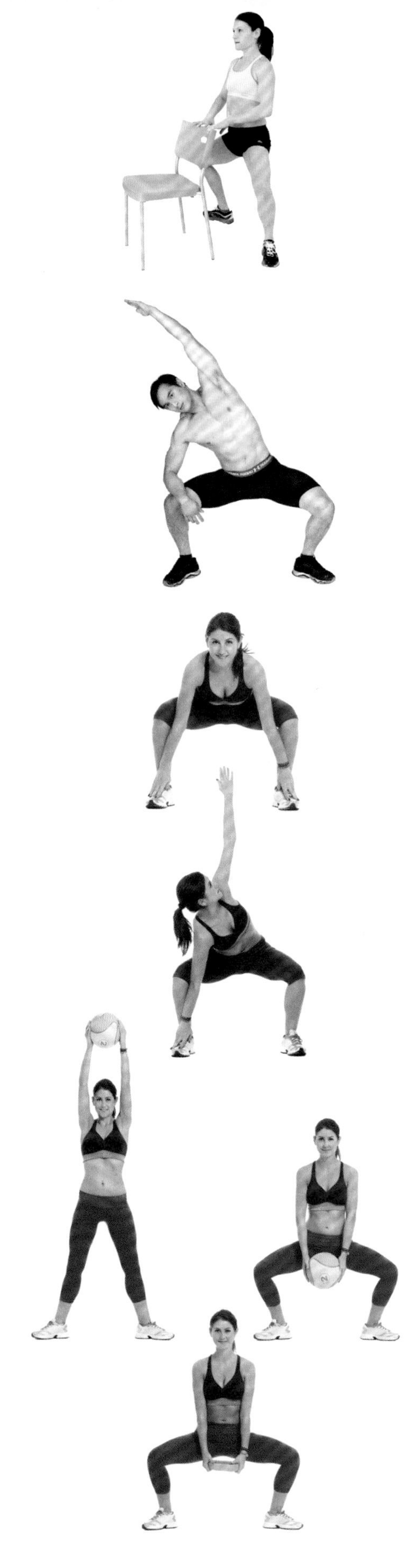

Split Squat

The Split Squat uses a staggered stance, with one foot placed forward of the other. This move is often confused with a lunge—the key difference between the two is your rear leg. In a split squat, you do not move your rear foot throughout the entire exercise. In a lunge, you engage your rear leg, using both legs at the same time. Like a regular squat, a split squat works your lower body, but places greater emphasis on the hamstrings, gluteus medius, and external obliques. Your back also remains more erect in a properly executed split squat.

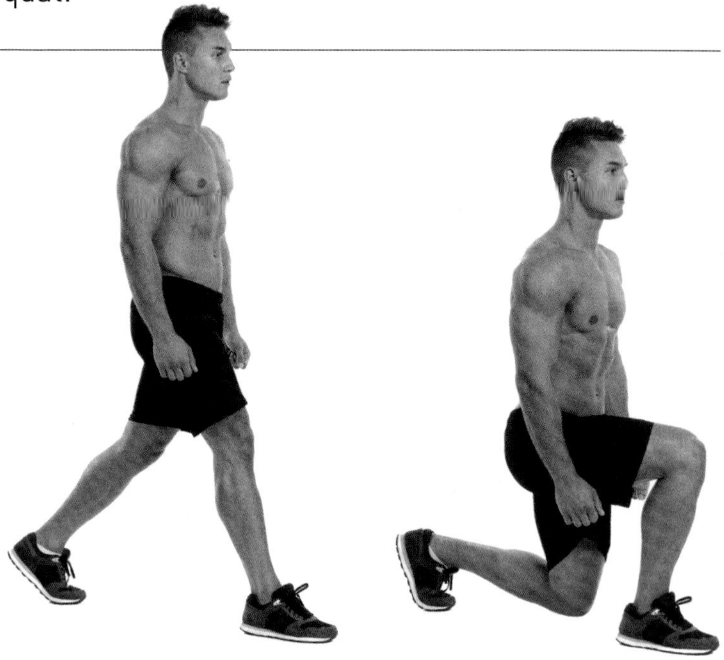

- Stand with hands on hips. Position feet far apart; one foot forward and other foot behind.
- Squat down by flexing knee and hip of front leg. Allow heel of rear foot to rise up while knee of rear leg bends slightly until it almost makes contact with floor. Return to original standing position by extending hip and knee of forward leg. Repeat for the desired repetitions, and then switch sides.

MUSCLE ANNOTATION KEY
- Black bold = primary
- Black = deep primary
- Gray bold = secondary
- Gray = deep secondary

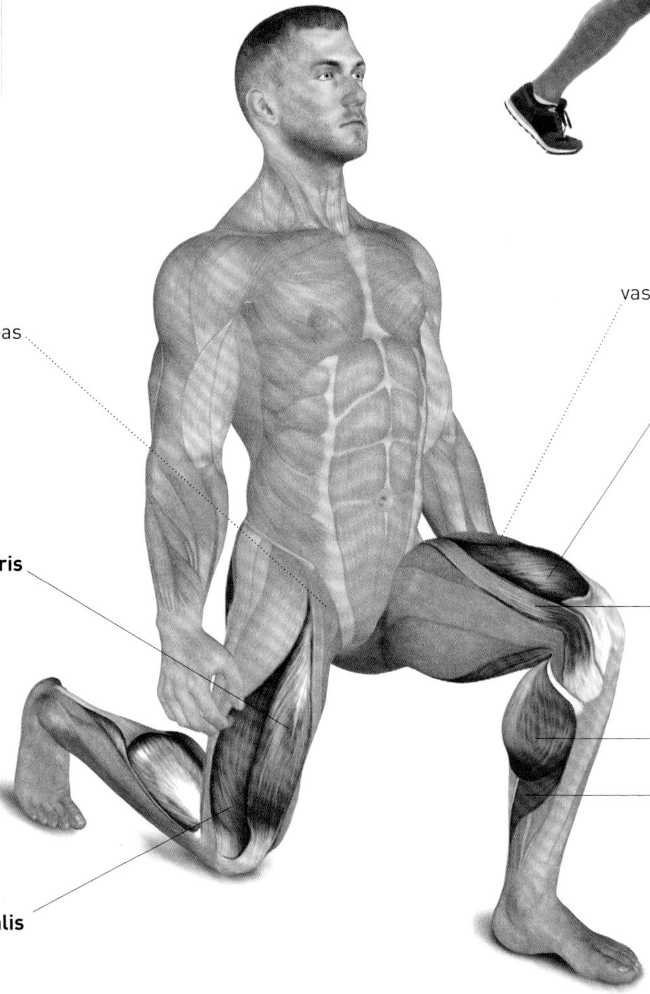

iliopsoas

rectus femoris

vastus lateralis

vastus intermedius

vastus medialis

sartorius

gastrocnemius

soleus

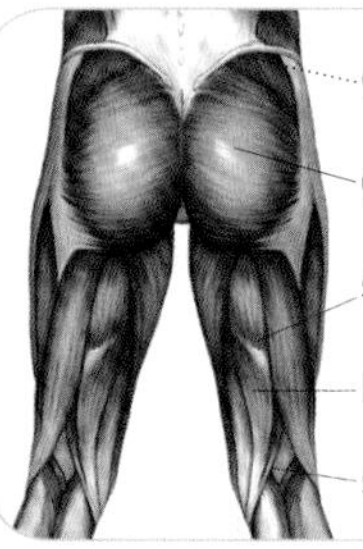

gluteus medius

gluteus maximus

semitendinosus

biceps femoris

semimembranosus

FIND YOUR FORM

Your knees should point in the same direction as your feet throughout movement, and your torso should remain upright as you lower into the squat.

030 Dumbbell Split Squat

Hold a pair of dumbbells in each hand, letting them hang at arm's length at your sides, your palms facing each other. Perform a Split Squat (#029), pause, and then push yourself back up to the starting position as quickly as you can. Switch legs, and repeat, continuing to alternate sides for the desired repetitions.

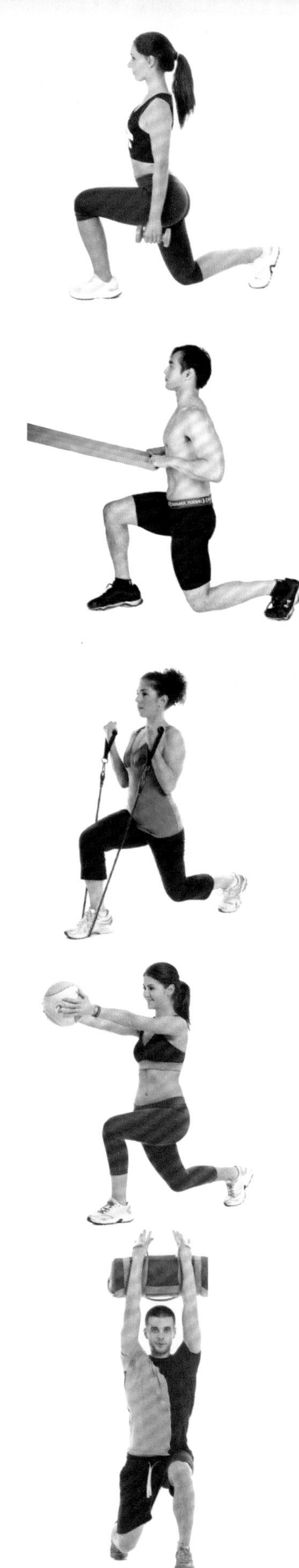

031 Split Squat with Band Row

Stand in a staggered stance, holding both ends of a resistance band or suspension cables in your hands. Bend one leg behind you to form a split squat while holding the cable taut. At the same time, bend your elbows as you pull both ends of the band in toward your body. Keeping the rest of your body stable and your abdominal muscles engaged, use both hands to pull the band even closer to your body. Smoothly return to starting position, and repeat for the desired repetitions. Switch sides and perform with the other leg behind.

032 Split Squat wit Band Curl

Holding both ends of a resistance band, perform a Split Squat (#029) while holding the band taut. At the same time, bend your elbows as you pull both ends of the band in toward your body. Keeping the rest of your body stable and your abdominal muscles engaged, use both hands to pull the band even closer to your body. Smoothly return to starting position, and repeat for the desired repetitions. Switch sides and perform with the other leg behind.

033 Medicine Ball Split Squat

Perform as you would a Split Squat (#029) while holding medicine ball with both hands at arm's length in front of you. Raise the ball to shoulder height as you descend, and bring it back down as you rise back up.

034 Overhead Sandbag Split Squat

Stand in a staggered stance, holding a sandbag with both hands at arm's length in front of you. Bend both knees into a split squat position as you simultaneously extend your arms over your head so that the sandbag flips behind you. Smoothly return to starting position, and repeat for the desired repetitions. Switch sides and perform with the other leg behind.

035

Bulgarian Split Squat

Also known as the Rear-Foot-Elevated Split Squat, the Bulgarian Split Squat calls for you to elevate your back, non-moving leg. This squat variation can be an antidote to the effects of too much time spent in front of a computer—sitting for long periods causes the hip flexor and quadriceps muscles to shorten. The Bulgarian Split Squat counteracts that by helping you to increase the strength and flexibility of your hip flexors and quadriceps, while not placing too much stress on your lower back.

- Stand in a staggered stance with your right leg behind you and he ball of your foot resting on an elevated surface, such as an aerobic step or weight bench. You can hold a weight such as a disc weight or medicine ball, or use just your body weight.
- Bend both knees into a split squat position.
- Smoothly return to starting position, and repeat for the desired repetitions. Switch sides and perform with the other leg behind.

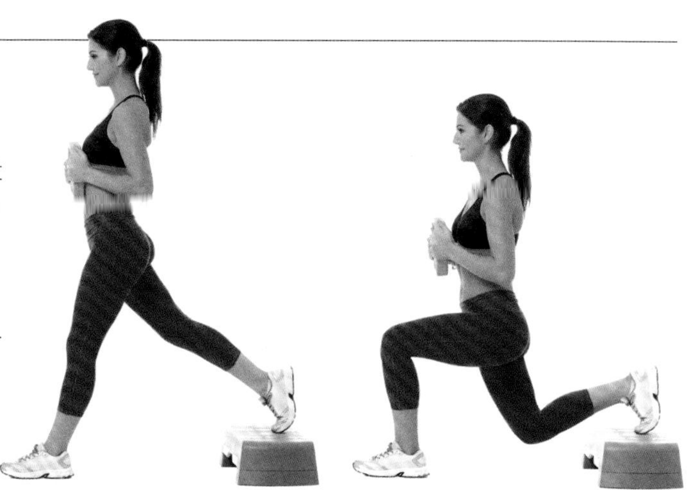

036

Swiss Ball Bulgarian Split Squat

Stand lunge-length in front of a Swiss ball. Rest the top of your right foot on the ball behind you. Lower your body until your front knee is bent at a 90-degree angle. Squeeze your thighs together to keep your balance. Switch legs, and perform on the other side.

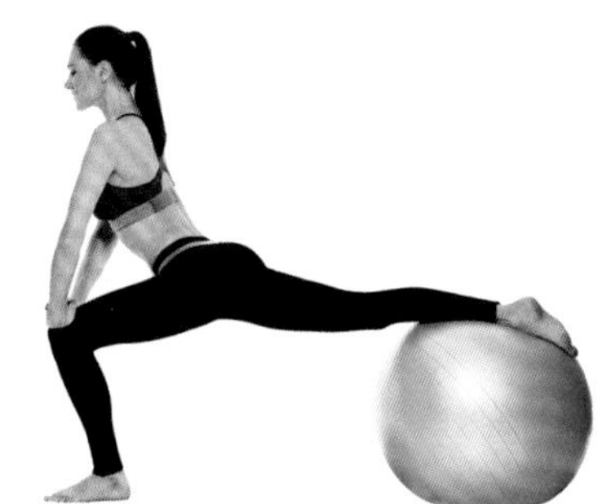

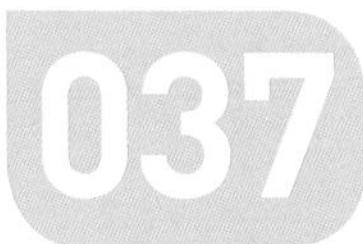

037

Bulgarian Split Squat with Overhead Press

Stand in a staggered stance with your elbows bent to form right angles. Perform a Bulgarian Split Squat (#035) as your raise both arms to shoulder height. Smoothly return to starting position, and repeat for the desired repetitions. Switch sides and perform on the other leg.

038

Bulgarian Split Squat with Dumbbell Overhead Press

Stand in a staggered stance holding a dumbbell in each hand. Perform a Bulgarian Split Squat (#035) as you extend the dumbbells over your head. Smoothly return to starting position, and repeat for the desired repetitions. Switch sides and perform on the other leg.

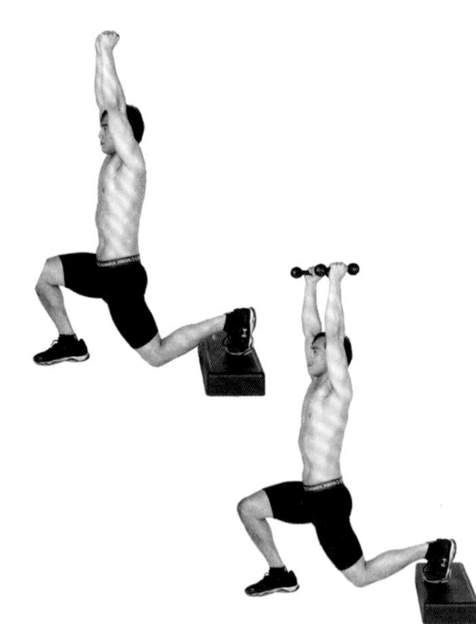

Wall Sit and Squat

A variation of the classic squat, the Wall Sit is a great way for exercise newbies to perfect their squatting form before advancing on to the more difficult versions of the squat. Aim for five sets of minute-long sits: with practice, you will gain core, back, and leg strength and hip and knee mobility, allowing you to squat lower.

- Stand with your feet planted beyond shoulder width and your toes turned out. Bend your knees very slightly and tuck your pelvis slightly forward, lift your chest, and press your shoulders downward and back.
- Place your hands on your thighs.
- Squat down until your thighs are parallel to the floor, keeping your weight on your heels.
- Push off with your heels at the bottom of the squat, squeezing your glutes and inner thighs to rise back to the starting position.

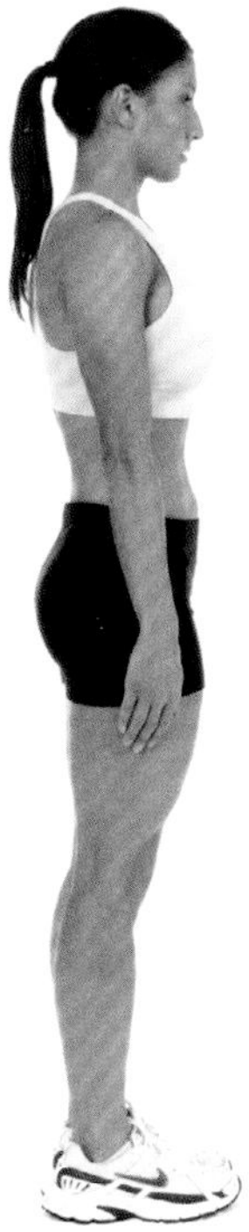

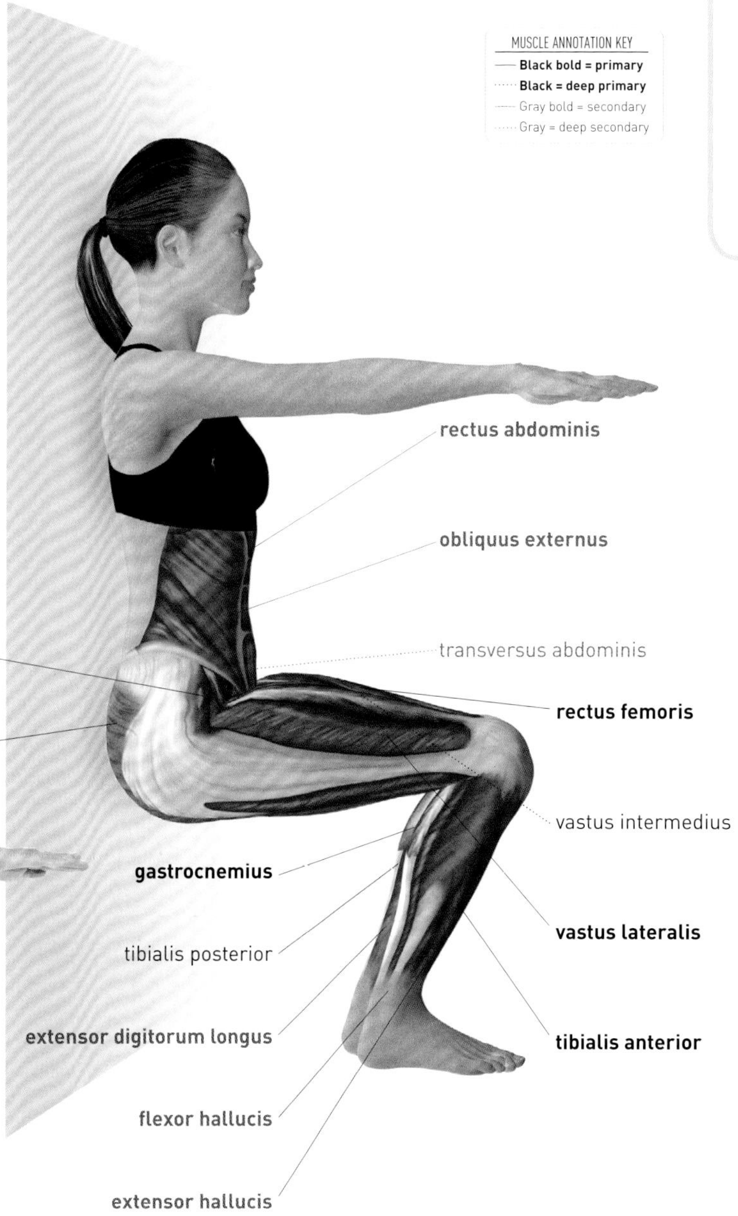

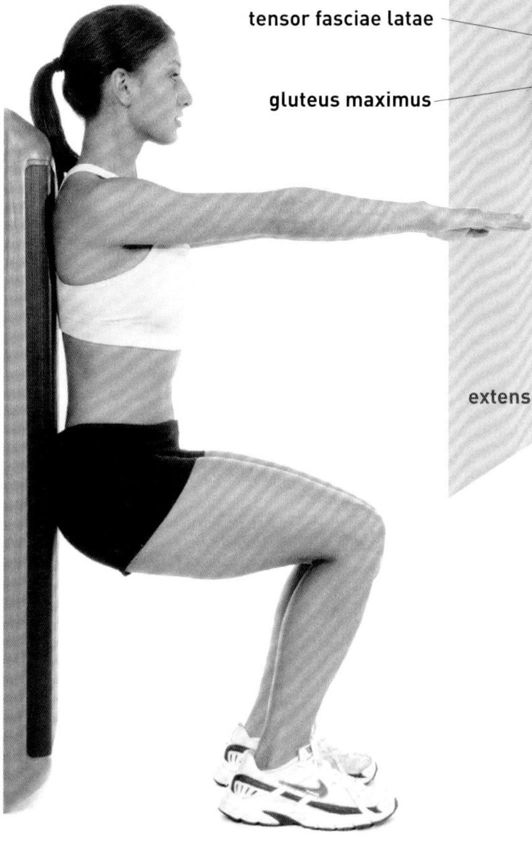

MUSCLE ANNOTATION KEY
Black bold = primary
Black = deep primary
Gray bold = secondary
Gray = deep secondary

rectus abdominis
obliquus externus
transversus abdominis
tensor fasciae latae
gluteus maximus
rectus femoris
vastus intermedius
gastrocnemius
tibialis posterior
vastus lateralis
extensor digitorum longus
tibialis anterior
flexor hallucis
extensor hallucis

FIND YOUR FORM

Keep your back straight, and do not allow your shoulders to round forward or your knees to come past your toes.

040 Swiss Ball Wall Squat

Place a Swiss ball against a wall and stand so that your back and shoulders are pinning it to the wall. Your feet should be about hip-width apart, but slightly ahead of your hips. Raise your arms straight out in front of you so that they are parallel to your thighs, and relax the upper torso. Keeping the ball pinned against the wall, slowly bend your hips and knees as you lower to a sitting position, rolling the ball down the wall with you as you sit. Hold for a count of 10, and then press back to the starting position, rolling the ball up the wall with your shoulders as you rise.

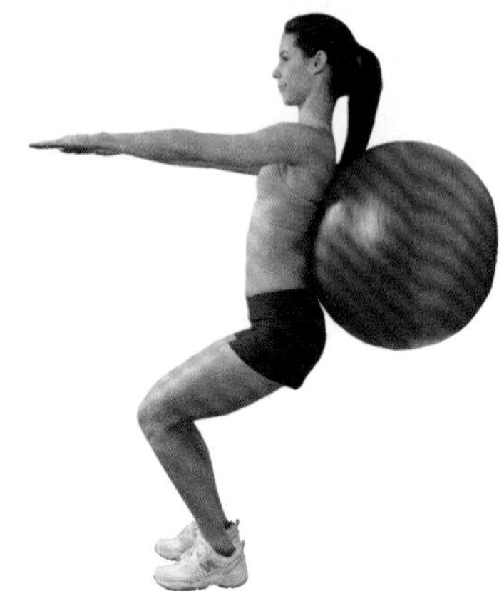

041 Swiss Ball Squat with Biceps Curl

Stand at a wall, with the Swiss ball against your back, grasping a dumbbell in each hand. Plant your feet slightly in front of your torso to prepare. Bend your knees, and lower toward the floor while curling the dumbbells toward your chest. As you lower into the squat position, keep the Swiss ball securely behind your back. Gradually straighten your arms and legs as you rise to stand. and release the dumbbells to your sides.

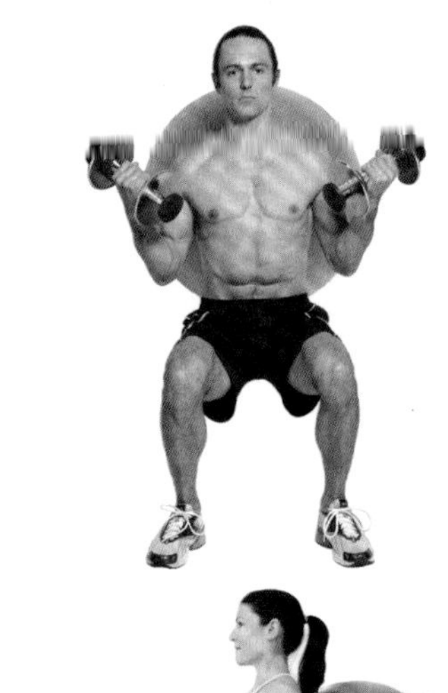

042 Single-Leg Swiss Ball Squat with Biceps Curl

Perform as you would a Swiss Ball Squat with Biceps Curl (#041), but while in the squatting and curling position, extend one leg, hold, and then release. Repeat on the other side.

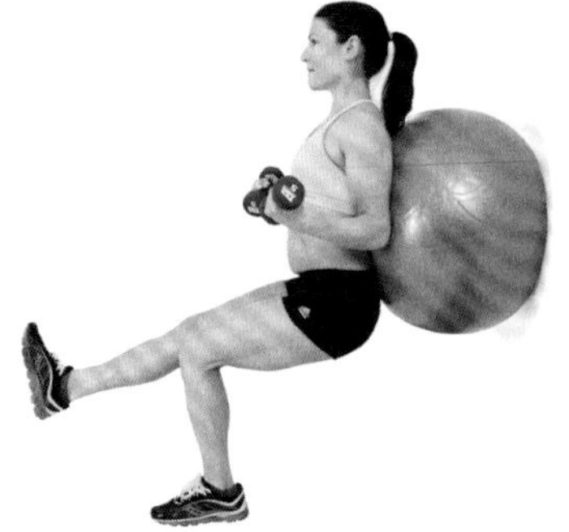

CHOOSING THE RIGHT SWISS BALL

A Swiss ball (also called a fitness ball, fitness ball, gym ball, physioball, and many other names) is a flexible, inflatable PVC ball with a host of fitness uses, including balance training, physical therapy, and many kinds of strength and cardio exercises. It is available in many sizes, from approximately 14 to 34 inches in circumference. If you want to get the most out of this piece of equipment, you must work with a ball of the correct size for your height. Exact sizes can vary from manufacturer to manufacturer, but this chart will give you a general guide to choosing the right size. Many come with their own pump—make sure to fill yours until it is firm, but still with a bit of give.

YOUR HEIGHT	BALL SIZE	BALL HEIGHT
Up to 4 feet 7 inches	Extra Small	14 inches
4 feet 7 inches to 5 feet	Small	18 inches
5 feet to 5 feet 6 inches	Medium	22 inches
5 feet 6 inches to 6 feet 1 inch	Large	26 inches
6 feet to 6 feet 8 inches	X Large	30 inches
Over 6 feet 8 inches	XX Large	33 inches

Forward Lunge

The lunge is an important group of exercises that strengthen your lower body and prepare you for everyday activities. There are many variations, but all will efficiently work your glutes, quadriceps, and hamstrings—and regularly engaging these large muscle groups can speed up your metabolism. Begin with the familiar Forward Lunge—just think of bending down to tie your shoelaces. This highly functional exercise closely mimics your walking pattern while challenging your balance. You must also effectively engage your core when properly executing it—to control the tilt of your pelvis as you flex one hip and extend the other, your hip, abdominal, and lower-back muscles must work synergistically.

- Stand with your legs and feet parallel and shoulder-width apart, and your knees bent very slightly. Tuck your pelvis slightly forwards, lift your chest, and press your shoulders down and back.
- Take a big step forward with your right leg, and start to shift weight forward so that your heel hits the floor first.
- Lower your body until your right thigh is parallel to floor and your right shin is vertical. Lightly tap your left knee to the floor while keeping your weight in your right heel.
- Press into your right heel to drive back up to the starting position.
- Switch legs, and repeat on the other side.

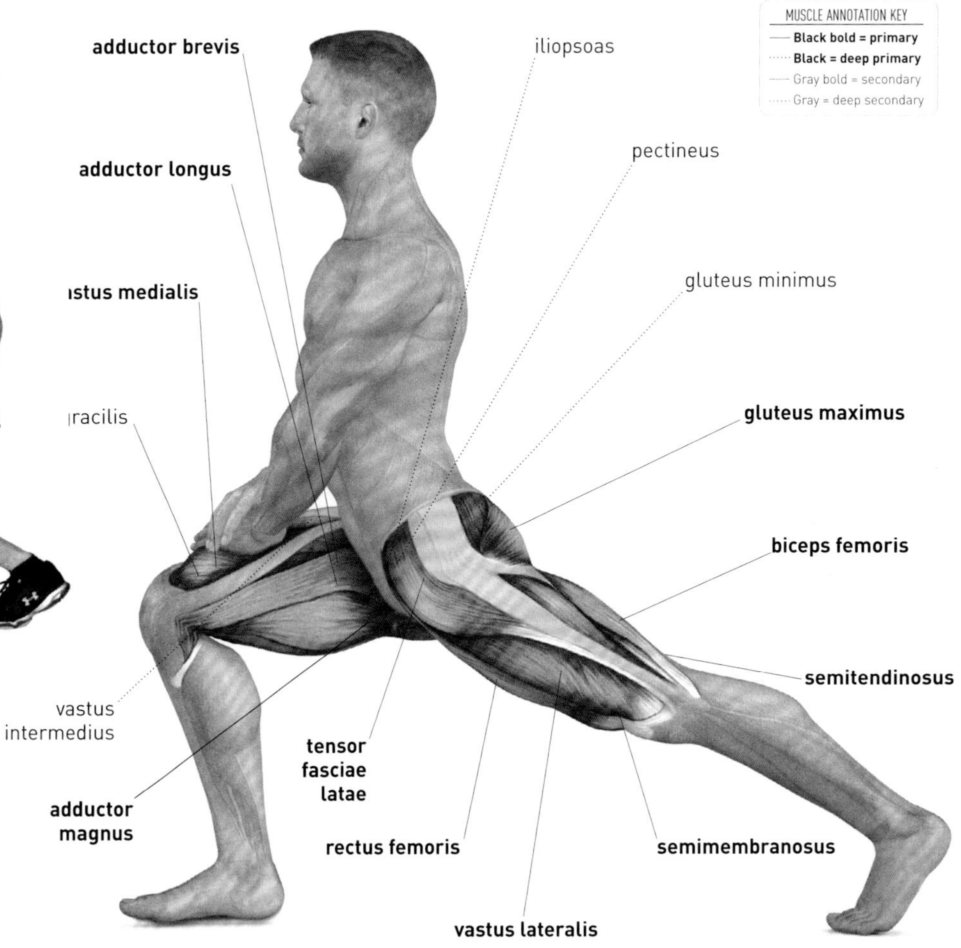

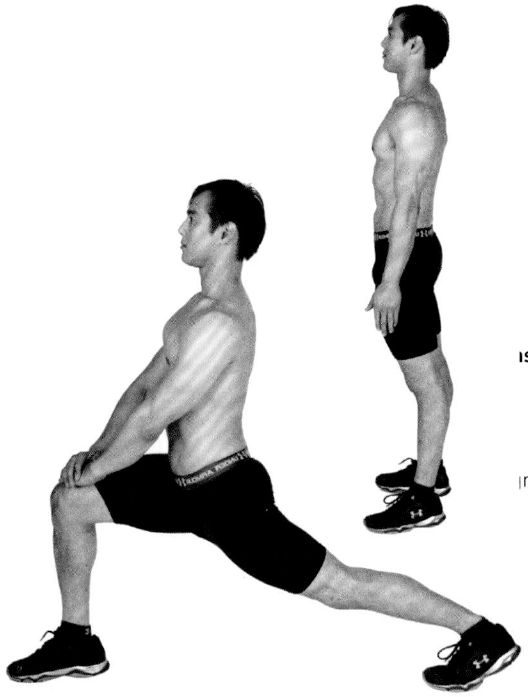

MUSCLE ANNOTATION KEY
Black bold = primary
Black = deep primary
Gray bold = secondary
Gray = deep secondary

adductor brevis
iliopsoas
adductor longus
pectineus
stus medialis
gluteus minimus
racilis
gluteus maximus
biceps femoris
semitendinosus
vastus intermedius
tensor fasciae latae
adductor magnus
rectus femoris
semimembranosus
vastus lateralis

FIND YOUR FORM

To help you maintain a straight upper body, relax your shoulder, and keep your chin up, gazing at a point in front of you. This will help you avoid looking downward and rounding your neck and upper back.

044 Forward Lunge with Twist

Perform as you would a Forward Lunge (#043), and then at the bottom of the movement, place your hands on the floor on the inside of your right foot, and then guide your right arm up toward the ceiling, twisting your torso. Return to the center, and repeat on the other side.

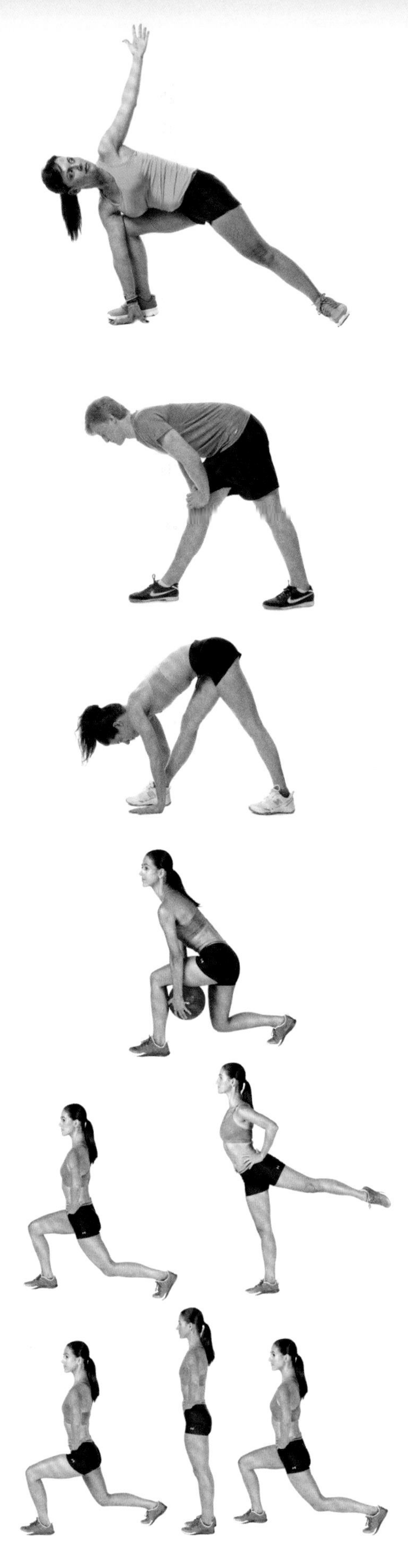

045 Straight-Leg Lunge

Stand with your legs and feet parallel and shoulder-width apart. Bend your knees very slightly and tuck your pelvis slightly forwards, lift your chest, and press your shoulders downward and back. Keeping both legs straight, take a big step forward with your right leg, and lean your torso forward over your right leg, placing your hands on your knee. Return to standing, and repeat on the other side.

046 Straight-Leg Lunge with Floor Touch

Perform as you would a Straight-Leg Lunge (#045), but rather than stopping at the knee, lean your torso forward as far as you are able, aiming to place your hands flat on the floor on either side of your front foot. Return to the starting position, and repeat on the other side.

047 Forward Lunge Pass Under

Stand with your feet together, holding a medicine ball a chest height. Take a big step forward with your left foot, and lower into a lunge. Hinge at the waist as you shift the ball into your right hand, bringing it beneath your left thigh to pass it to your left hand. Return to the starting position, and then repeat on the other side.

048 Forward Lunge with Rear Leg Raise

Perform a Forward Lunge (#043), your right leg forward. As you straighten your right leg, hinge forward at the hips and lift your straightened left leg off the floor behind you until it's about parallel to the floor. Return to the starting position, and then repeat on the other side.

049 Tick-Tock Lunge

Perform a Forward Lunge (#043), and then return to the starting position. Perform a Reverse Lunge (#056). Return to the starting position, and then repeat on the opposite legs.

050

Twisting Lunge

Stand with your feet shoulder-width apart and your arms extended at shoulder height, palms down. Perform a Forward Lunge (#043), twist your torso to right, and reach your right hand back to touch your left heel while extending your left arm straight up. Return to the starting position, and repeat on the opposite side.

051

Diagonal Lunge

Perform as you would a Forward Lunge (#043), but instead of moving in a straight line, step out on a diagonal. Return to the starting position, and then repeat on the other side.

052

Diagonal Jumpers

Perform as you would a Forward Lunge (#043) with your right leg in front. Then, straighten both legs. Jump up to switch legs so that your left leg is in front. Take a moment to find your balance. Bend both knees to sink down into another lunge. Straighten your knees and then keep repeating for the desired repetitions.

053

Dumbbell Lunge

Stand up straight with a tight core, holding dumbbells at your sides, and perform as you would a Forward Lunge (#043)

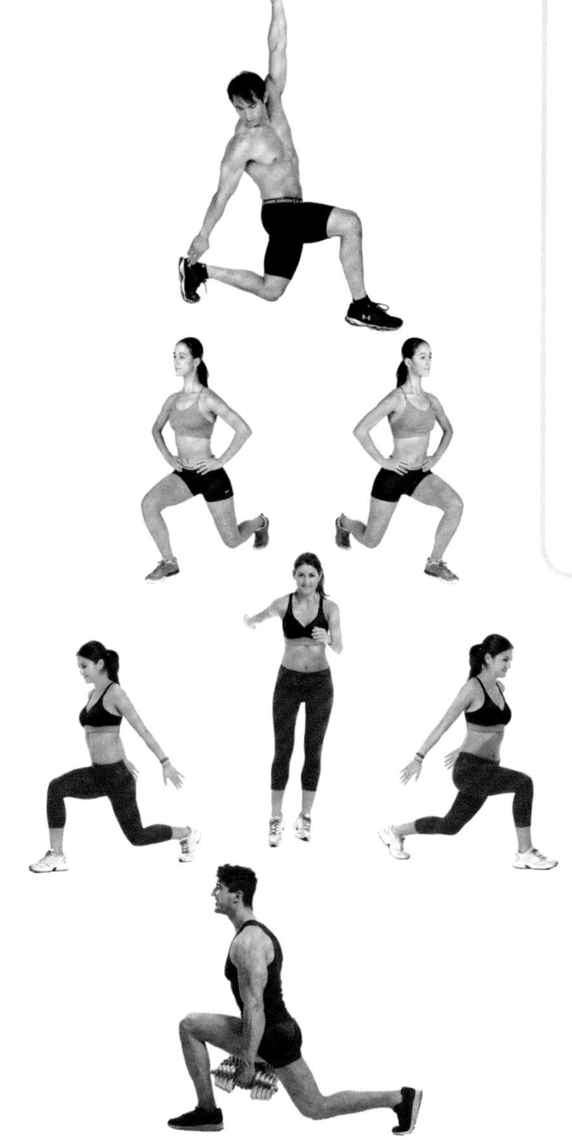

054

Barbell Lunge

The Barbell Lunge is one of the most effective exercises for improving coordination and upping athleticism. Executed properly, it will help you to strengthen the muscles needed for many real-life movements like sprinting, jumping and climbing stairs. When attempting this move, caution should be exercised as well as your muscles—it requires a great deal of balance. It is also safest to perform this lunge inside a squat rack.

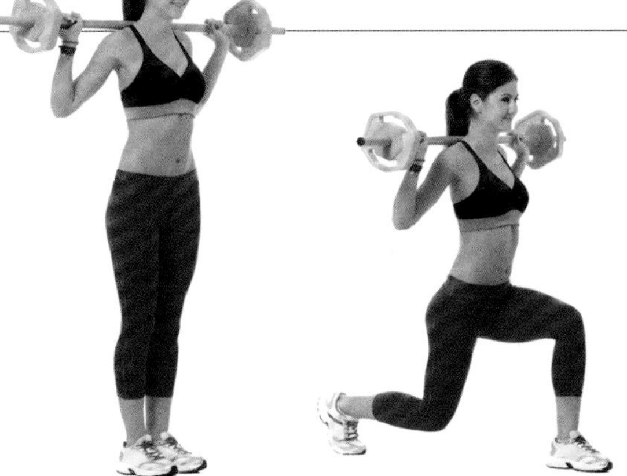

- Stand holding a barbell across your shoulders with an overhand grip, and your feet about shoulder-width apart.
- Keeping your head up, back straight, and chest high, step one foot forward, bending your knees, and bring your trailing knee almost to the floor.
- Push yourself back up to the starting position with one strong, controlled thrust.
- Repeat the movement stepping forward with the other foot.

Walking Lunge

Like the Forward Lunge, the Walking Lunge is a dynamic stretch that stabilizes your knees while building strength in your thigh muscles, both front and back. The Walking Lunge also efficiently works your glutes to firm and lift your butt, and the forward progression adds cardio intensity.

- Stand with your legs together and your arms hanging at your sides.
- Take a large step forward with your left leg.
- Lower your right knee to the floor, and then forcefully push off your left foot to return to the standing position. Repeat on the other side, and continue to alternate your leading leg as you move forward for the desired steps.

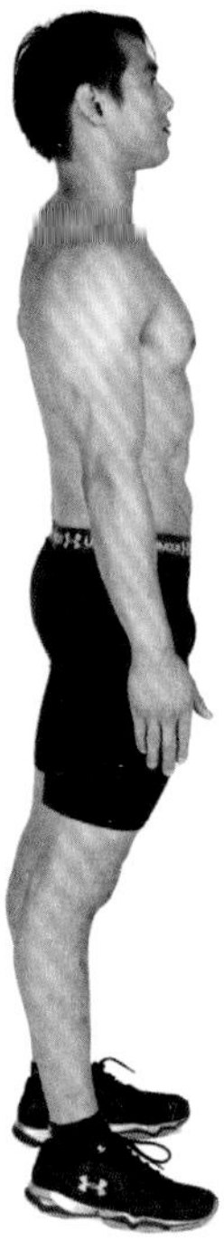

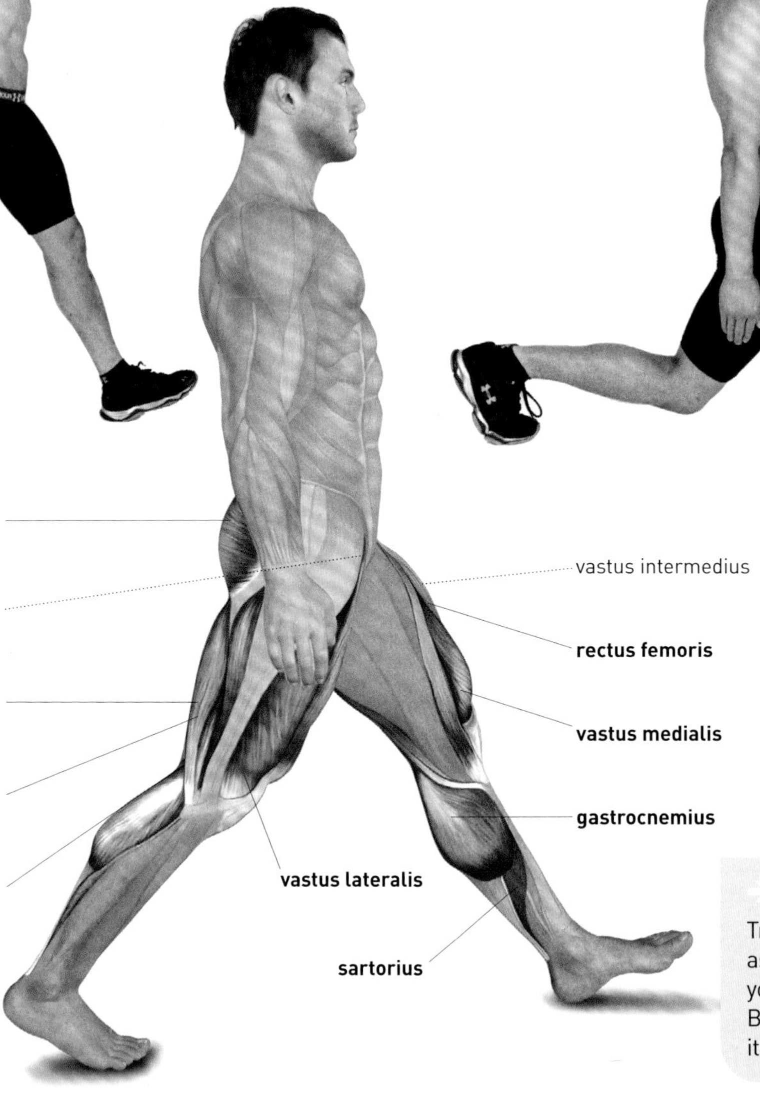

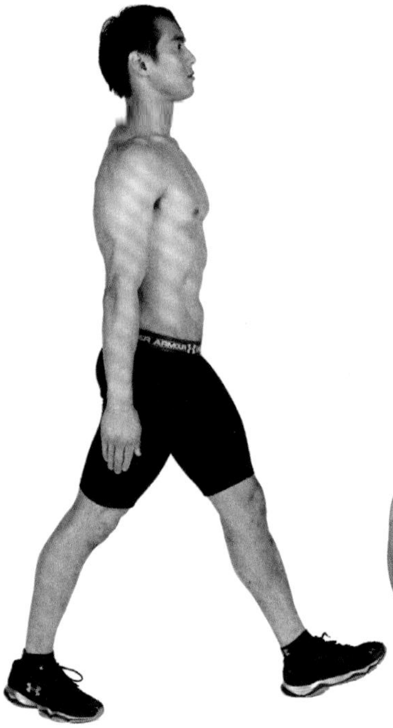

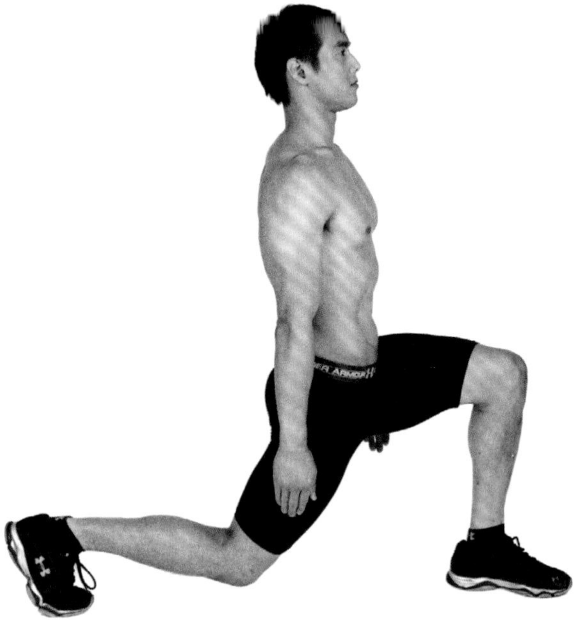

gluteus maximus

iliopsoas

biceps femoris

semitendinosus

semimembranosus

vastus lateralis

sartorius

vastus intermedius

rectus femoris

vastus medialis

gastrocnemius

MUSCLE ANNOTATION KEY
- **Black bold = primary**
- Black = deep primary
- Gray bold = secondary
- Gray = deep secondary

FIND YOUR FORM

Try to drop your back knee as close to the ground as you can without touching it. Bend your front knee so that it is directly over your ankle.

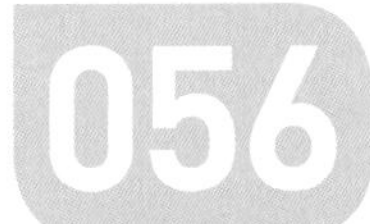

Dumbbell Walking Lunge

Stand with your legs together and your arms at your sides, a dumbbell in each hand, and perform as you would a Walking Lunge (#055).

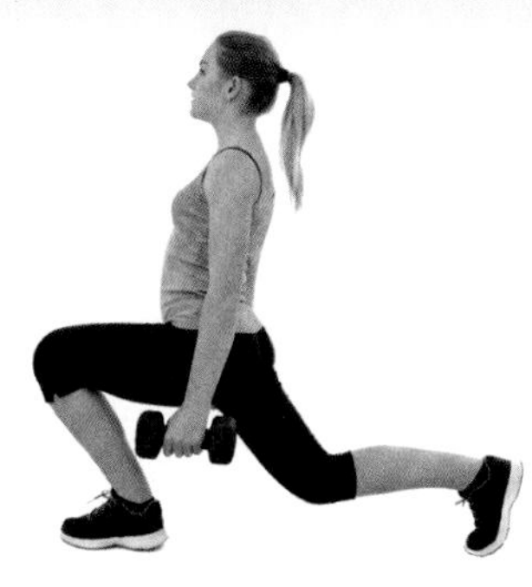

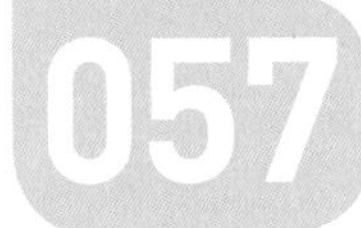

Reach-and-Twist Walking Lunge

Stand with feet about hip-width apart and your torso facing forward. Hold a weighted medicine ball in both hands. Lunge your left foot forward. Begin to bend both knees, lowering your whole body into the lunge. At the same time, raise the medicine ball until it is over your left shoulder. In a single motion, rise up to stand, bring the ball back to center, and then perform the lunge and reach in the other direction. Continue to lunge and move the ball from side to side as you walk forward.

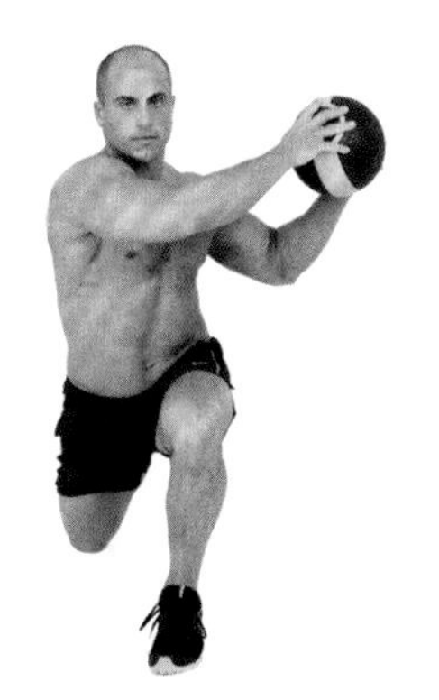

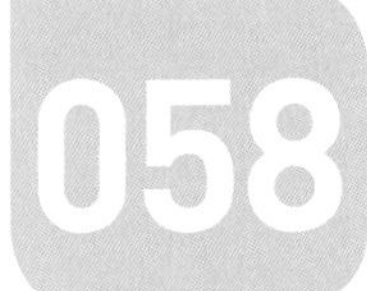

Jumping Lunge

The quick pace of this exercise intensifies the already hard-working lunge, demonstrating how the principles of plyometrics can add intensity to a basic exercise.

- Stand upright with your feet hip-width apart and your arms at your sides. With your right leg, take a big step forward.
- Bend both legs to lower into a deep lunge, and then, straighten both legs.
- Lifting your arms overhead, jump up to switch legs so that your left leg is in front. Take a moment to find your balance.
- Bend both knees to sink down into another lunge. Straighten your knees, and then keep repeating for the desired time or repetitions.

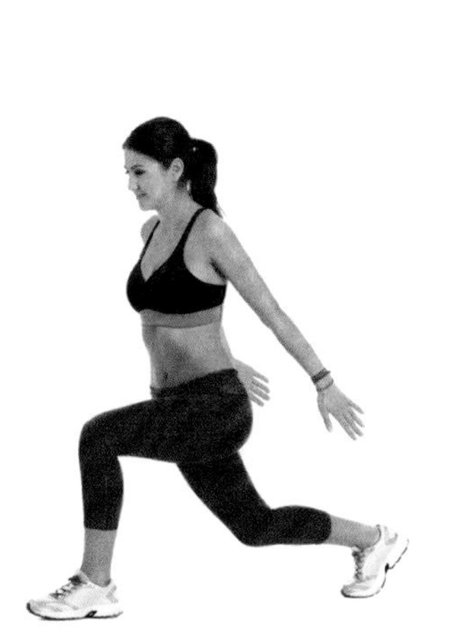

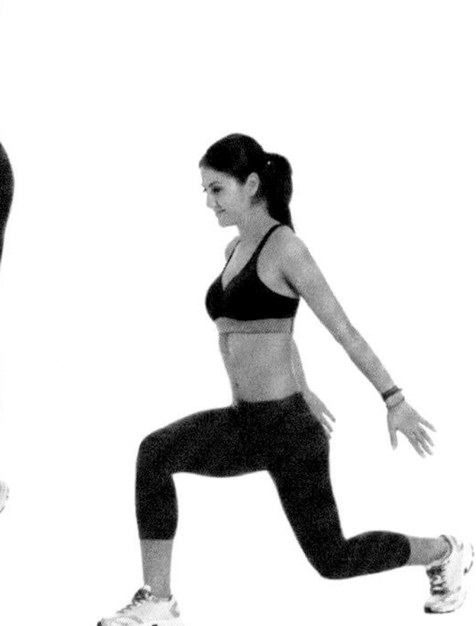

UP THE INTENSITY WITH PLYOMETRIC MOVEMENTS

Probably one of the easiest—and arguably one of the most efficient—ways to up the intensity of your workout regimen is to include plenty of plyometric moves. The plyometrics method, also known as jump training, calls for you to focus on quickly moving a muscle from extension to contraction in an explosive manner, such as in repeatedly alternating jumps and squats. Used by athletes and martial artist, to improve performance, plyometric exercises can increase power, speed, and strength.

Reverse Lunge

Like the Forward Lunge, the Reverse Lunge is an excellent lower-body exercise. Some proponents prefer this version over its opposite, because its backward momentum keeps your body in the optimal lunge position—your weight is on your heel with your knee above your ankle. Also known as the Step-Back Lunge, this lunge variation offers your body a challenge by moving you backward—a direction you probably don't move in very often. This is a great exercise to prepare you for sports and other activities that require speed and power, particularly sprinting, but it is also the less difficult of the two basic lunges, and it is often a good option for anyone with a balance problem.

- Stand with your hands on your hips and your feet shoulder-width apart.
- Take a big step backward, bending your knees as you do so.
- When your front thigh is roughly parallel to the floor, push through your front heel to return to the starting position.
- Switch legs, and repeat on the other side.

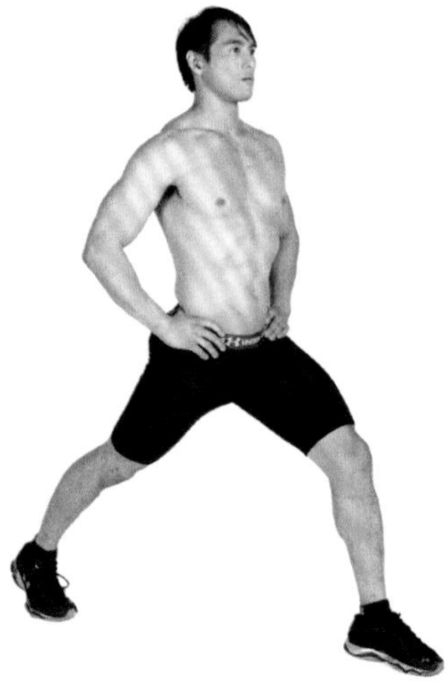

FIND YOUR FORM

To fully engage your glutes, focus on pressing the heel of your front foot into the floor as you lift up.

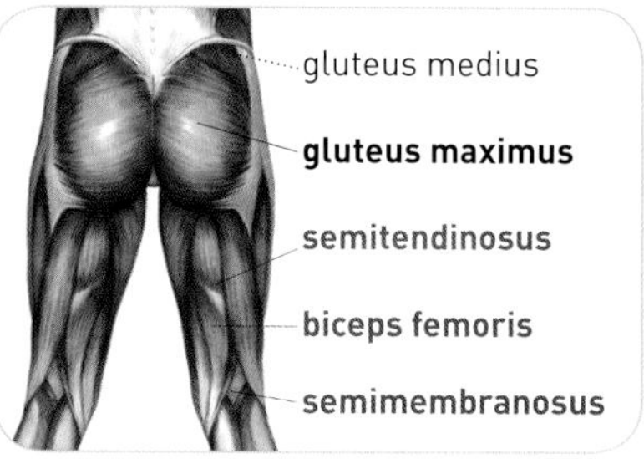

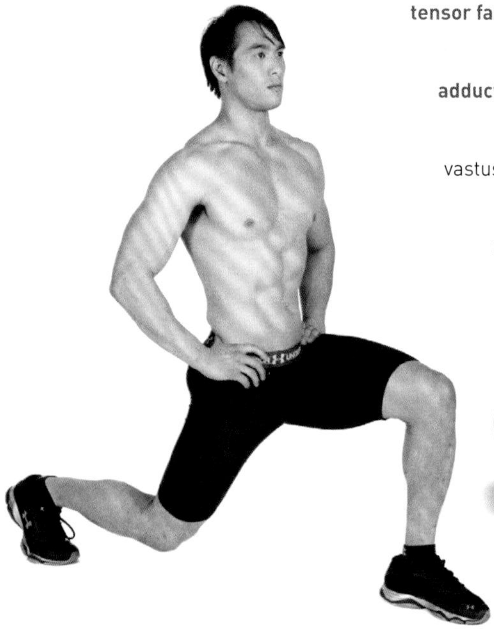

gluteus medius
gluteus maximus
semitendinosus
biceps femoris
semimembranosus

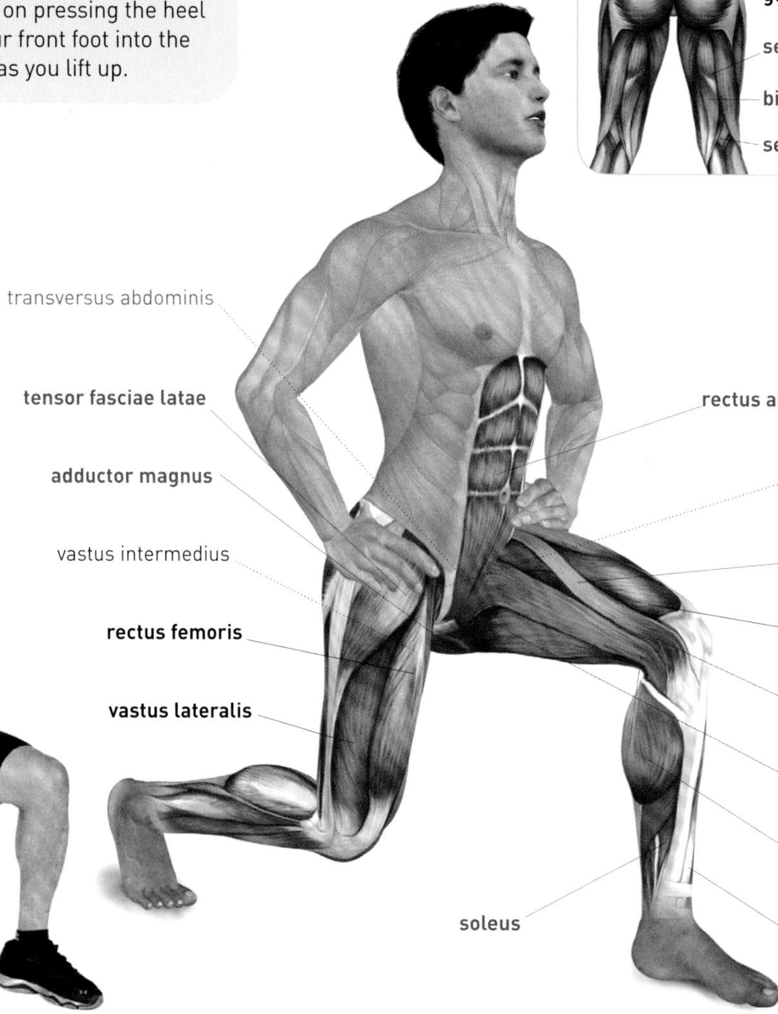

MUSCLE ANNOTATION KEY
Black bold = primary
Black = deep primary
Gray bold = secondary
Gray = deep secondary

transversus abdominis
tensor fasciae latae
adductor magnus
vastus intermedius
rectus femoris
vastus lateralis
rectus abdominis
iliopsoas
sartorius
vastus medialis
gracilis
adductor longus
gastrocnemius
soleus
flexor digitorum

060 Dumbbell Reverse Lunge

To add resistance, perform a Reverse Lunge (#059) while holding a dumbbell in each hand.

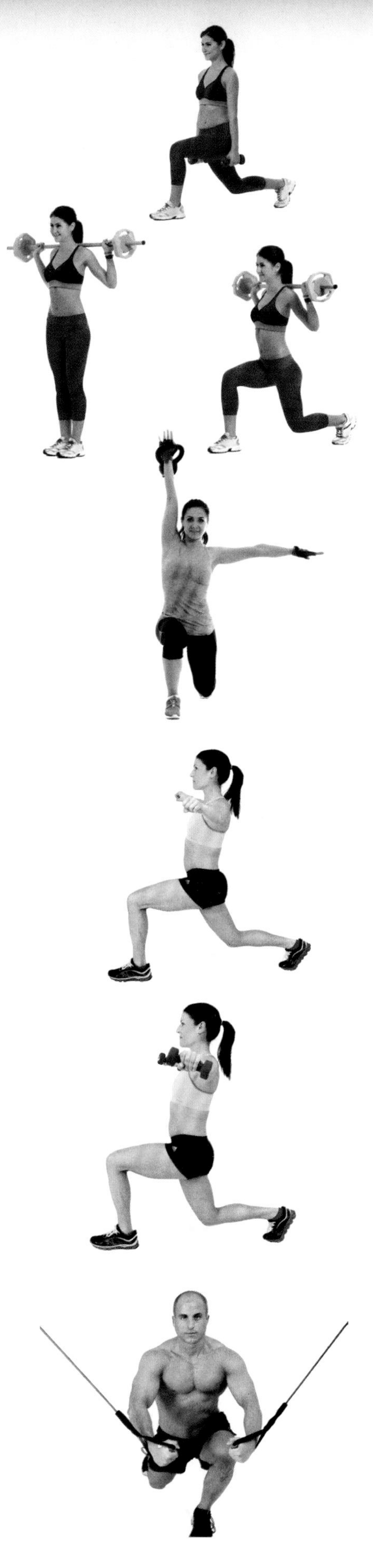

061 Barbell Reverse Lunge

Holding a barbell across your shoulders with an overhand grip, perform a Reverse Lunge (#059). Press through your heel and glutes, and explosively ascend back up to the starting position. Repeat a full set on one side and then switch to the opposite side, and repeat.

062 Kettlebell Overhead Reverse Lunge

Hold a dumbbell in your right hand, and extend your left arm straight out to the side. Press the kettlebell overhead, then with the kettlebell locked out directly above you, perform a Reverse Lunge (#059), lowering your left knee until it nearly touches the floor. Flex through your hips again to raise your torso back up to a standing position. Repeat with alternating legs and arms.

063 Lateral-Extension Reverse Lunge

Stand with your feet hip-width apart and your arms at your sides or on your hips, and perform a Reverse Lunge (#059) as you raise your arms to the side until they are level with your shoulders. Return to starting position by extending the hip and knee of your left leg and bringing your right leg forward to meet your left. Repeat with alternating legs and arms.

064 Dumbbell Lateral-Extension Reverse Lunge

To add resistance, perform a Lateral-Extension Reverse Lunge (#063) while holding a dumbbell in each hand.

065 Reverse Lunge with Chest Press

Stand with your feet hip-width apart. Loop a resistance band around a stable object, and grasp a handle in each hand. Raise your arms to hold both bands perpendicular to your body, slightly taut. Step your left leg behind you. Perform a Reverse Lunge (#059), while at the same time lowering both arms, feeling resistance on the bands. Gradually straighten your legs, and raise your arms to your sides to return to starting position Step your left leg forward, and repeat on the other side.

066

Reverse Lunge Knee-Up

Perform as you would a Reverse Lunge (#059), but instead of returning to standing position, in one explosive motion, straighten your front leg to jump up and draw your back leg up in front of you so that your thigh is parallel to the floor. Return to the Reverse Lunge stance, and repeat for the desired repetitions. Repeat on the other side.

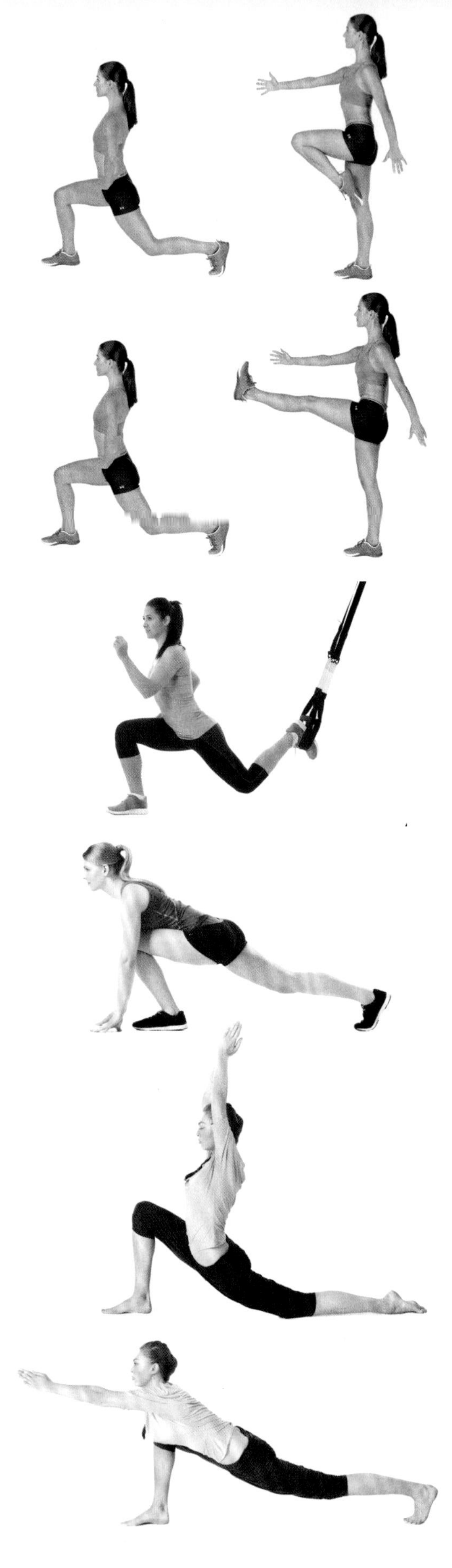

067

Reverse Lunge and Kick

Perform as you would a Reverse Lunge (#059), but instead of returning to standing position, kick your back leg out in front of you until you can touch your toes with your opposite hand. Return to standing position, and repeat on the other side.

068

Suspended Reverse Lunge

Standing in a staggered stance, face away from the anchor, and suspend your back foot in both foot cradles below the anchor point. Lower into a lunge, keeping your torso erect until both knees form 90-degree angles. Drive back up by pushing through your front heel.

069

Low Lunge

Stand with your feet hip-width apart. Bend your knees, and step back with your right foot, keeping your legs in line with your hips. Press the ball of your right foot on the floor, and contract your thigh muscles, as your bring your hands to either side of your left foot. Return to standing position, and then repeat on the opposite side.

070

Crescent Lunge

Perform a Low Lunge (#069), and at the bottom of the movement, drop your back knee to the floor. Bring your hands onto your front knee, and make sure the knee is directly over your ankle. Inhale, and raise your arms above your head, keeping your arms in line with your ears. Lower your arms, return to standing position, and then repeat on the opposite side.

071

Low Lunge with Reach

Perform a Low Lunge (#069), and at the bottom of the movement, bring your hands to the front knee. Inhale, and reach forward with the same-side hand as the extended leg.

072 Lateral Lunge

The Lateral Lunge introduces a new plane of movement to lunge or squat exercises. Rather than a forward or backward motion, which takes place in the sagittal plane that divides the body into left and right, the side-to-side motion moves you in the frontal plane, which divides the body into back and front portions. A Lateral Lunge also calls for each leg to work independently, so that your dominant leg cannot take on a greater share of the work. This kind of lunge has many variations that you can add to your workout regimen. Just perform as many reps as possible for one to two minutes on each side, or plug one of its variations into a high-intensity circuit.

- Stand upright with your arms outstretched in front of you, parallel to the floor.
- Step out to the left. Squat down on your right leg, bending at your hips, while maintaining a neutral spine. Begin to extend your left leg, keeping both feet flat on the floor.
- Bend your right knee until your thigh is parallel to the floor, and your left leg is fully extended.
- Keeping your arms parallel to the floor, squeeze your glutes, and press off your right leg to return to the starting position, and repeat. Perform the desired reps, and then repeat on the other side.

FIND YOUR FORM

Keep your chest up, your shoulders down, and your upper arms parallel to the floor throughout the exercise. and be sure to engage your glutes as you lunge.

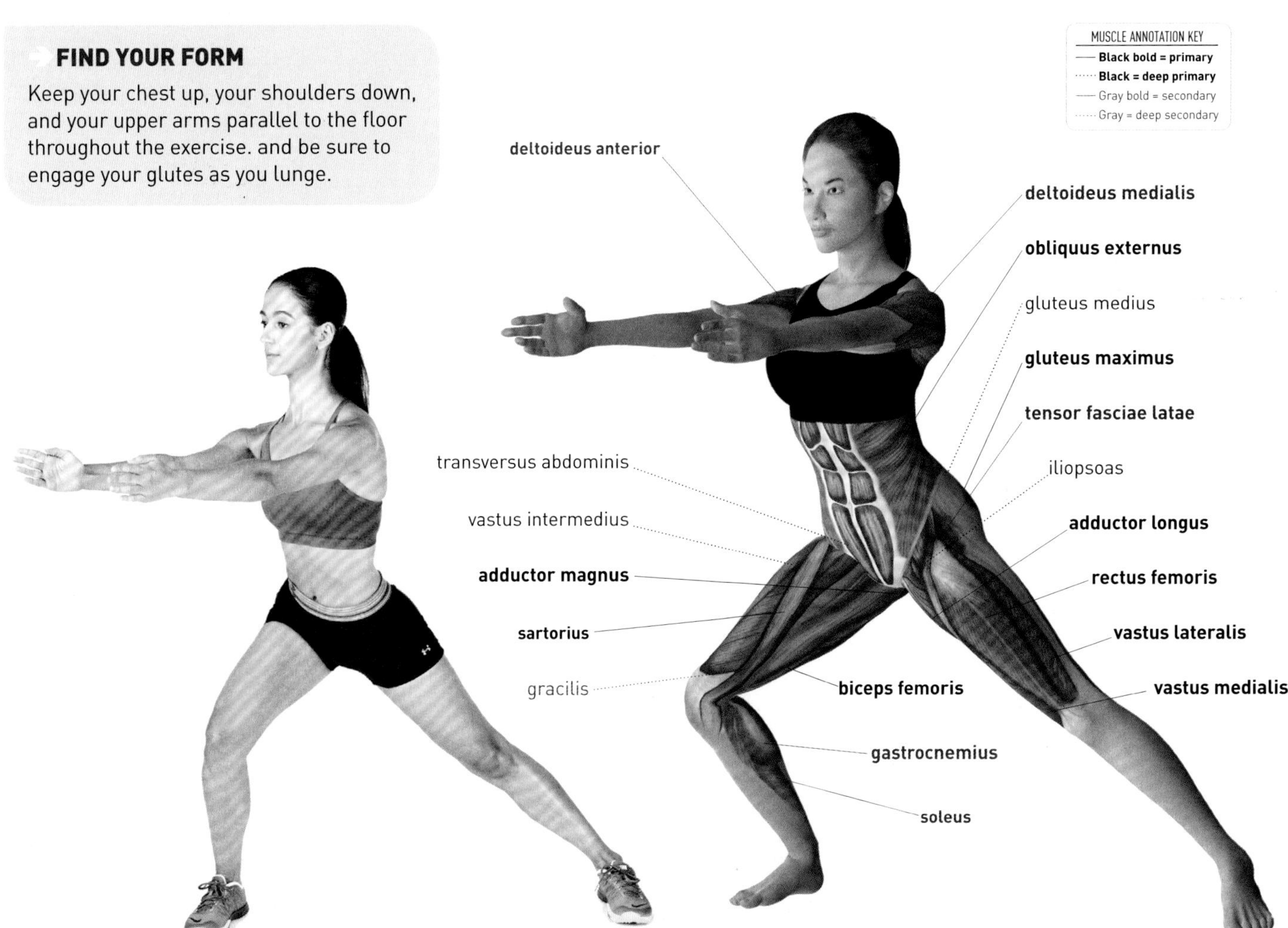

073

Curtsy Lunge

Stand upright with your feet together and your arms outstretched in front of you, parallel to the floor. Take a big step back with your right leg, crossing it behind your left leg. Bend both knees, and lower your body until your front thigh is parallel with the floor. Return to the starting position, and repeat on the other side.

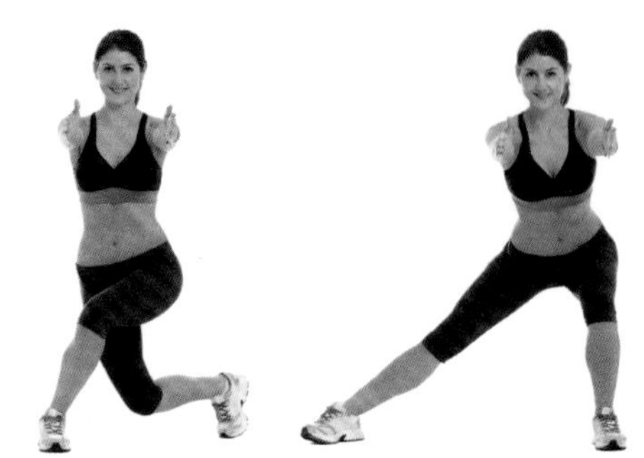

074

Clock Lunge

This exercise combines the three basic lunges into one. Stand with your legs and feet parallel and shoulder-width apart, and your knees bent very slightly. Tuck your pelvis slightly forward, lift your chest, press your shoulders down and back, and then perform a Forward Lunge (#043). Return to standing position, and then perform a Lateral Lunge (#072). Return to standing position, and then perform a Reverse Lunge (#059). Return to standing position, and repeat in the opposite direction.

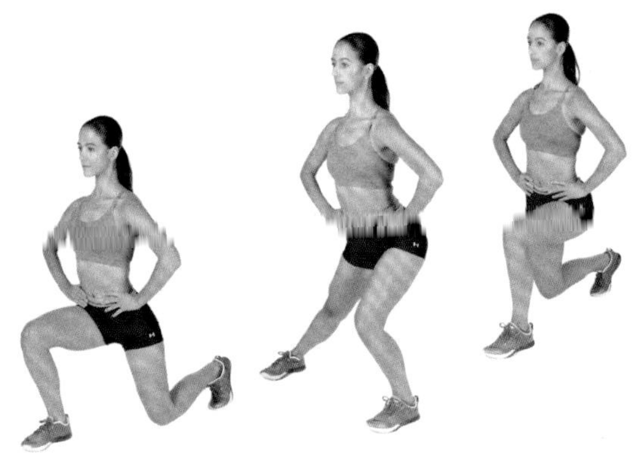

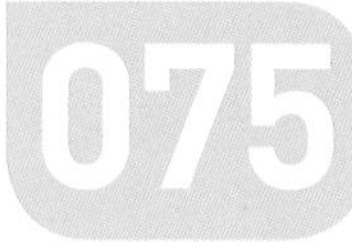

Lateral-Extension Lateral Lunge

Stand with your feet hip-width apart and your arms at your sides, a dumbbell in each hand. Take a big step to the left, performing a Lateral Lunge (#072), and at the same time, raise both arms so that they are parallel to the floor, forming a straight line. Smoothly and with control, return to the starting position. Repeat on the other side.

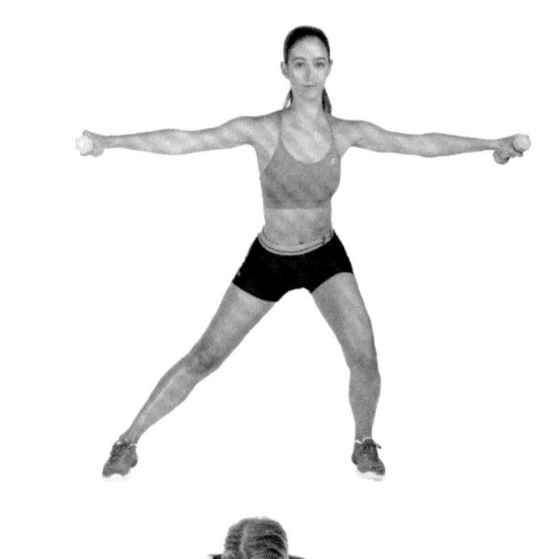

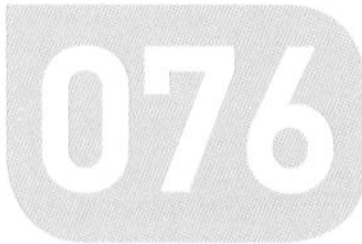

Side Lunge Stretch

From the Sumo Squat (#022), drop your hands onto the floor in front of you, transferring some of your weight onto your arms. Shift your body over to the right, staying as low as possible, bending your right knee, and extending and straightening your left leg. Return to the center, switch sides, and repeat.

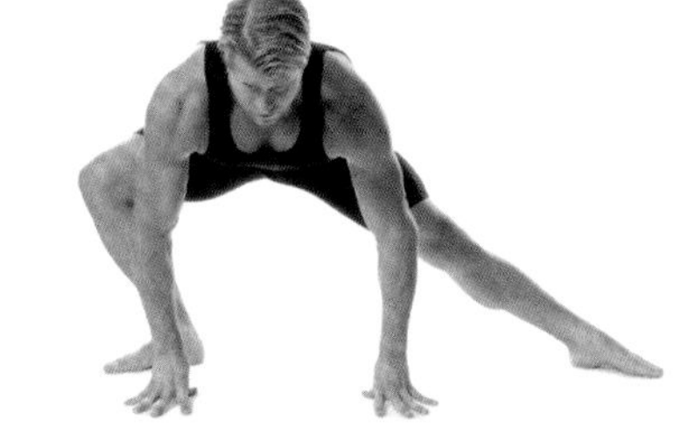

Single-Leg Lateral Lunge with Lift

Grasp a dumbbell in each hand with palms facing each other. Perform a Lateral Lunge (#072) on your left leg as you lean your torso slightly forward until the weights are at knee level. As you straighten your left leg, lift your right leg out to the side until it is almost parallel to the floor. Lower your right leg back to the lateral lunge, and then return to standing. Repeat on the other side.

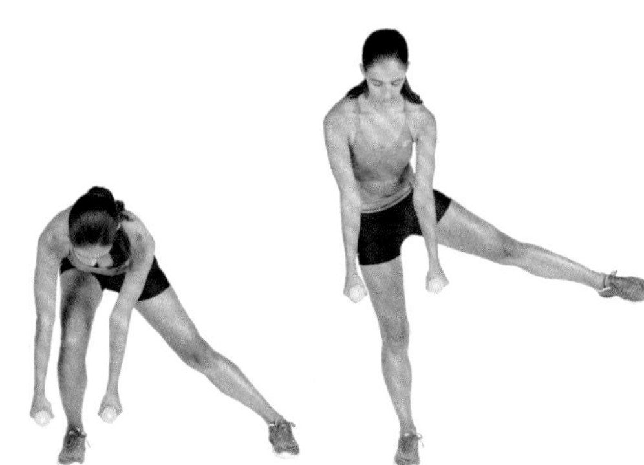

078 Alternating Touchdown Lunge

Perform a Lateral Lunge (#072) to the right, keeping your back straight and chest high, bring your left arm across your body to touch your right toes. Reverse the movement, and return to standing position. Repeat on the other side, and continue alternating sides.

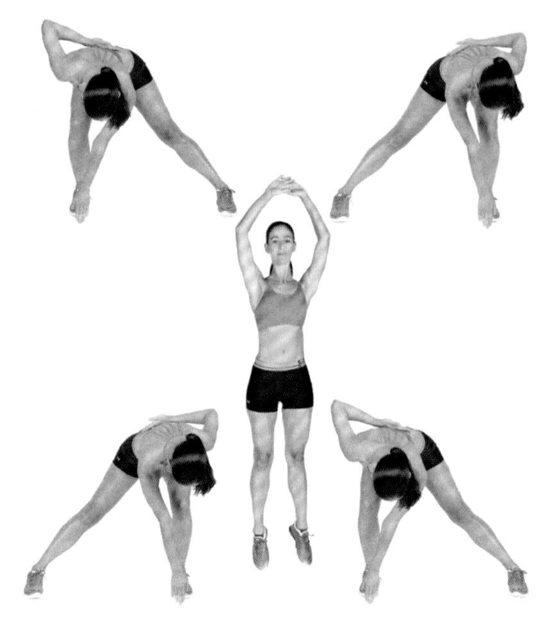

079 Plyo Touchdown Switch

Perform a Lateral Lunge (#072) to the left, keeping your chest high as you simultaneously reach your right hand to your left toes. Push through your left foot to jump back up to the starting stance, and then repeat on the opposite side. Continue quickly alternating sides.

080 Straddle Adductor Lunge

Spread your feet widely apart, and bend your knees. Clasp your hands in front of you, and distribute your weight evenly between your feet. Bend forward at a 45-degree angle to the floor so that your hips are behind your heels. Alternate leaning from side to side.

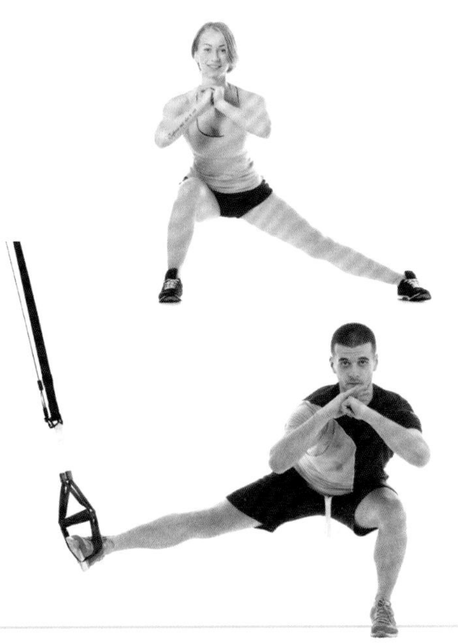

081 Suspended Adductor Lunge

Place one foot on its side in the foot cradle, and face to the side with your leg straight out to the side. Keeping your chest up, bend your standing leg, and push your butt back as you sink down into a lunge so that the suspended leg slides out to the side as you sit back and down. Driving through your standing heel, return to standing, pulling the suspended leg back in toward your standing leg. Perform the desired reps, and then repeat on the opposite side.

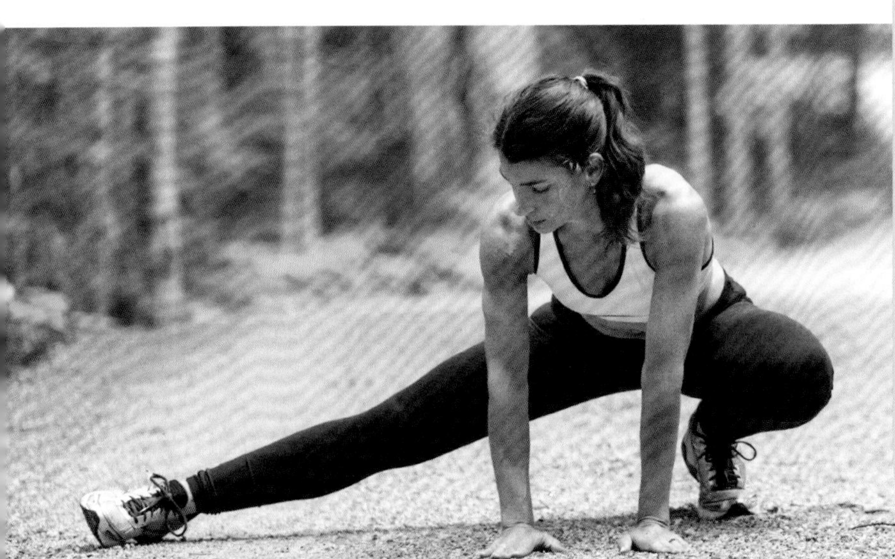

ADDUCTION AND ABDUCTION

Your muscles and joints function in a variety of ways as you work out or just move through your daily life—and exercise names often refer to these movements. The term *abduction* refers to movement away from the body; the contraction of an abductor muscle moves a limb away from the midline of the body or from another part. *Adduction* is toward the body; the contraction of an adductor muscle moves a limb toward the midline of the body or toward another part.

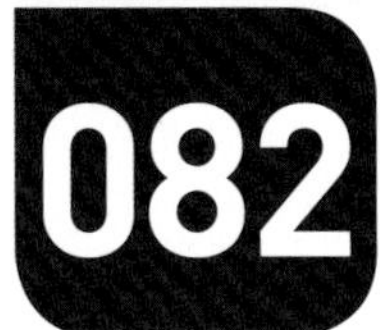

Forward Bend

Moving through daily life requires quite a bit of bending, whether you are reaching down to pick up your child or retrieving your dropped car keys. The Forward Bend and its variations prepare you to do those everyday movements with ease and efficiency, and they also get you in shape for high-intensity activities like gymnastics and martial arts. Bending exercises can strengthen muscles and joints while helping your to become more flexible by stretching and opening tight areas of your body. The Forward Bend particularly targets the hamstrings muscles and the spine.

- Stand tall, with your arms at your sides.
- Raise your arms toward the ceiling.
- Exhale, and bend forward from your hips, sweeping your arms to the sides with your palms facing the floor. While you lower your torso, keep your back flat, and tuck your abdominals in toward your spine. Lengthen your spine as much as possible.

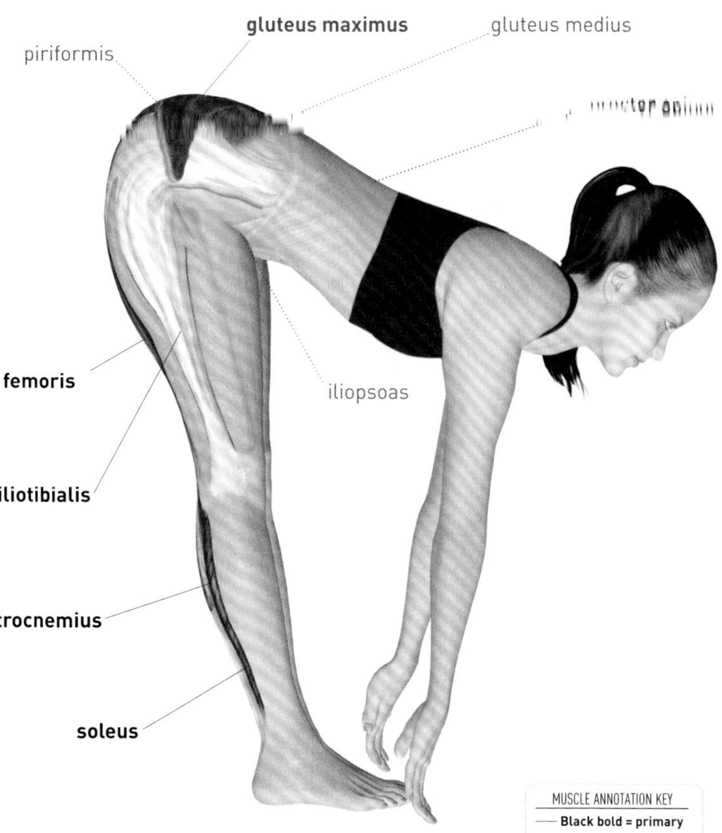

piriformis
gluteus maximus
gluteus medius
biceps femoris
iliopsoas
tractus iliotibialis
gastrocnemius
soleus

MUSCLE ANNOTATION KEY
— **Black bold = primary**
······ **Black = deep primary**
— Gray bold = secondary
······ Gray = deep secondary

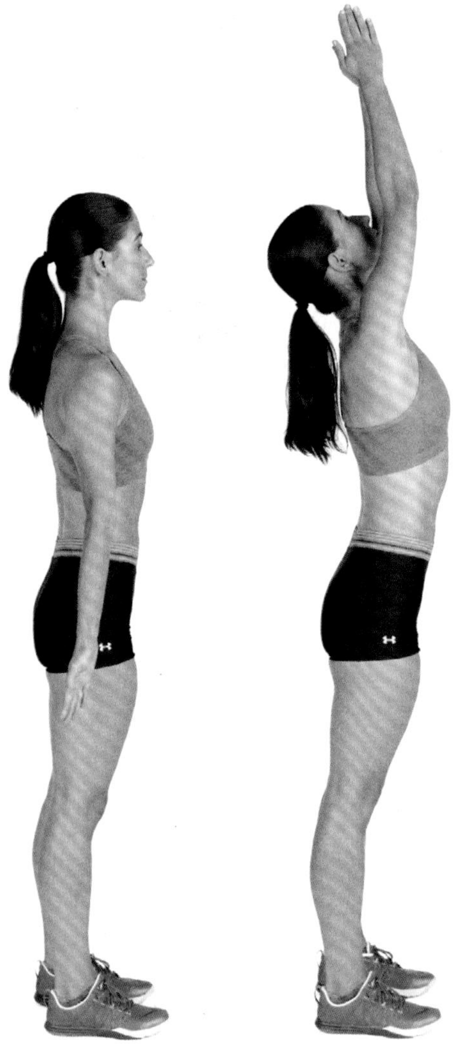

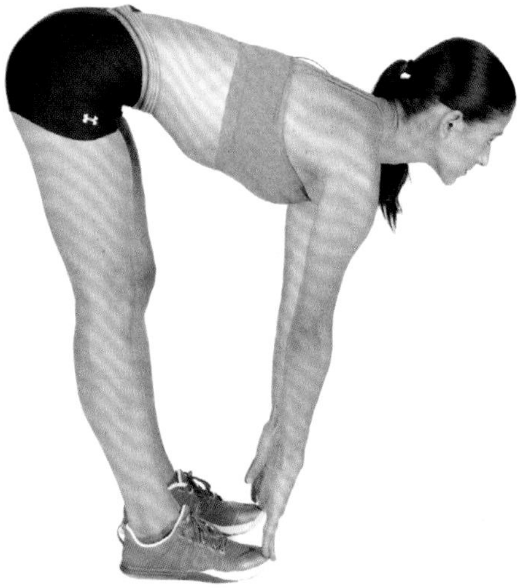

FIND YOUR FORM

Make the stretch long and smooth, and avoid bouncing as you reach your fingers toward your toes—reach down only as far as you can comfortably extend.

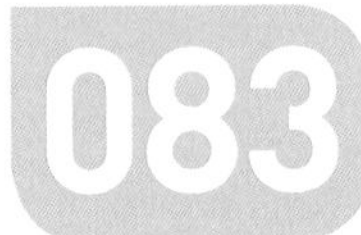

Deep Forward Bend

Perform a Forward Bend (#082), and then fold your torso and abdominals onto the front of your legs, aiming your forehead toward your shins. Grasp the backs of your ankles, and contract your thigh muscles to try to straighten your knees as much as possible. Hold for the desired time, and then release.

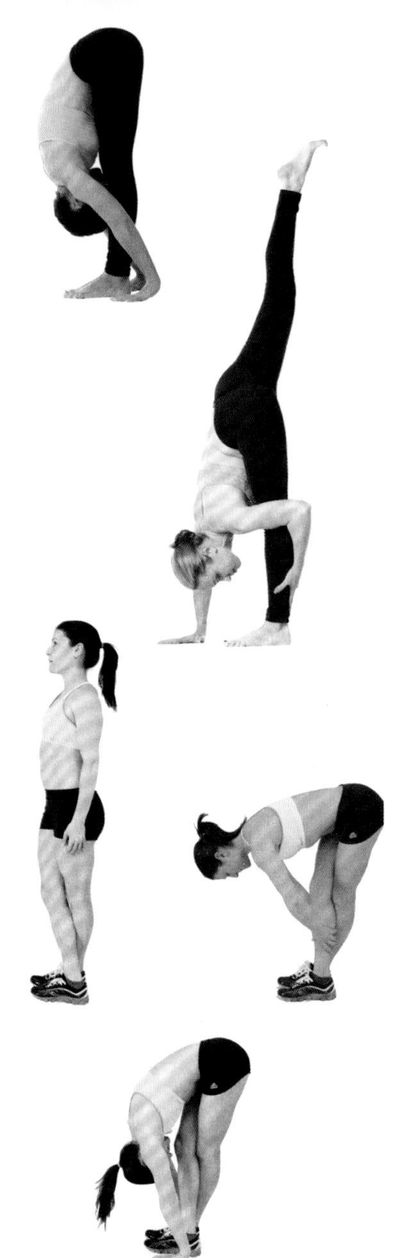

Standing Split

Stand tall, and shift your weight onto your left foot. Bend forward with your back flat, simultaneously raising your right leg behind you. Square your shoulders, and reach your fingertips toward the floor. Inhale, hold your right ankle with your right hand, and lift your heel toward the ceiling. Maintain balance with your right palm on the floor. Hold for the desired time, and then release. Switch sides and repeat.

085

ITB Forward Bend

Stand upright, with your arms along your sides. Cross one foot in front of the other. Bending at your waist, grasp your legs at the shins. Hold for the desired time, and then release, slowly rolling up, and repeat twice. Switch sides and repeat.

ITB Floor Touch

Stand upright, with your arms along your sides. Cross one foot in front of the other. Bending at your waist, gradually reach toward the floor with your hands. Hold for the desired time, and then release, slowly rolling up, and repeat twice. Switch sides and repeat.

WHY WORRY ABOUT YOUR ILIOTIBIAL BAND?

The iliotibial tract or band, commonly known as the ITB or IT band, is a thick band of fibrous tissue that runs down the outside of the thigh, beginning at the iliac crest and extending to the outer side of the shinbone, just below the knee joint. The ITB also attaches to the gluteal muscles and the tensor fascia latae, the muscle on the outside of your hip that moves your leg outward. The ITB functions in coordination with several of the thigh muscles to extend, abduct, and laterally rotate the hip. It also contributes to lateral knee stabilization. In order to work out at high intensities—running and jumping, in particular—it is essential to keep the ITB in shape. Iliotibial band syndrome, usually shortened to IT band syndrome or simply ITBS, is common in runners, and it occurs when the ITB thickens and rubs the knee bone, producing inflammation. Certain structural factors may make you more susceptible, such as a difference in length between one leg and the other.

087 Wide-Legged Forward Bend

Stand tall, and then take a large step—about 3 to 4 feet—to the side. Your feet should be parallel to each other. Exhale, and bend forward from your hips, keeping your back flat. With your elbows straight, place your fingertips on the floor. With another exhalation, place your hands on the floor in between your feet, and lower your torso into a full forward bend, bending your elbows and placing your forehead on the floor. Hold for the desired time, and then straighten your elbows and raise your torso while keeping your back flat to return to the starting position.

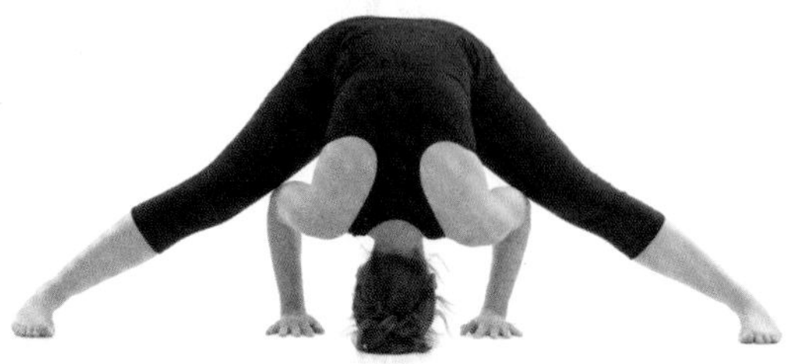

088 Wide-Legged Half Forward Bend

Stand tall, and then take a large step—about 3 to 4 feet—to the side. Your feet should be parallel to each other. Exhale, bending forwards until your torso is nearly parallel to the floor. Place your hands on the floor, making sure that your lower back is straight. Hold for the desired time, and then release.

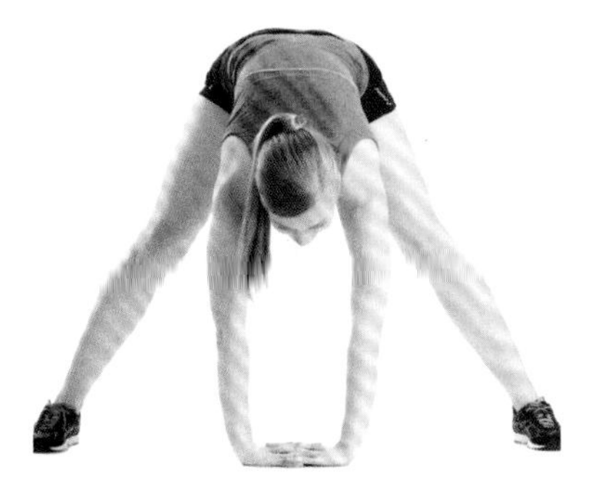

089 Alternating Toe Touches

Perform the Wide-Legged Half Forward Bend (#088), and then, keeping your back flat, touch your toes to your left foot. Return to standing position, and repeat on the other side. Continue alternating right and left toe touches.

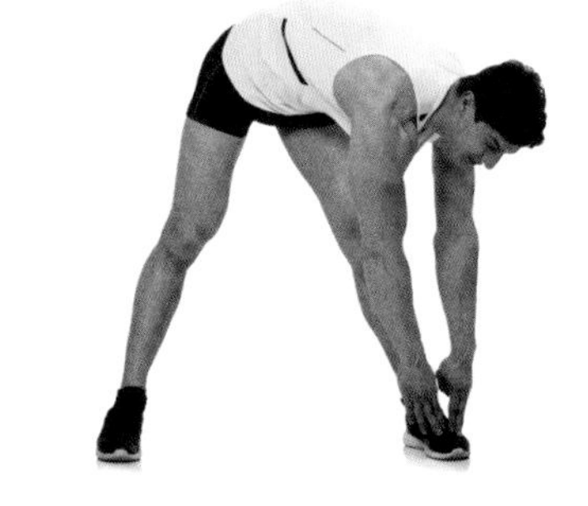

090 Seated Forward Bend

Sit on the floor as straight as possible with your back flattened and your legs extended in front of you. Lean forward, lowering your abdominals toward your thighs and grasping the soles of your feet with both hands.

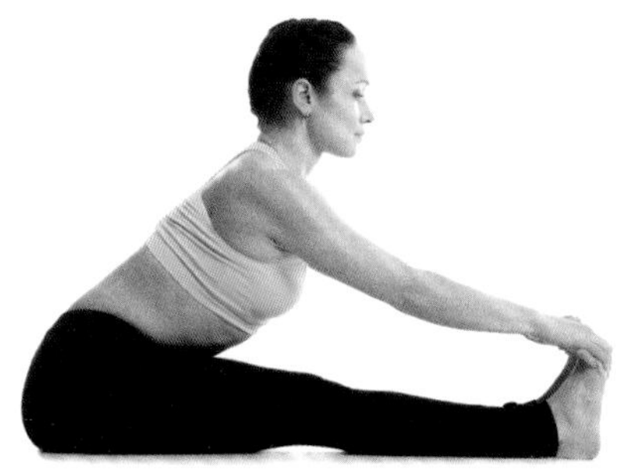

091 Single-Leg Seated Forward Bend

Sit on the floor as straight as possible with your back flattened and your legs extended in front of you in parallel position, and then bend your right leg until it is turned out, with the bottom of your right foot resting at your left inner thigh just above the kneecap. Rest your hands on your knee, and bend from your waist to lean forward over your left leg. Grasp the inside of your left foot with your right hand. Use your left hand to guide your torso to the left. Return to the starting position, and then repeat on the other side.

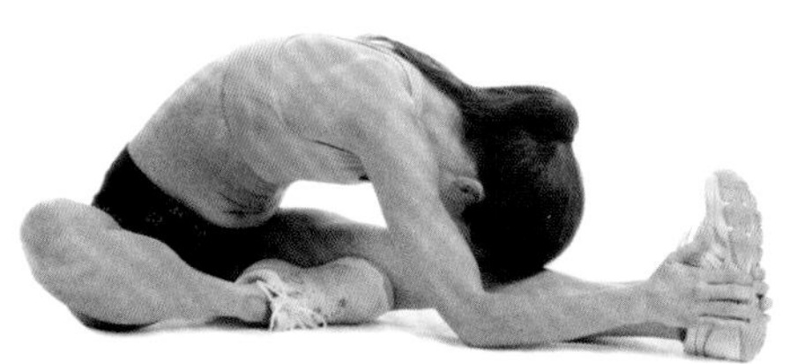

092 Side Bend

The Side Bend does a lot with a little—this simple move strengthens and stretches the spinal stabilizer muscles, including the erector spinae, latissimus dorsi, and obliques. A functional flexibility exercise, the Side Bend helps improve your performance of daily movements, like reaching into a high cabinet, or sport movements, like shooting a basketball. It will also improve your balance and general range of motion.

- Stand with your feet together, keeping your neck, shoulders, and torso straight.
- Raise both arms above your head and clasp your hands together, palms facing upward.
- Leaning from your hips, drop your torso to the left.
- Return to the starting position, and then lean your torso to the right. Keeping a smooth flow, continue alternating sides.

FIND YOUR FORM

Elongate your arms and shoulders as much as possible, avoid dropping to the side too quickly—be sure to move with control

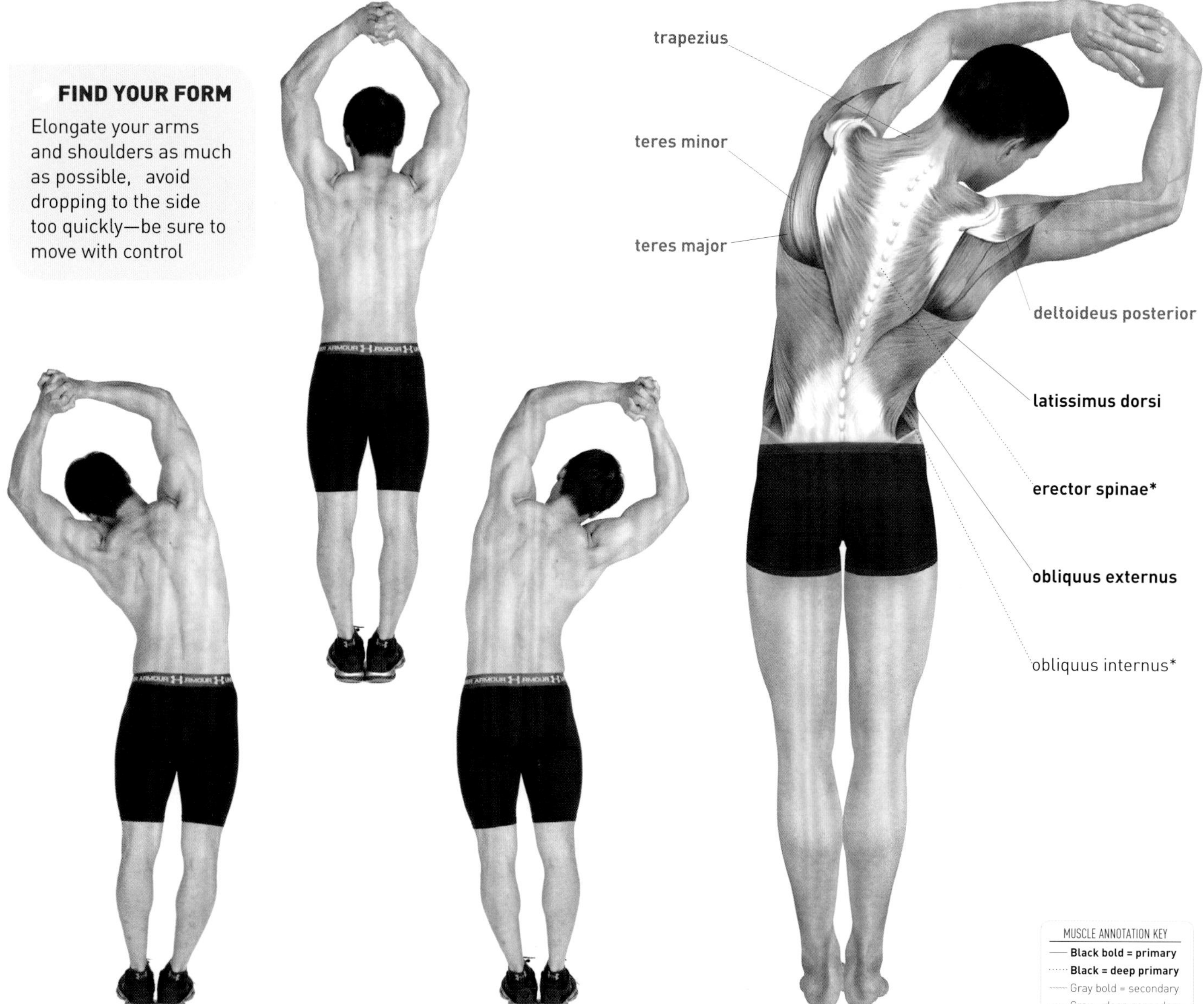

093

Side Bend Squat

Spread your feet widely apart, and bend your knees into a squat. Let your arms hang straight down at your sides. Leaning from your hips and moving with control, slowly drop your torso to the right, while at the same time extending your left arm straight up toward the ceiling. Return to the starting position, and then lean your torso to the left, while raising your right arm. Keeping a smooth flow, continue alternating sides.

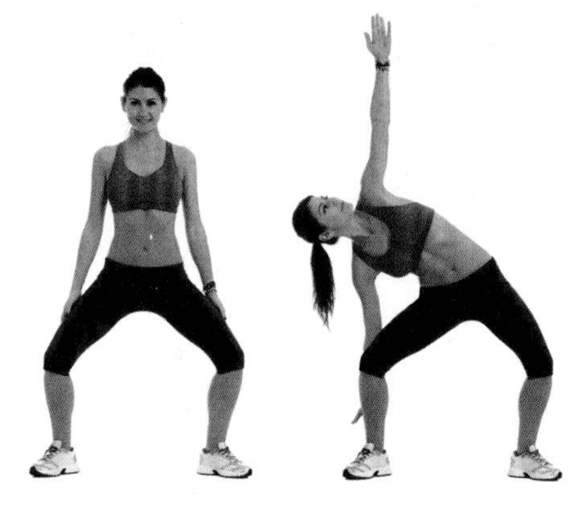

094

Dumbbell Side Bend

Stand with your feet hip-width apart and your arms at your sides, a dumbbell in each hand. Leaning from your hips, drop your torso to the right, lowering the weight toward your right knee. Pause, and then slowly return to the starting position, and then lean your torso to the left, lowering the weight toward your left knee. Keeping a smooth flow, continue alternating sides.

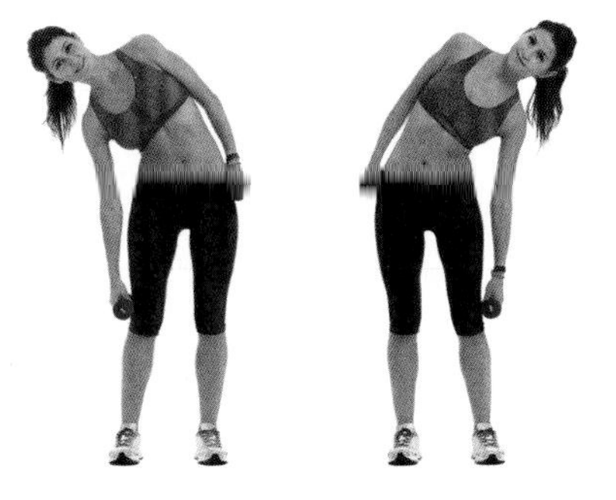

095

Dumbbell Side Crunch

Stand with your feet hip-width apart, a dumbbell in each hand. Raise your right arm straight up toward the ceiling. Lift your right knee while bending to the right to bring your right elbow and knee together, doing a side crunch. Straighten your spine as you bring your right foot to the floor, lowering your arm to return to the starting position, and then lift your left knee while bending to the left to bring your left elbow and knee together. Keeping a smooth flow, continue alternating sides.

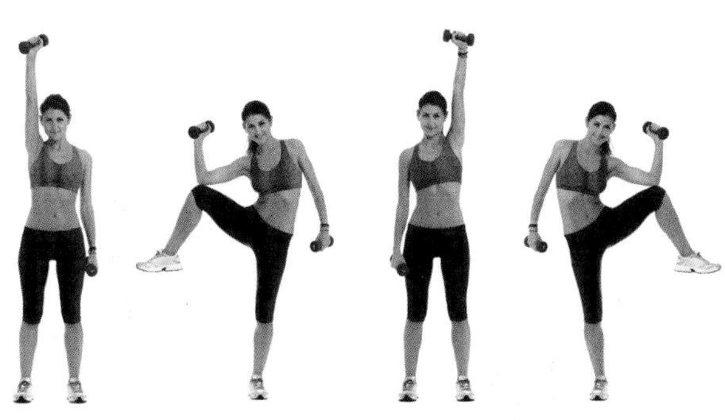

096

Windmill

With your right arm by your side and your feet shoulder-width apart, stand with your left hand raised overhead. Push your left hip out to the left and slightly bend your knees while lowering your torso to the right as far as possible. Pause, then return to the starting position. Complete the desired repetitions, and then repeat on the other side.

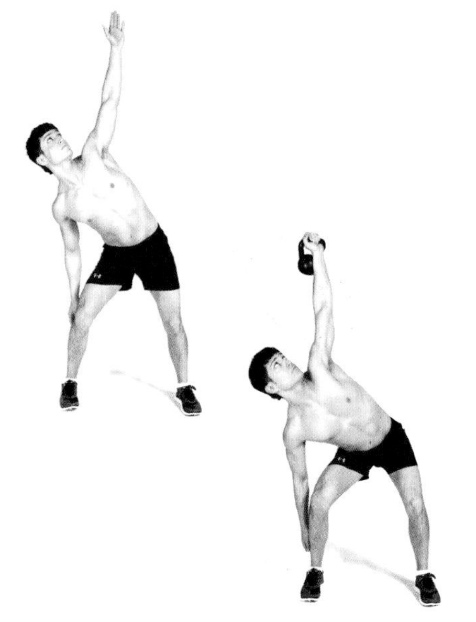

097

Kettlebell Windmill

With your right arm by your side and your feet shoulder-width apart, stand with a kettlebell in your left hand raised overhead. Perform as you would a Windmill (#096).

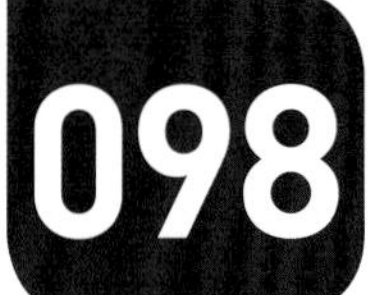

Lateral Step-Over

The Lateral Step-Over is great exercise to help you improve lateral quickness and increase your agility. Perform it as a drill to really focus on your coordination, starting at half speed and, as the footwork becomes familiar, working up to moving as quickly as you can while maintaining good form. You can also vary the height and width of your obstacle—try setting up small cones or a low step to start out, eventually stepping over higher benches or bars.

- Stand next to an obstacle like a step or flat bench.
- Raise the knee of the leg closest to the bench, and then lower your foot down to the floor on the opposite side of the bench.
- Lift the opposite leg to meet the other, bringing your feet together.
- Reverse the motion until you are standing with both feet together in the starting position. Repeat in continuous motion for the desired time or reps.

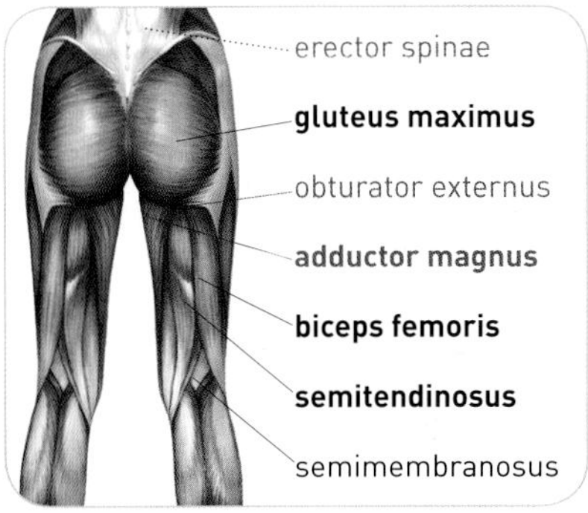

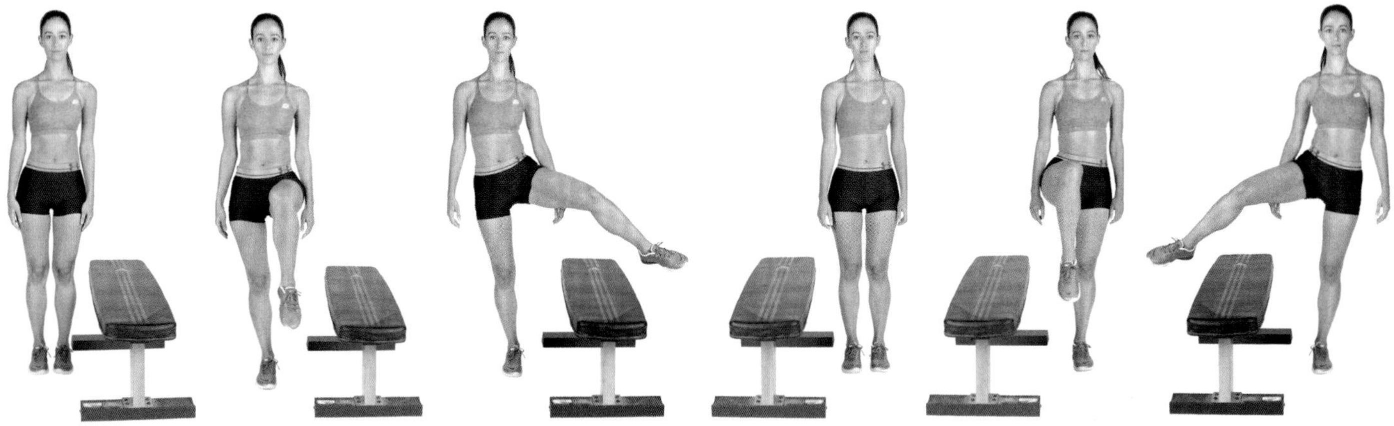

erector spinae
gluteus maximus
obturator externus
adductor magnus
biceps femoris
semitendinosus
semimembranosus

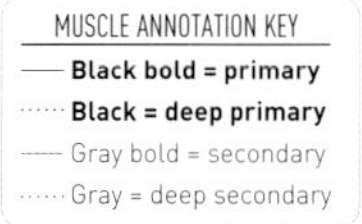

MUSCLE ANNOTATION KEY
Black bold = primary
Black = deep primary
Gray bold = secondary
Gray = deep secondary

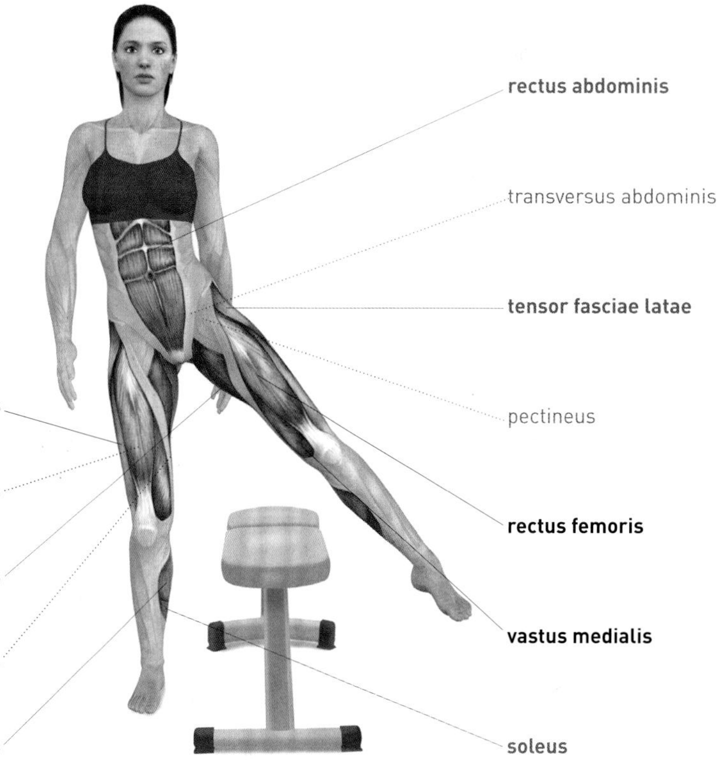

rectus abdominis
transversus abdominis
tensor fasciae latae
pectineus
rectus femoris
vastus medialis
soleus
vastus lateralis
vastus intermedius
adductor longus
gracilis
gastrocnemius

FIND YOUR FORM

Keep facing forward throughout the exercise. When stepping over the bench, be sure to raise your leg, and then rotate your thigh outward—avoid just turning your torso to step over the bench.

099 Resisted Side Steps

Stand with your feet shoulder-width apart, with a resistance loop or a resistance band tied around your ankles. Tuck your pelvis slightly forward, lift your chest, and press your shoulders downward and back. Keeping your head up and shoulders back, place your hands on your hips, and step sideways as far as you can while keeping your knees slightly bent and your posture tall. Bring the opposite foot inward to meet the other foot, moving with control. Continue to step to the side for one to three sets of the desired repetitions, then repeat in the other direction.

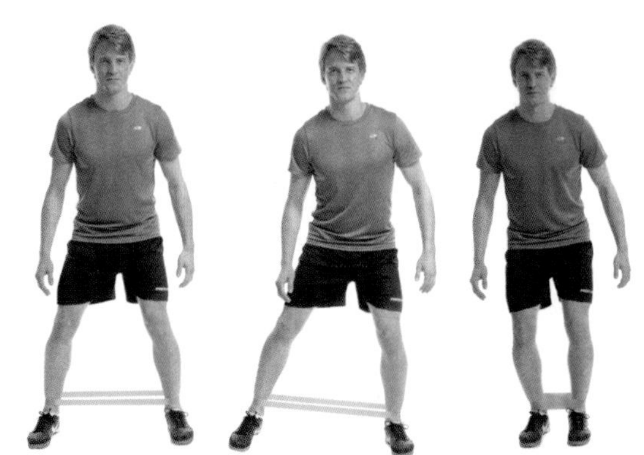

100 Resisted Crossover Steps

Stand with your feet shoulder-width apart, with a resistance loop or a resistance band tied around your ankles. Tuck your pelvis slightly forward, lift your chest, and press your shoulders downward and back. Step out until with your left foot until you feel moderate tension in the band, and then cross your left foot over your right. Next, step your right foot in front of your left, and then step your left foot out, for a total of at least three steps with both feet to the left. Return to the starting position, and then begin crossing right over left in the opposite direction. Repeat all moves for the desired sets and reps.

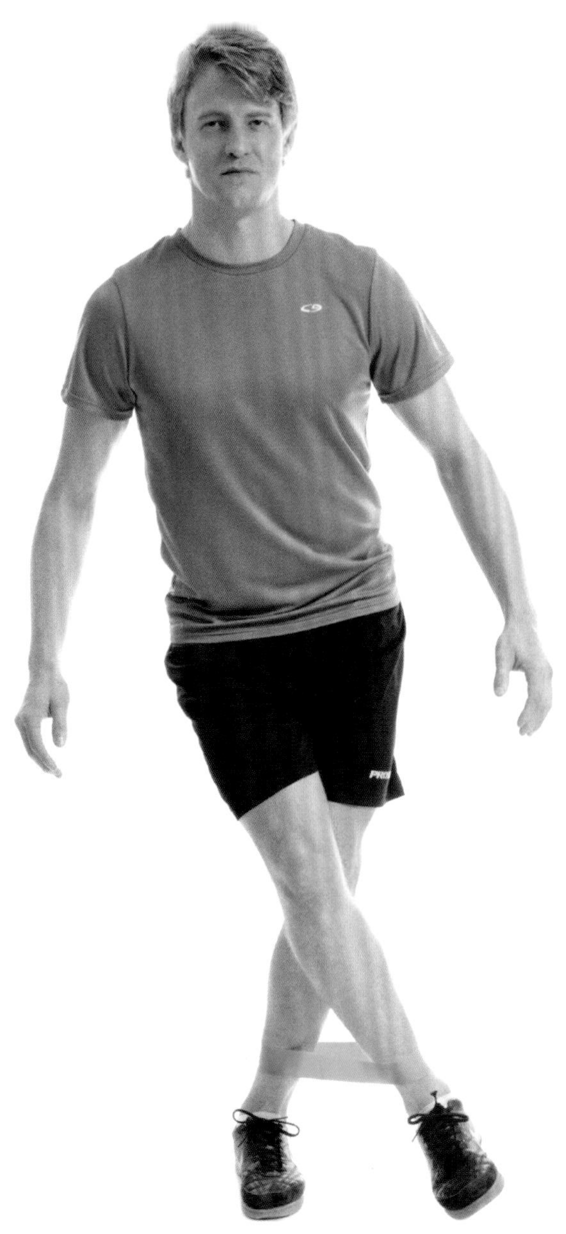

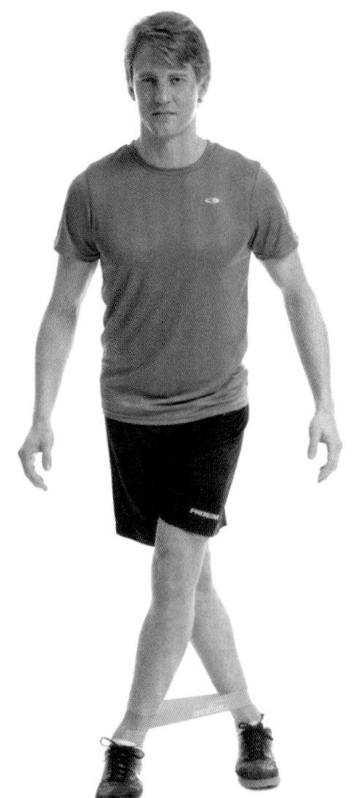

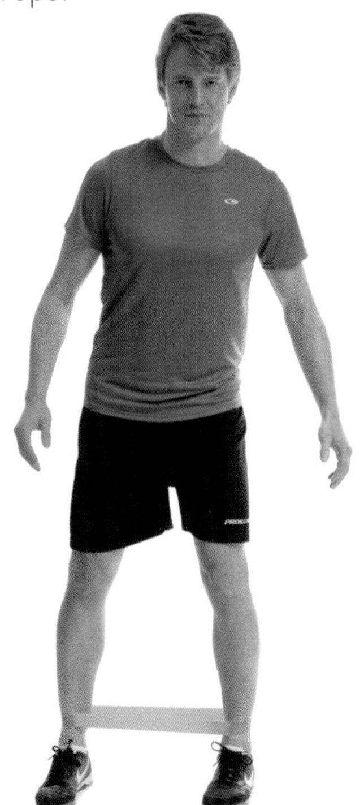

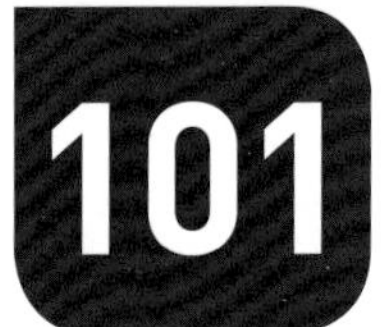

Step-Up

As part of a strength and conditioning program, the Step-Up effectively tones and sculpts your lower-body muscles, especially your quads, glutes, hip flexors, and hamstrings. It is also a great balance move for improving stability in your pelvis and legs, and adds a strong dose of cardio to a workout. Start with a step or box high enough so that you must bend your knee to at least a 90-degree angle, and build up to higher boxes or benches as your strength and stamina improve.

- Stand in front of a step, bench or other platform.
- Step onto the bench with your right leg, making sure your foot is flat against the bench.
- Lean forward slightly. and push yourself upward through the heel of your right foot, so that your left leg comes up to the bench.
- Step down with the right leg, and then repeat the same sequence with the left leg. Continue stepping up and down, alternating sides.

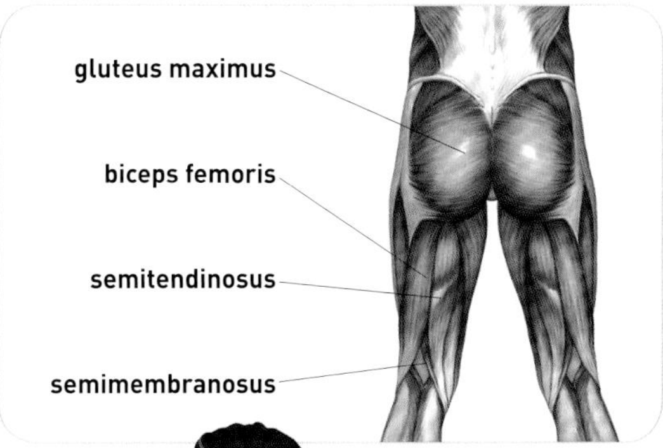

gluteus maximus

biceps femoris

semitendinosus

semimembranosus

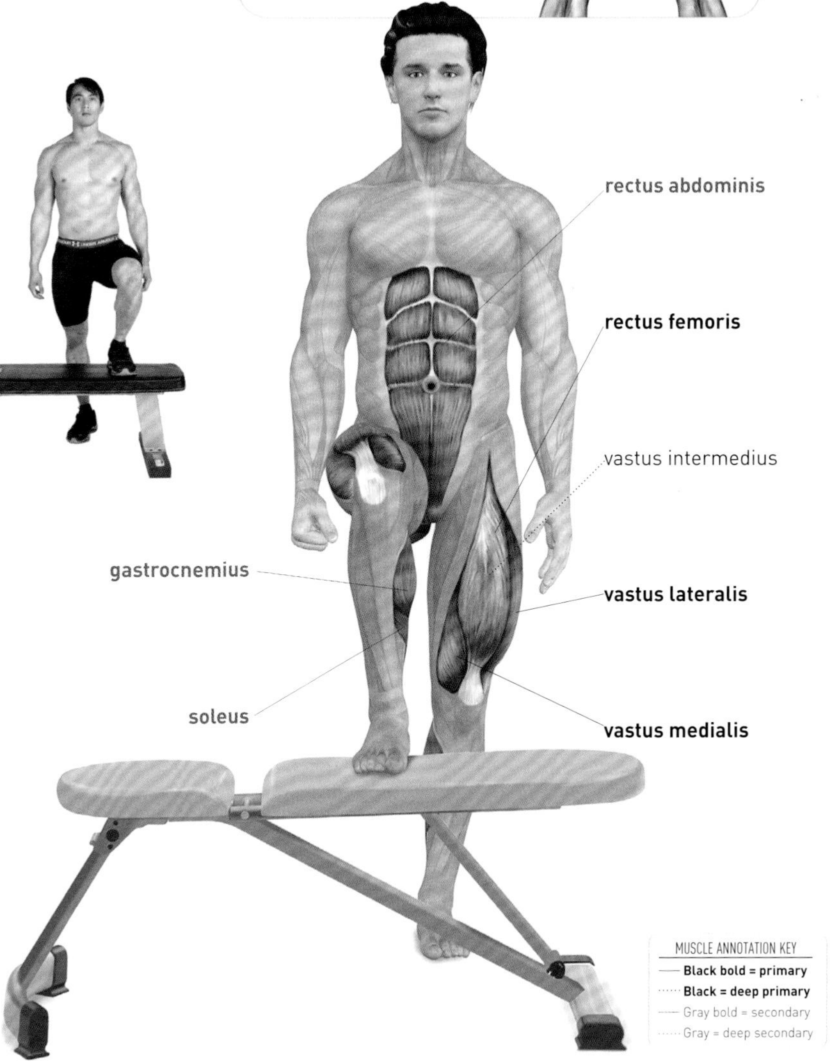

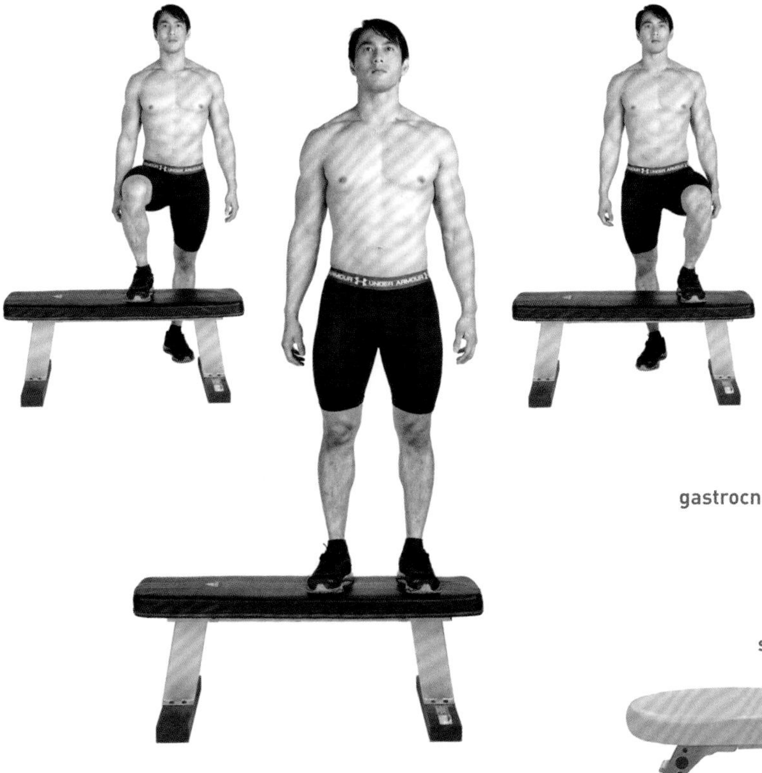

rectus abdominis

rectus femoris

vastus intermedius

gastrocnemius

vastus lateralis

soleus

vastus medialis

FIND YOUR FORM

Push through the working heel, keeping that foot planted. Avoid hyperextending your knee past your toes, or moving faster than you can while still maintaining control.

MUSCLE ANNOTATION KEY
— Black bold = primary
····· Black = deep primary
— Gray bold = secondary
····· Gray = deep secondary

102 Alternating Step-Up with Knee Lift

Perform as you would the Step-Up (#101), but at the top of the movement, when both feet are on the step, raise one knee as high as you can. Lower your knee, step down, and repeat on the other side.

103 Step-Up with Knee Lift and Overhead Extension

Perform as you would a Alternating Step-Up with Knee Lift (#102), but as you raise your knee, simultaneously extend the opposite arm straight toward the ceiling. Lower your knee and arm, step down, and repeat on the other side.

104 Dumbbell Step-Up

Holding a dumbbell in each hand with your arms at our side, perform the Step-Up (#101). Continue stepping up and down, alternating sides for the desired reps.

105 Lateral Step and Curl

Stand with your feet hip-width apart and your arms at your sides, a dumbbell in each hand. Position a step beside your right foot. Step to the right, placing your right foot on the step. Simultaneously bend your elbows, curling the dumbbells into your chest. Lowering the dumbbells, bring your left leg onto the step. Curl the dumbbells into your chest as you step your right leg off of the step. Release the dumbbells as you step down with your left leg to return to the starting position with the step to your right.

106 Curling Step and Raise

Stand with your feet hip-width apart and your arms at your sides, a dumbbell in each hand. Position a step beside your left foot. Place your left foot on the step Shift your weight onto your left foot. Bend your elbows, curling the dumbbells toward your chest. At the same time, raise your right knee as your foot comes off the floor. Lowering the dumbbells, cross your right leg over your left leg, which should bend slightly as you lower your right leg to the floor, left of the platform. Simultaneously bend your left leg slightly. Step your left leg onto the floor so that you are in starting position on the other side of the step. Repeat on the other side, and continue to alternate sides for the desired reps.

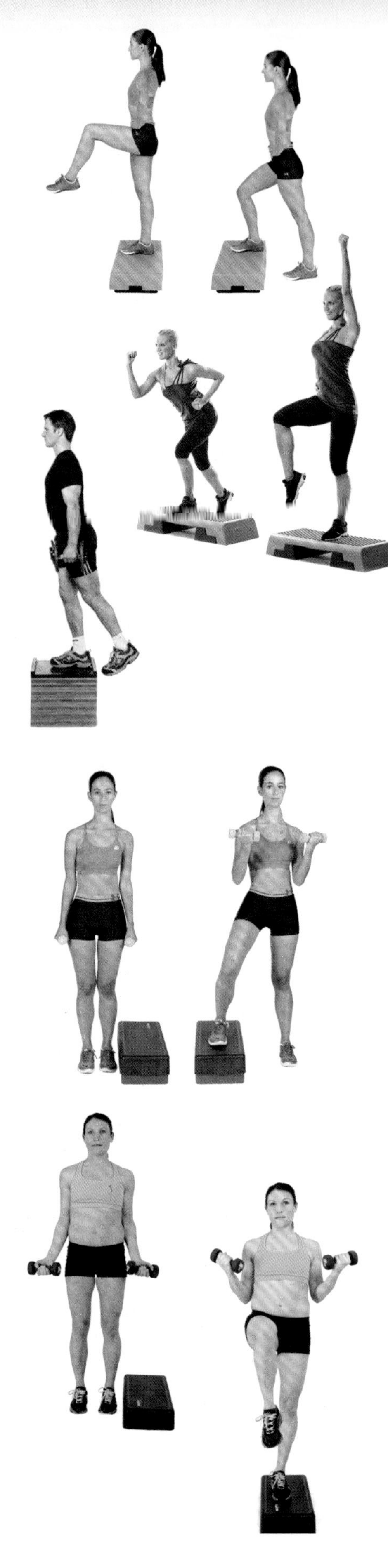

107

Medicine Ball Crossover Step-Up

Stand with your feet hip-width apart, holding a medicine ball in front of your chest. Position a high step and a lower step beside your left foot. Cross your right leg over your left, resting it on the step. Shift your weight onto your right foot to step up. Rest your left foot on the lower step. Again cross your right leg over your left to step down onto the floor. Step your right leg onto the floor so that you are standing to the left of the step. Repeat in the other direction.

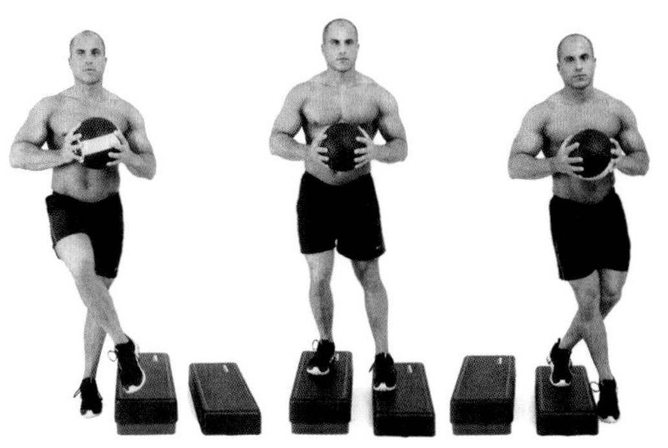

108

Crossover Bench Step-Up

Stand to the right of a bench. Cross your right leg in front of your left, and step on to the bench. Push through the stabilized right heel on the bench to raise yourself up. Bring your left leg up on to the bench, then perform the motion in reverse to step down. Repeat for the desired repetitions, and the repeat on the opposite leg.

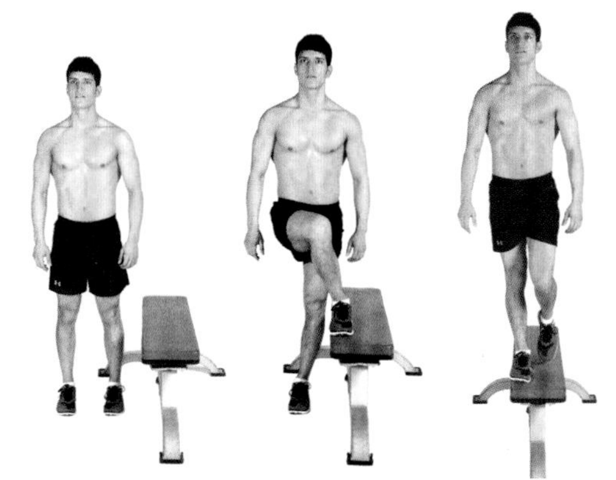

109

Side Step-Up Shuffle

Stand with your left foot on a low box or step and your right foot on the floor about two feet to the right of the box. Bend your knees slightly, keep your chest up, and bend your arms to 90 degrees, keeping your elbows close to your body. Push off your left foot, and jump to your left, landing with your right foot on the box and your left foot on the floor, knees bent. Push off your right foot to jump back to the starting position.

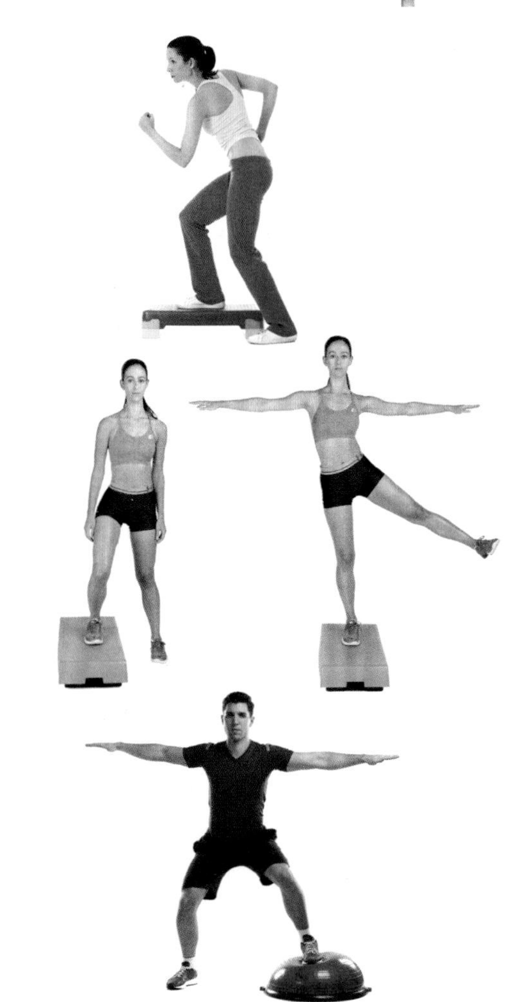

110

Side Step-Up with Lateral Leg Raise

Stand to the right of a bench or step. Step on to the bench with your right leg, and push up. As you bring your left leg up, power it out to the left, and raise your arms to shoulder height. Keep your focus and feet forward. Step down to the same side to complete one rep.

111

BOSU Triple Squat Lateral Step-Up

With the platform side down, stand to the side of a BOSU trainer with your right foot on top. Squat down, and then step onto the dome with your left foot, lowering into another squat. Next, step to the other side of the BOSU, and squat, repeating the side-to-side sequence for the desired repetitions.

Step-Down

High-intensity workouts often call for moves, such as jumping and running, that can be hard on the knees. Including in your routine exercises that strengthen the muscles that support this joint is wise. The Step-Down is particularly effective at working the vastus medialis. This muscle, one of the quadriceps, runs along the inside portion of your front thigh, closest to your kneecap. When your vastus medialis muscle is weak, it is unable to support the knee cap in proper alignment.

- Stand facing forward on a step with feet together and hands on hips.
- Bend your right leg. Simultaneously step your left leg downward, flexing the foot to rest on your heel.
- Without rotating your torso or knee, press upward through your right leg to return to the starting position. Switch legs, and repeat, continuing to alternate legs for the desired repetitions.

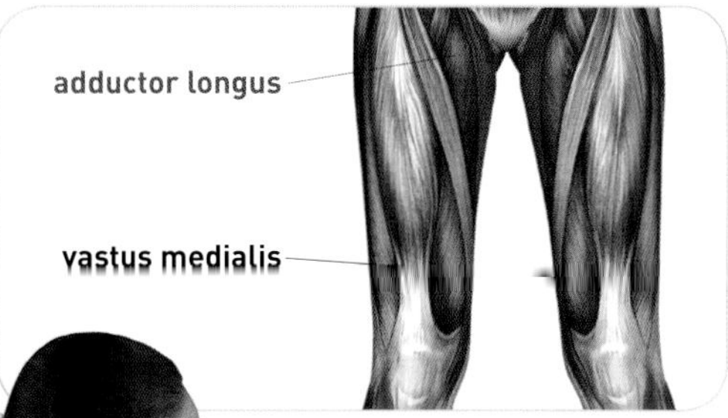

adductor longus
vastus medialis

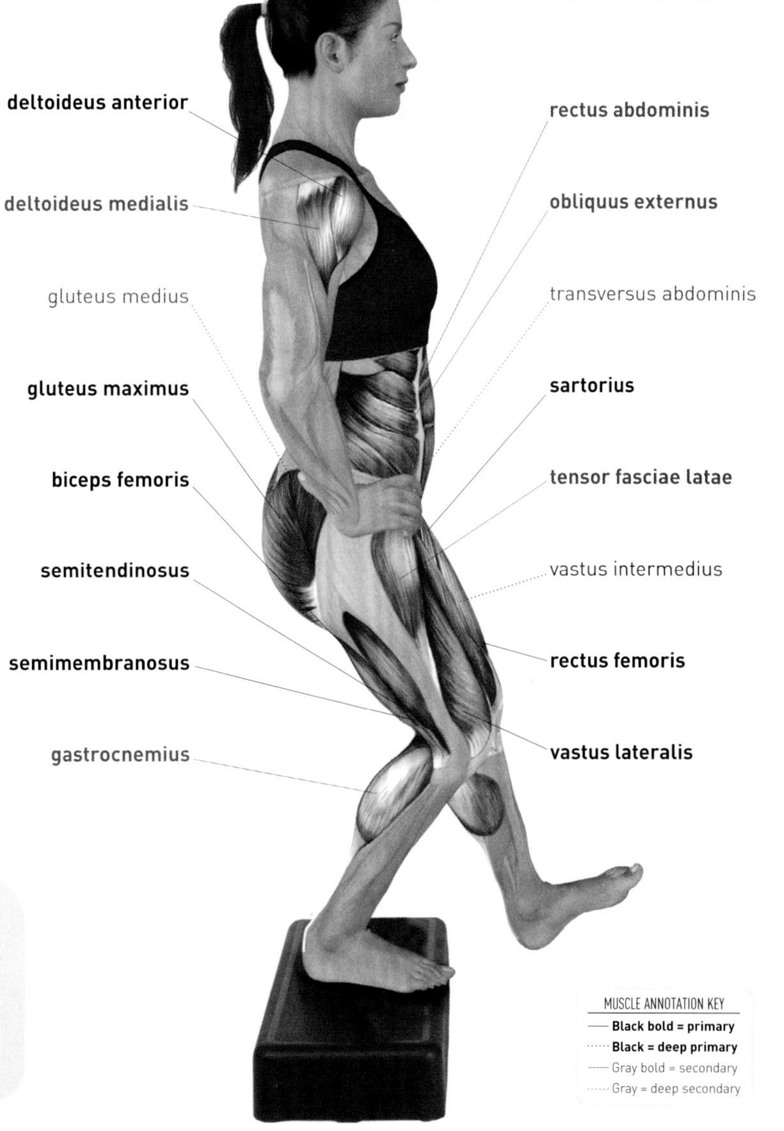

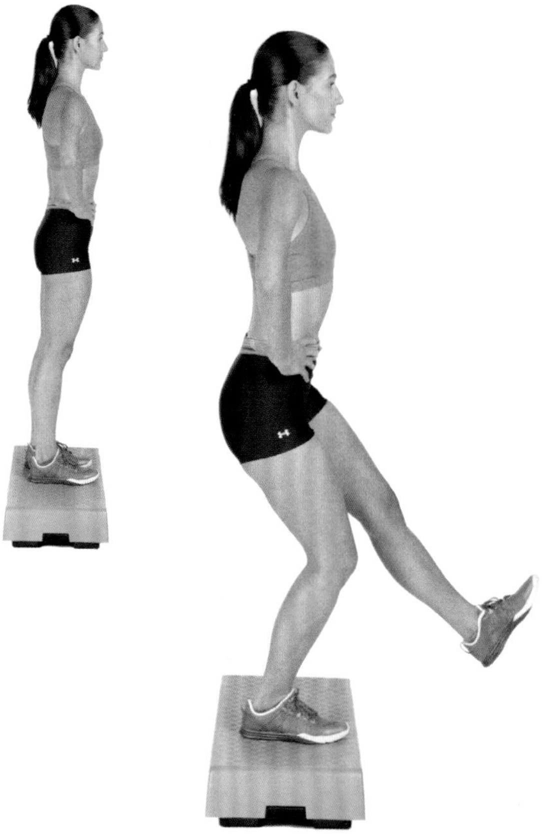

deltoideus anterior
deltoideus medialis
gluteus medius
gluteus maximus
biceps femoris
semitendinosus
semimembranosus
gastrocnemius
rectus abdominis
obliquus externus
transversus abdominis
sartorius
tensor fasciae latae
vastus intermedius
rectus femoris
vastus lateralis

FIND YOUR FORM

Never rush this movement—concentrate on activating the vastus medialis, pushing through the ball of the foot on your working, elevated leg throughout the contraction. Avoid allowing your knee to twist inward; instead, keep it in line with your middle toe

MUSCLE ANNOTATION KEY
— **Black bold = primary**
······ Black = deep primary
— Gray bold = secondary
······ Gray = deep secondary

113 Lateral Step-Down

Like the Step-Down, the Lateral Step-Down is a highly functional exercise that strengthens your muscles to prepare them for high-intensity workouts, as well as daily life. This version of a step-down move strengthens your quadriceps, along with your glutes, hip abductors, and hip adductors and promotes the smooth coordination of your hip and leg muscles.

- Stand up straight on a firm step or block
- Plant your left foot firmly close to the edge, and allow your right foot to hang off the side.
- Flex the toes of your right foot.
- Lift your arms out in front of you for balance, keeping them parallel to the floor.
- Lower your torso as you bend at your hips and knees, dropping your right leg toward the floor.
- Without rotating your torso or knee, press upward through your left leg to return to the starting position.
- Performed the desired reps, and then repeat on the other side.

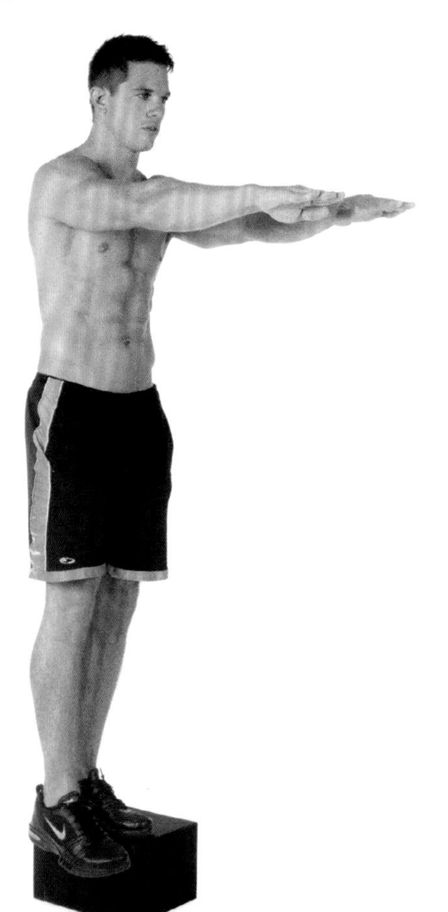

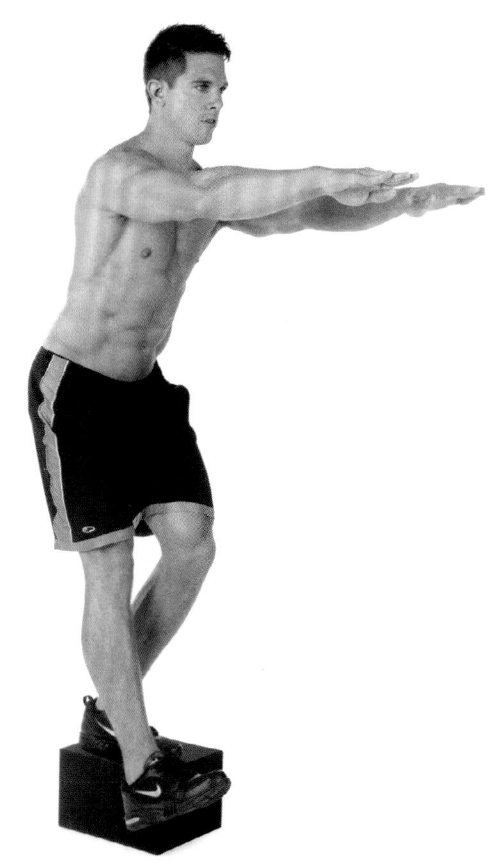

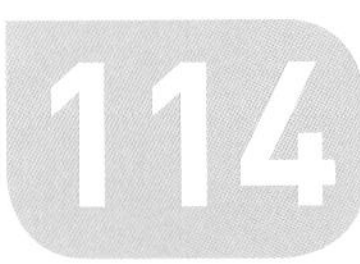

114 Medicine Ball Lateral Step-Down

Grasp a medicine ball in both hands, and perform as you would the Lateral Step-Down, but as you drop your right leg toward the floor, simultaneously extend the weight forward so that at the bottom of the movement the weight and your arms are fully extended from your torso and balance is achieved. Return to the starting position by extending your hip and knee and elevating your torso, while at the same time drawing the weight back toward your chest to the starting position. Performed the desired reps, and then repeat on the other side.

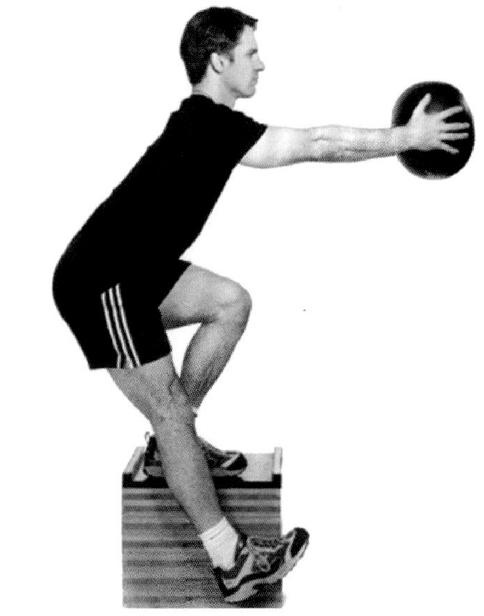

Toe-Ups

You rely on the gastrocnemius muscles on the backs of your calves for everyday movement, especially walking, and for high-intensity activities, such as jumping and running. The shape and insertion points of these diamond-shaped muscles are largely a result of genetics, so changing the look of them through exercise can be hard, if not impossible. Yet, exercises like the Toe-Up can help you target these stubborn muscles, along with the other major calf muscle, the soleus, and keep them strong and ready for action. It can also keep your Achilles tendon supple and injury-free.

- Stand with your legs and feet parallel and shoulder-width apart in front of a step. Bend your knees very slightly and tuck your pelvis slightly forwards, lift your chest and press your shoulders downward and back.
- Position the ball of your right foot on the step.
- With your knees straight, bring your hips forward.
- Release, switch feet, and repeat on the other side.

FIND YOUR FORM

Engage each head of your calf muscles by gently and slowly rolling from your big toe to your small toe and back again, shifting your body weight over your toes as you go. Perform a few calf stretches during your cardiovascular workout—this will help relieve calf tightness and stress throughout your workout.

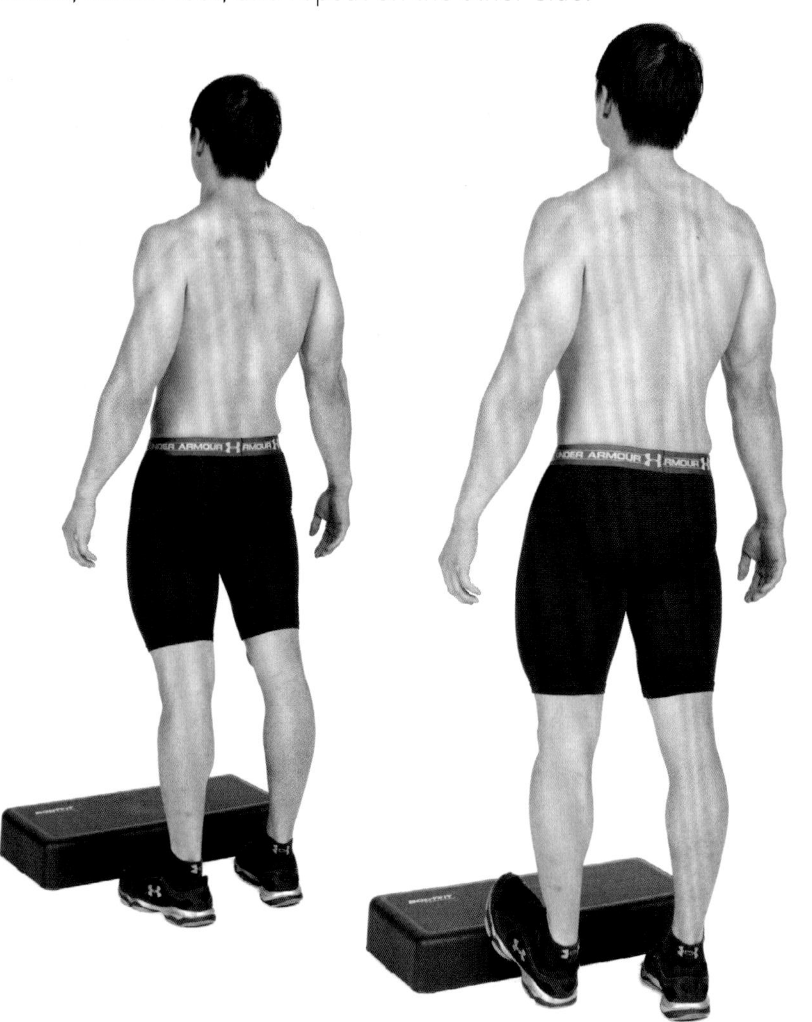

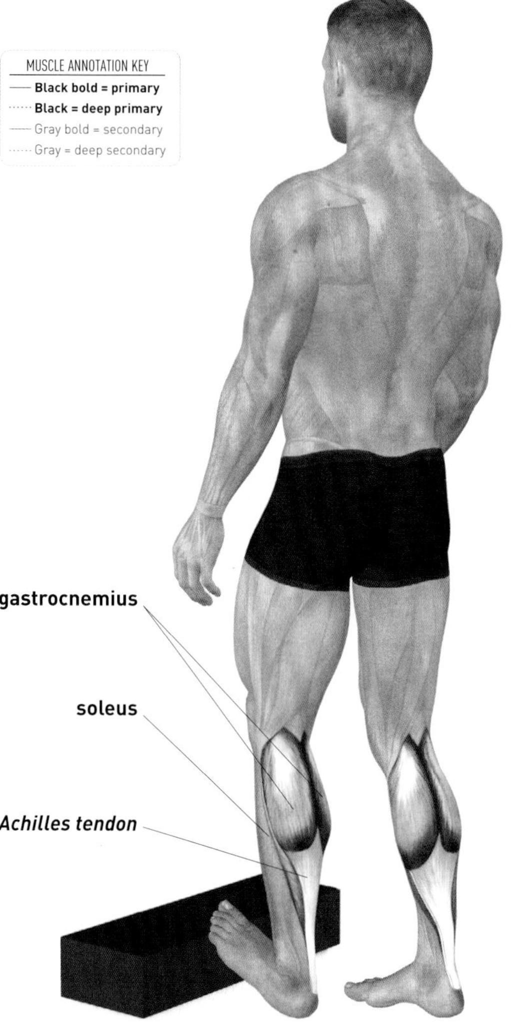

116 Heel Drop

Stand on a step with your legs and feet parallel and shoulder-width apart. Bend your knees very slightly and tuck your pelvis slightly forward, lift your chest and press your shoulders downward and back. Position your left foot slightly in front of your right, and place the ball of your right foot on the edge of the step. Drop your right heel down while controlling the amount of weight on the right leg to increase or decrease the intensity of the stretch in the right calf. Release, switch feet, and repeat on the other side.

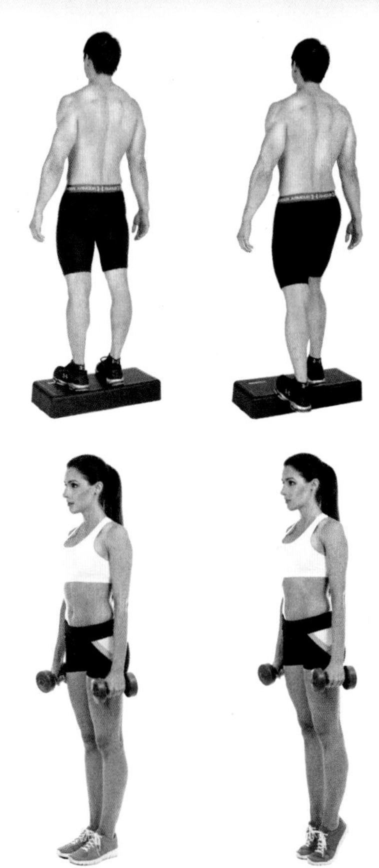

117 Heel Raise

Stand with your arms at your sides (you can hold a hand weight or dumbbell in each hand with palms facing inward).Keeping the rest of your body steady, slowly raise your heels off the floor to balance on the balls of your feet. Hold for 10 seconds, and then continue for the desired repetitions.

118 Heel Raise with Overhead Press

The Heel Raise exercise, also known as the Calf Raise, targets the same muscles as the Toe-Up, including the gastrocnemius, soleus, and tibialis posterior of the calf. In this version, the Heel Raise with Overhead Press, you simultaneously perform an overhead pressing motion to add some upper-body emphasis to this lower-body classic.

- Stand with your feet hip-width apart and your arms at your sides, a dumbbell or hand weight in each hand.
- Raise your arms, bending your elbows and lifting until the dumbbells are at ear height.
- Bring the weights overhead as you lift your heels off the floor to stand on your tiptoes. Balance for a few seconds, if desired.
- Lower your heels to the floor and bring your arms back to starting position. Continue for the desired repetitions.

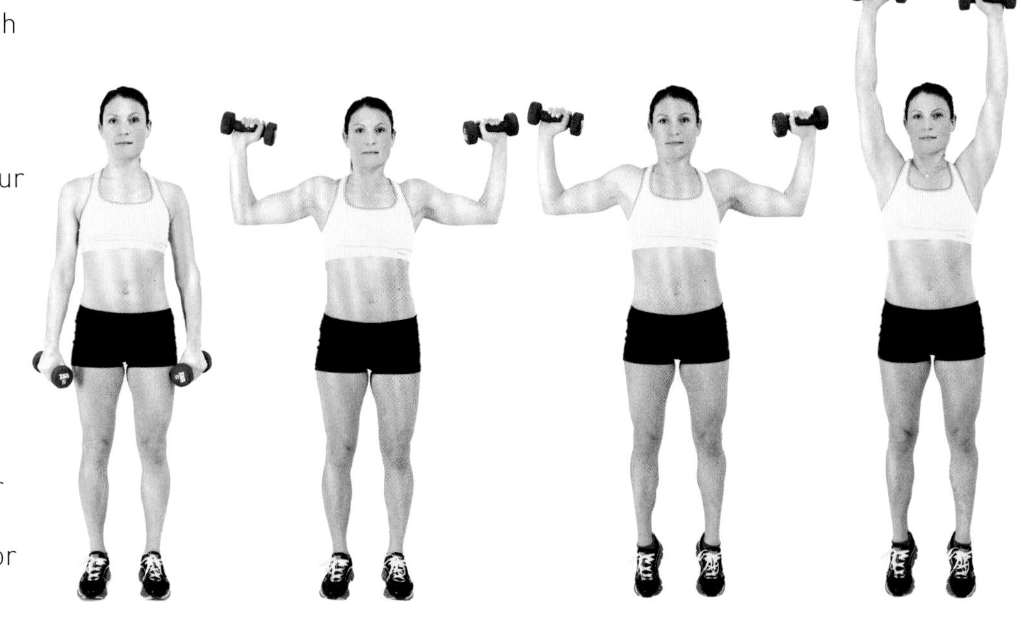

Running in Place

Running has earned its place as a top high-intensity cardio workout. But you don't need to hit the streets to reap its benefits. The Running in Place exercise does the same work, but you can do it anywhere and in any weather. The key is keeping your heart rate up. These days there are plenty of fitness trackers with heart rate monitors that give you the numbers you need. To determine your optimal range, first calculate your target zone by subtracting your age from 220 and multiplying by 70 percent. For example, if you are 30 years old, your would subtract 30 from 220 to get 190. You would then multiply 190 by .70 to get a target heart rate of 133 beats per minute.

- Stand tall, and begin by warming up with a light jog. lifting your feet only an inch or two off the ground, hopping from foot to foot. To warm up your upper body, give yourself a few bear hugs.
- Increase your speed, and lift your knees higher, alternating periods of high intensity with periods of recovery.

FIND YOUR FORM

Be sure to move your [illegible] place—the more you move every bit of your body, the more calories you'll burn and the more effective the cardio workout.

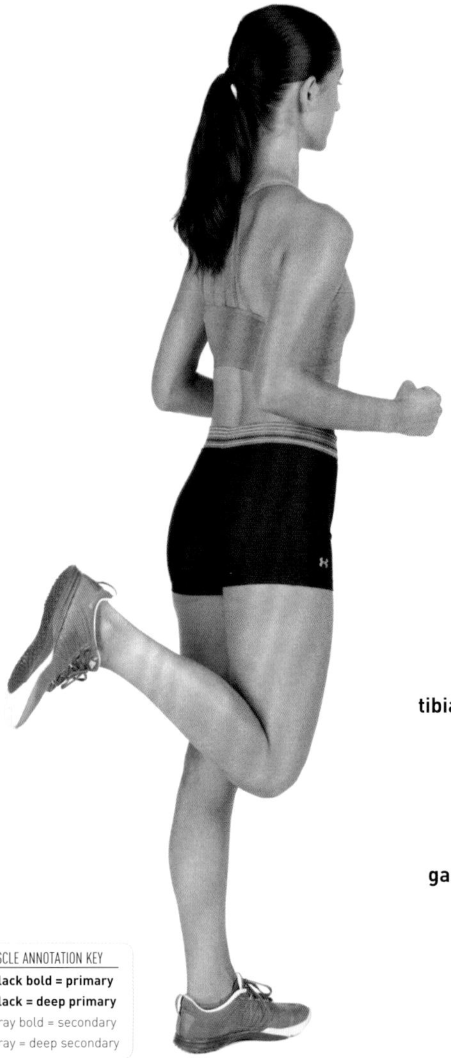

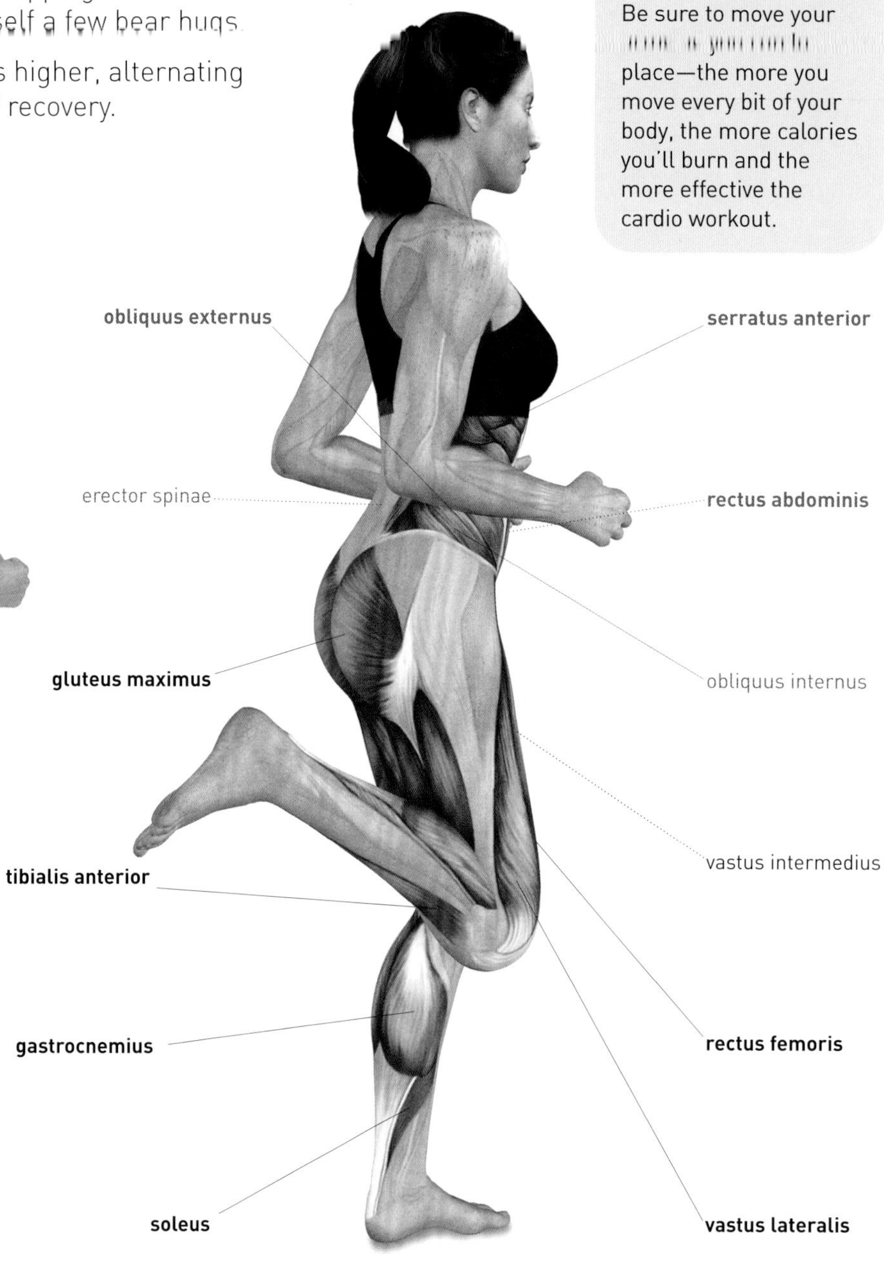

obliquus externus
erector spinae
gluteus maximus
tibialis anterior
gastrocnemius
soleus
serratus anterior
rectus abdominis
obliquus internus
vastus intermedius
rectus femoris
vastus lateralis

MUSCLE ANNOTATION KEY
— Black bold = primary
····· Black = deep primary
— Gray bold = secondary
····· Gray = deep secondary

120 Skipping

Go ahead and indulge your inner child, and skip on down the road. Skipping may seem like a frivolous pursuit—and it's certainly fun—but it also gives you a great cardio workout. Runners can use this activity as a dynamic warm-up session, too.

- Stand with your feet hip-width apart. With your upper arms pressed to your sides, bend your elbows to 90 degrees. Drive your right knee and left arm up while exploding upward off your left leg.
- Land on your left leg, and then immediately drive your left knee and right arm up while pushing off of your right foot.
- With each skip, propel yourself upward as high as possible and aim your knee toward your chest. Continue skipping until you have covered the desired distance.

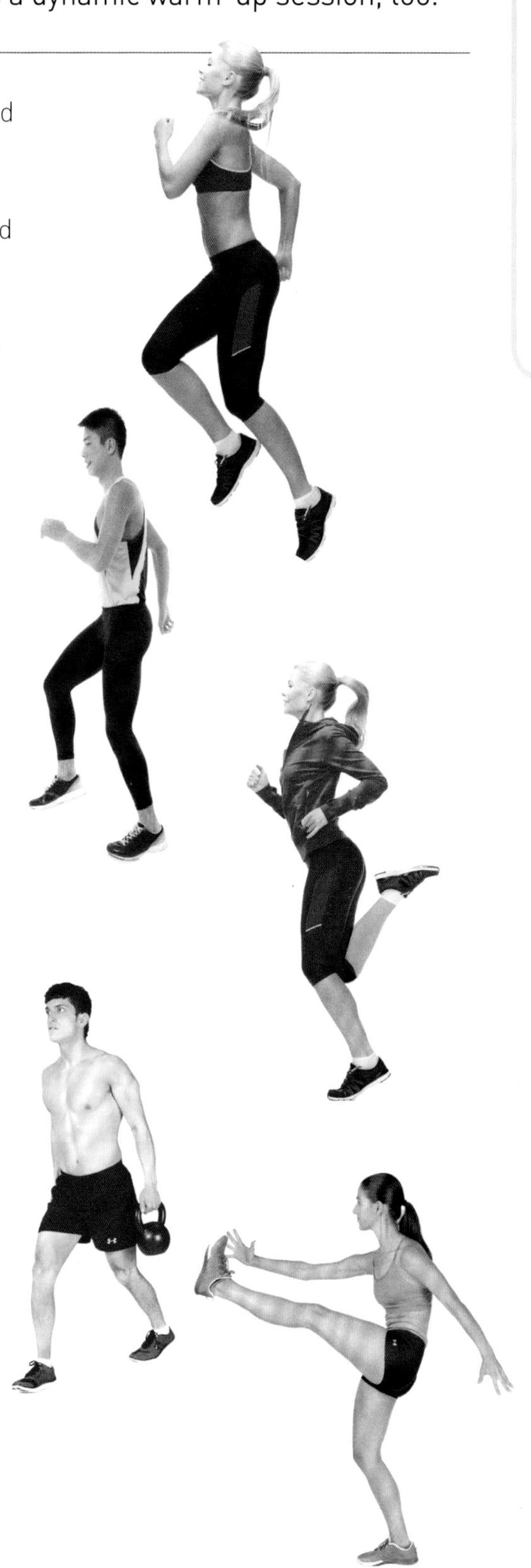

121 Backpedaling

Stand with your feet hip-width apart. With your upper arms pressed to your sides, bend your elbows to 90 degrees. Run backward with short, quick steps, pumping your arms up and down and landing on the balls of your feet. Keep your chest up, and continue backpedaling until you have covered the desired distance.

122 Butt Kicks

Begin in a standing position, and then begin jogging in place. Kick your heels up as high as you can, aiming toward your glutes. Continue jogging and lifting your heels high, while increasing your speed until you have covered the desired distance or ran for the desired time.

123 Farmer's Walk

Stand with your feet shoulder-width apart, holding a pair of kettlebells or dumbbells in each hand with your arms by your sides. Walk rapidly for a predetermined distance or time (for example, the length of the gym or 20 seconds) while holding the weights. Lower the weights, rest, and repeat for the desired sets.

124 Monster Walk

Begin in a standing position, and then walk in place, kicking each leg out straight in front of you. As you elevate your leg, attempt to touch your foot with the opposite hand. Continue alternating sides until you have covered the desired distance or walked for the desired time.

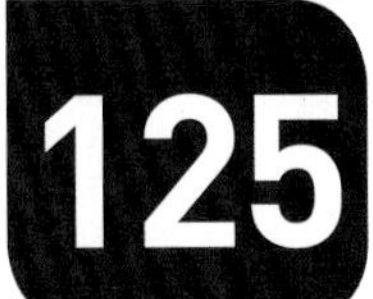

High Knees

The high knees exercise combines the action of jogging in place with exaggerated knee lifts. It is a versatile move that can serve as a dynamic cardio warm-up, especially for runners—but it can help improve running form for any athlete—and it also helps build speed, power, and flexibility.

- Stand tall with your hands either on your hips or down by your sides.
- Raise up one knee as high as you are able, aiming it toward your chest, and then return to the starting position.
- Alternate legs while increasing your speed as you jog in place.

FIND YOUR FORM

Avoiding pushing solely off your toes—push off from your entire foot, and build up in speed as you go.

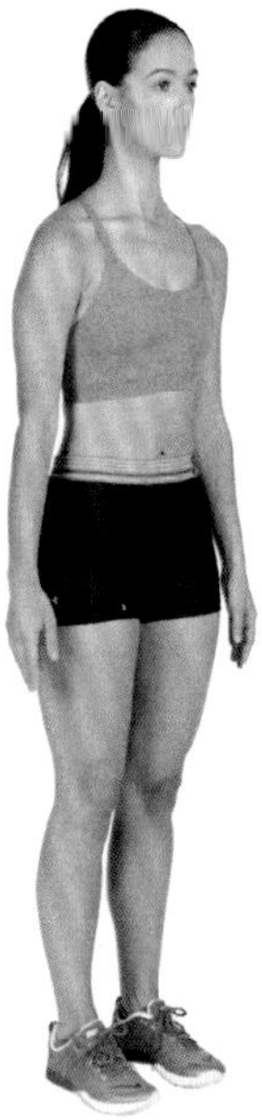

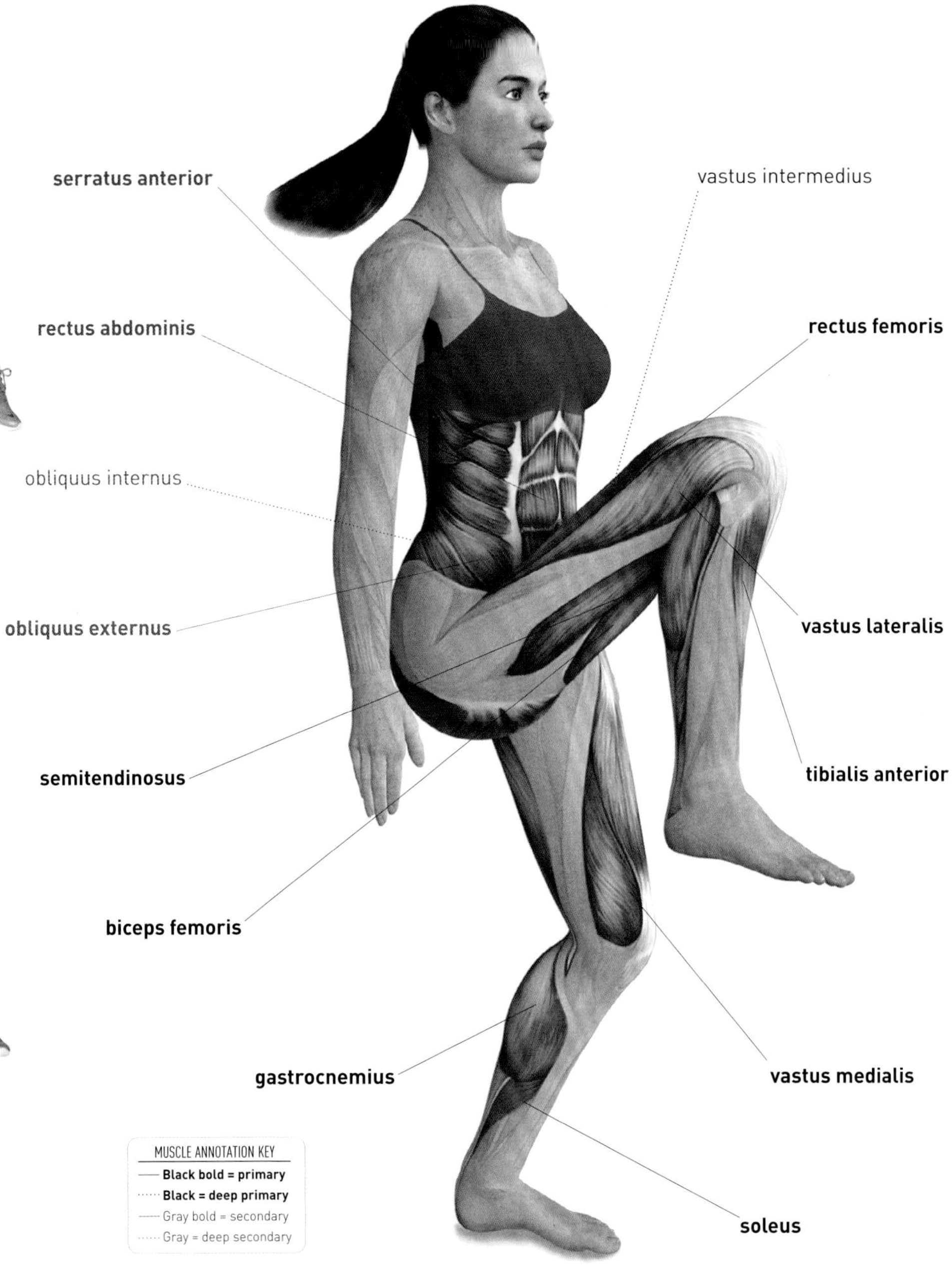

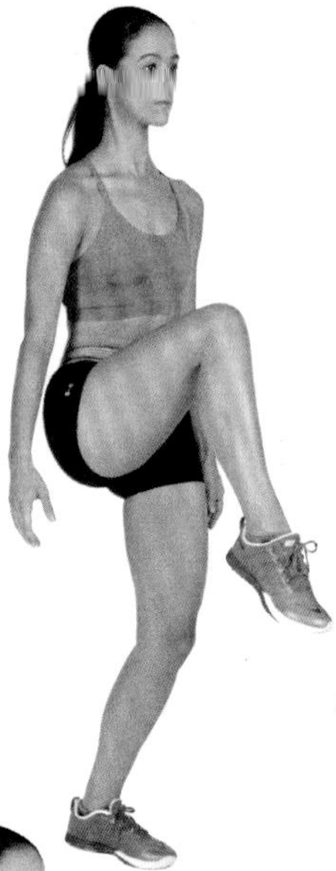

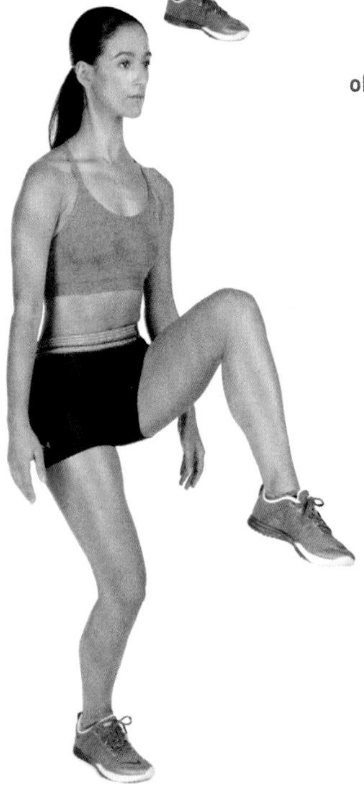

serratus anterior
rectus abdominis
obliquus internus
obliquus externus
semitendinosus
biceps femoris
gastrocnemius
vastus intermedius
rectus femoris
vastus lateralis
tibialis anterior
vastus medialis
soleus

MUSCLE ANNOTATION KEY
Black bold = primary
Black = deep primary
Gray bold = secondary
Gray = deep secondary

126 High Knees March

Stand tall with your feet slightly apart, your weight on the balls of your feet. Raise up one knee as high as you are able, keeping your toes up. Drive your leg back toward the floor, taking a step forward. Repeat the movement with your right leg. Continue to march until you have covered the desired distance.

127 High Knees March with Arm Raise

Perform as you would the High Knees March (#120), but as you raise your knee, extend the opposite arm overhead.

128 Swiss Ball Marching

Stand tall holding a Swiss ball overhead. Drive your right knee upward while lowering the ball to touch it to your knee. Drive your right leg back to the floor, taking a step forward as you raise the ball back overhead. Repeat with the left leg, and continue to march until you have covered the desired distance.

129 Steam Engine

Stand with your feet hip-width apart, and interlock your fingers behind your head. Drive your right knee upward while twisting your torso to touch your left elbow to your right knee. Pause at the top of the movement, and then return your right foot to the floor. Repeat with your left leg, and continue to alternate knees until your muscles fatigue.

130 Twisting Knee Raise

Stand with your feet hip-width apart, and raise both arms, bending your elbows up and facing your palms forward. Perform as you would the Steam Engine (#129).

131 Knee Raise with Lateral Extension

Stand with your feet hip-width apart and your arms at your sides, a dumbbell in each hand. Shifting your weight onto your left leg, raise your right knee, while lifting your arms until the weights are slightly below shoulder height. Find your balance, and then keeping your arms and upper body stationary, extend your right leg out to the side. Hold, and then lower your arms, and return your right leg to the starting position. Repeat on the other side. Continue alternating sides for the desired repetitions.

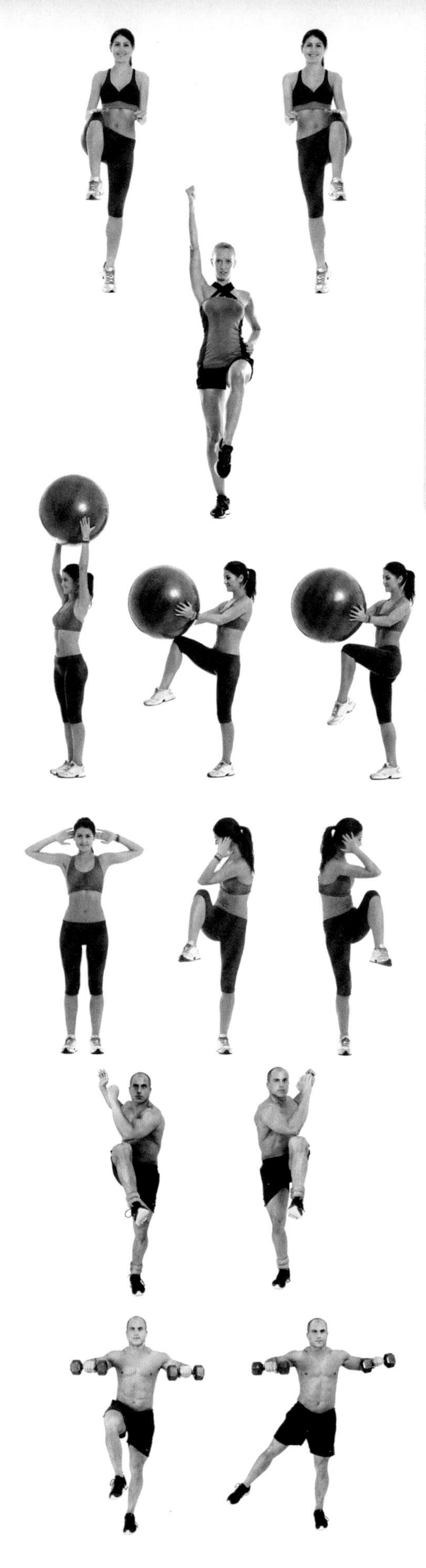

132 Obstacle Course Warm-Up

Obstacle course challenges are a fun way to get your heart going while training for speed, power, agility, and coordination. You can purchase obstacle course kits that supply you with cones and discs that you can easily set up at home or in your yard, or you can use everyday objects like paper plates and buckets. The Obstacle Course Warm-Up starts you out with this boot camp–style training, moving you through a course of small disc training cones as you step, hop, jog, and perform Jumping Jacks.

- Set up seven small objects on the floor to form a triangle and a square.
- Taking small, quick steps, step around all of the objects in the triangle.
- Stand in front of the square and jump forward to land in the middle of the square. Complete a jumping jack.
- Jump forward to land outside the square. Jog back to the beginning of the course, and repeat.

FIND YOUR FORM

Keep a steady pace as you move through the course, and take small steps, focusing on coordination.

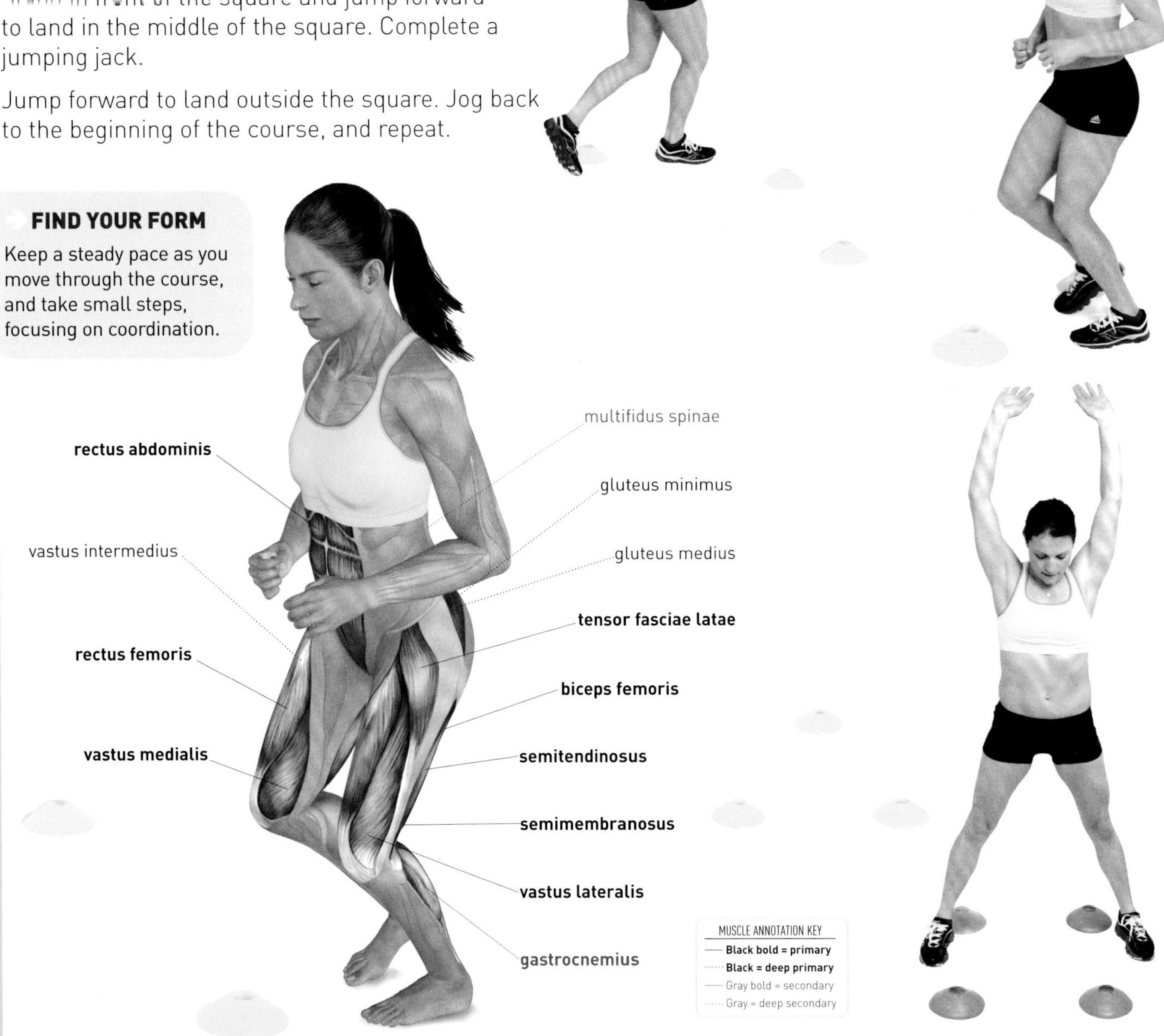

133 Obstacle Course Challenge

The Obstacle Course Challenge ups the intensity, adding high cones and aerobic steps to the small disc cones. You also add resistance, holding a medicine ball as you move through the course for added strength training.

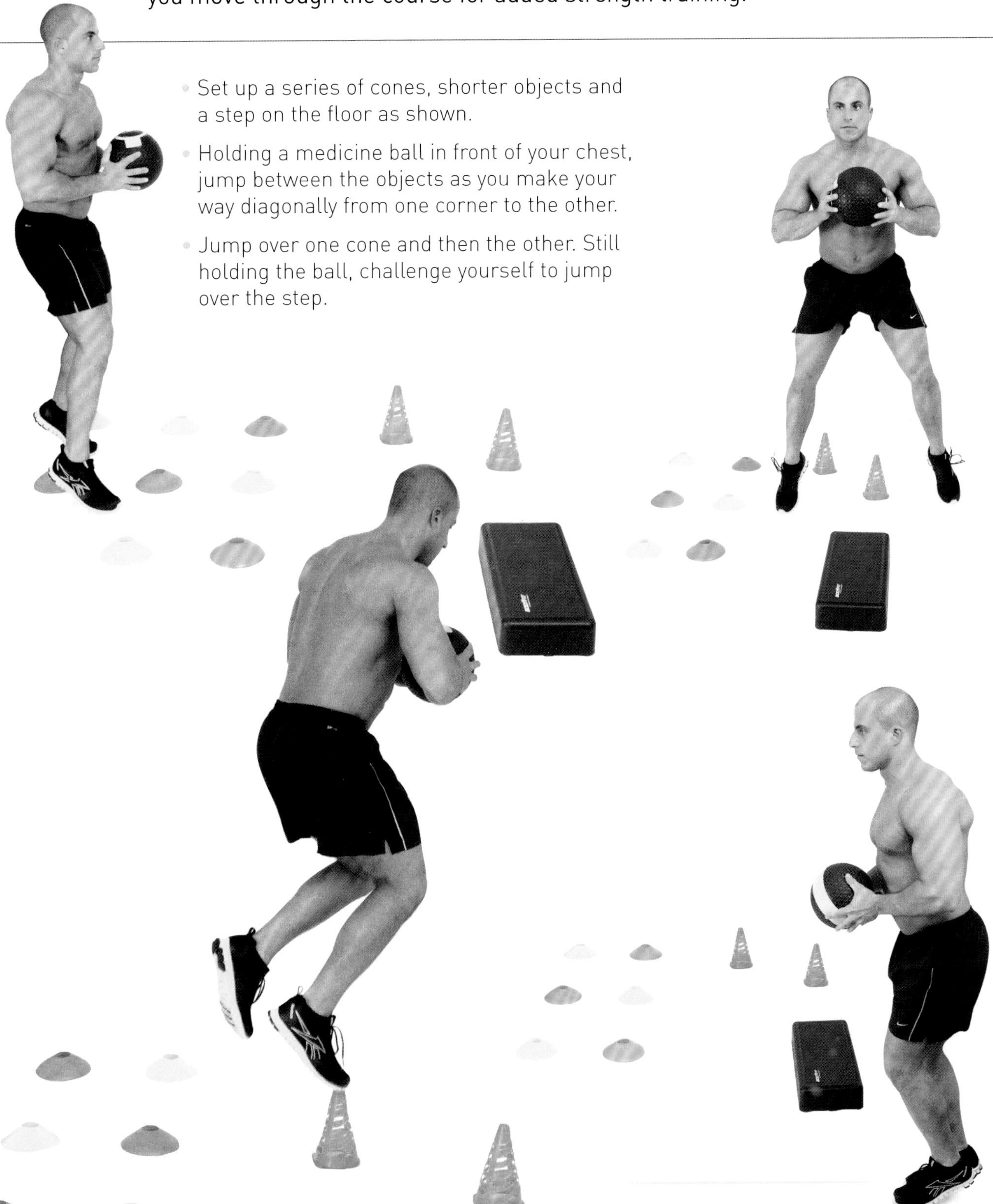

- Set up a series of cones, shorter objects and a step on the floor as shown.
- Holding a medicine ball in front of your chest, jump between the objects as you make your way diagonally from one corner to the other.
- Jump over one cone and then the other. Still holding the ball, challenge yourself to jump over the step.

Straight Kick

Kicking exercises can be part of a great aerobic workout and form the foundation of many high-intensity sports, like kickboxing and other forms of martial arts. Combining kicks with punches provides a full-body, calorie-burning workout and is a fantastic way to release stress. Try using kickboxing pads or punching bags to burn even more calories and to fully engage your core. To get started, try the Straight Kick (also known as the Front Kick), which will help you to learn the action and hone your balance, and then move on to more complex moves, like Roundhouse and other martial arts moves.

- Stand with your hands on your hips, in a staggered stance, with your left foot forward.
- Kick upward, shifting your weight to your left foot as your right foot leaves the floor.
- End back in the staggered stance, and continue kicking for the desired repetitions.
- Switch sides, and continue kicking with the left foot.

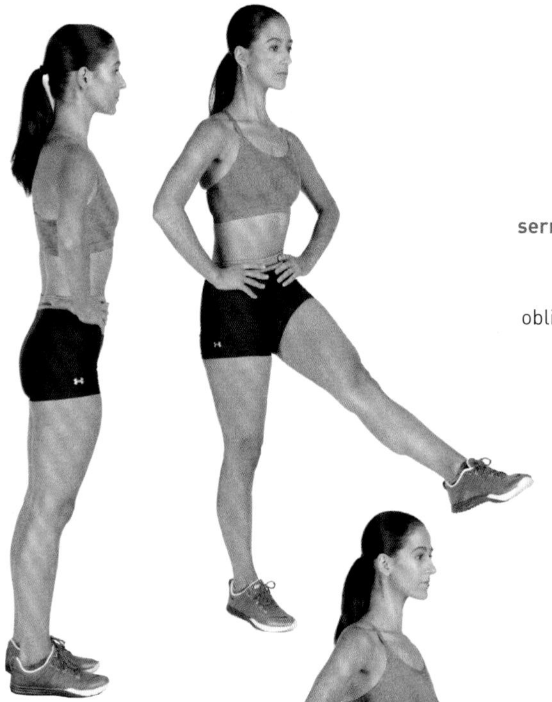

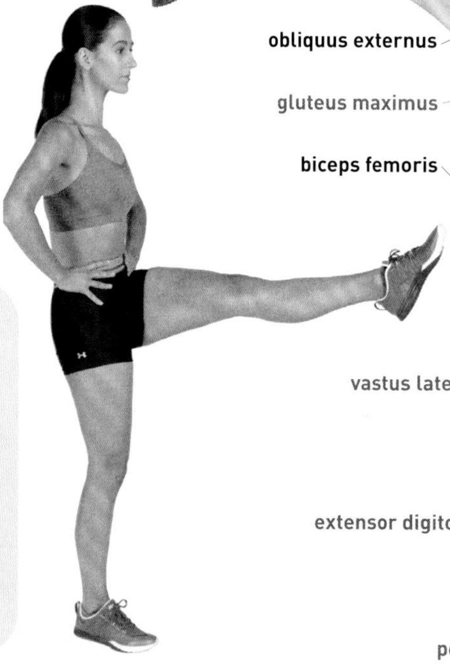

MUSCLE ANNOTATION KEY
Black bold = primary
Black = deep primary
Gray bold = secondary
Gray = deep secondary

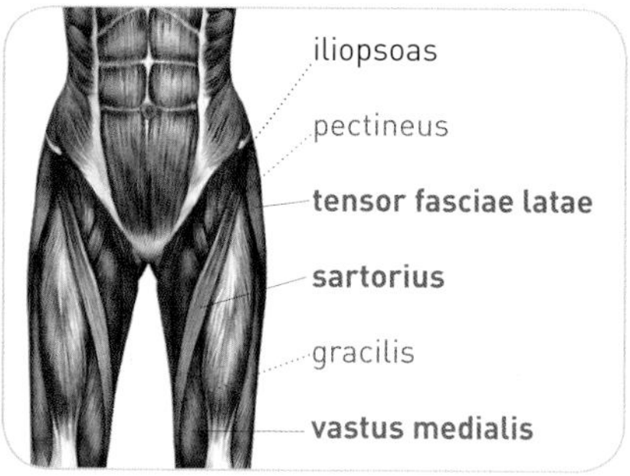

iliopsoas
pectineus
tensor fasciae latae
sartorius
gracilis
vastus medialis
serratus anterior
obliquus internus
obliquus externus
gluteus maximus
biceps femoris
semimembranosus
semitendinosus
adductor longus
adductor magnus
vastus intermedius
vastus lateralis
rectus femoris
extensor digitorum
tibialis anterior
peroneus
soleus

FIND YOUR FORM

Perform this kick with your upper body straight and balanced, beginning in a staggered stance. If you assume the correct starting position, you will appear to be leaning forward, and you should feel a slight stretch in your hamstrings.

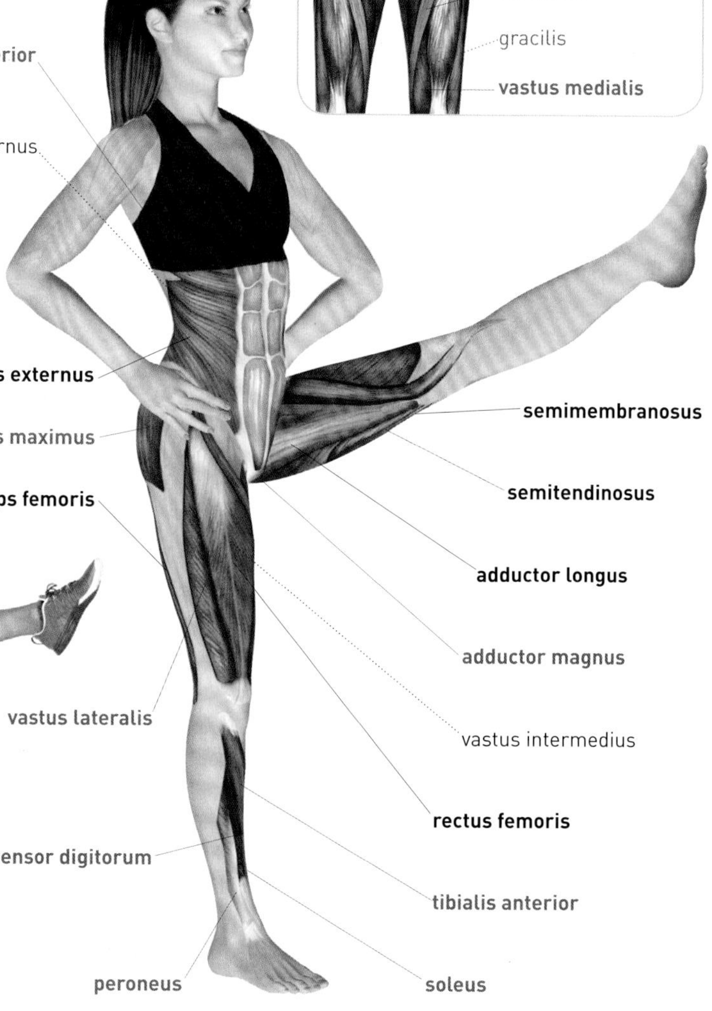

135

Kick with Toe Touch

Stand with your right hand on your hip, and extend your left arm straight up toward the ceiling. Kick upward, shifting your weight to your left foot as your right foot leaves the floor. At the same time, reach your left arm to touch the toes of your right foot. Bring your right foot to the floor as your raise your right arm, and then repeat, kicking with your left leg and reaching with your right. Continue alternating legs.

136

Kick with Arm Reach

Perform as you would a Straight Kick (#134), but as you raise your leg, extend the opposite arm straight out, engaging all your arm muscles. Switch sides, and continue kicking with the opposite foot.

137

Switch Kick Punch

Assume a boxing stance with your fists up and your left foot forward and your right foot back and to the right, your knees slightly bent. Bracing your core, kick your right foot in front of you, leg straight, while punching your left fist toward your foot. Quickly return to start, place your right foot in front of your left, and repeat on the other side. Continue alternating.

138

Martial Arts Kick

Assume a boxing stance with your fists up and your left foot forward and your right foot back and to the right, your knees slightly bent. Raise your right knee toward your chest. Rotate your hips and left foot, and kick your right leg to the side, pushing through the heel while punching with your right arm. Quickly bring your right leg down, placing it staggered in front of your left. Bring your right arm back in. Repeat with your left leg and arm to complete one rep.

139

Roundhouse Kick

Assume a boxing stance with your fists up and your left foot forward and your right foot back and to the right. Pivoting slightly on your left foot, swing your right leg up, and snap your foot at the top, aiming for a waist-high, shoulder-height, or head-height target before bringing it down. Repeat with your left leg to complete one rep.

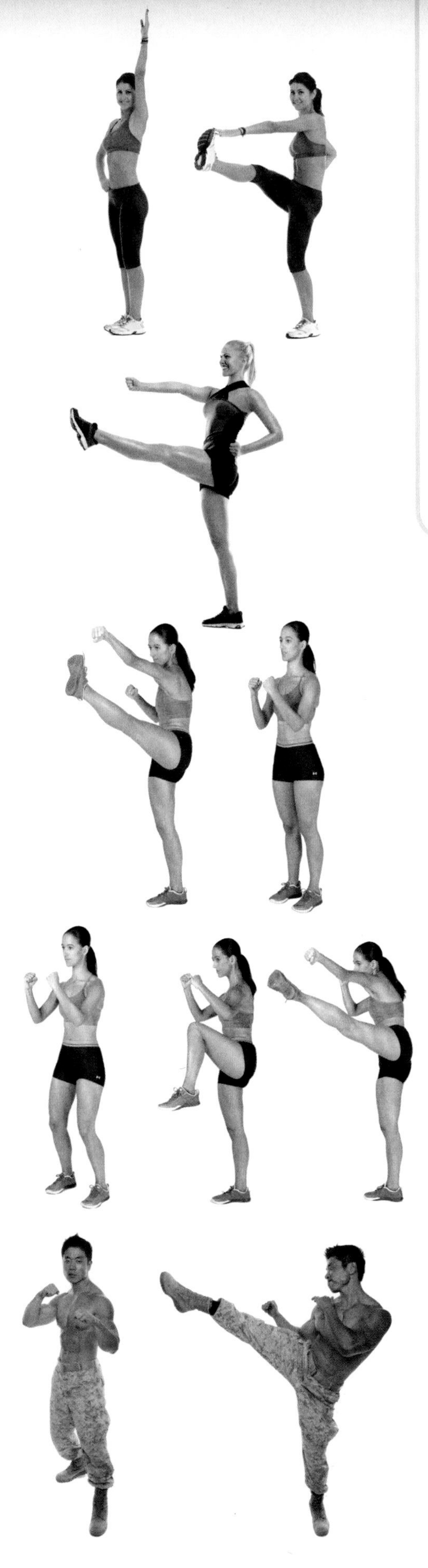

140 Side Kick

Like a Straight Kick, the Side Kick(also known as a Lateral Kick) works to strengthen your lower body while giving you a cardio workout and preparing you for more complex compound kick exercises. The lateral movement of your legs in this version adds emphasis to your oblique muscles.

- Stand with feet hip-width apart and your arms at your sides.
- Kick your right leg out to the side, keeping it in line with your torso and shifting your weight to your left foot as your right foot leaves the floor. At the same time, extend both arms out to the side until the are at shoulder height, parallel to the floor.
- Return to the starting position, and repeat on the other side, and then continue alternating legs.

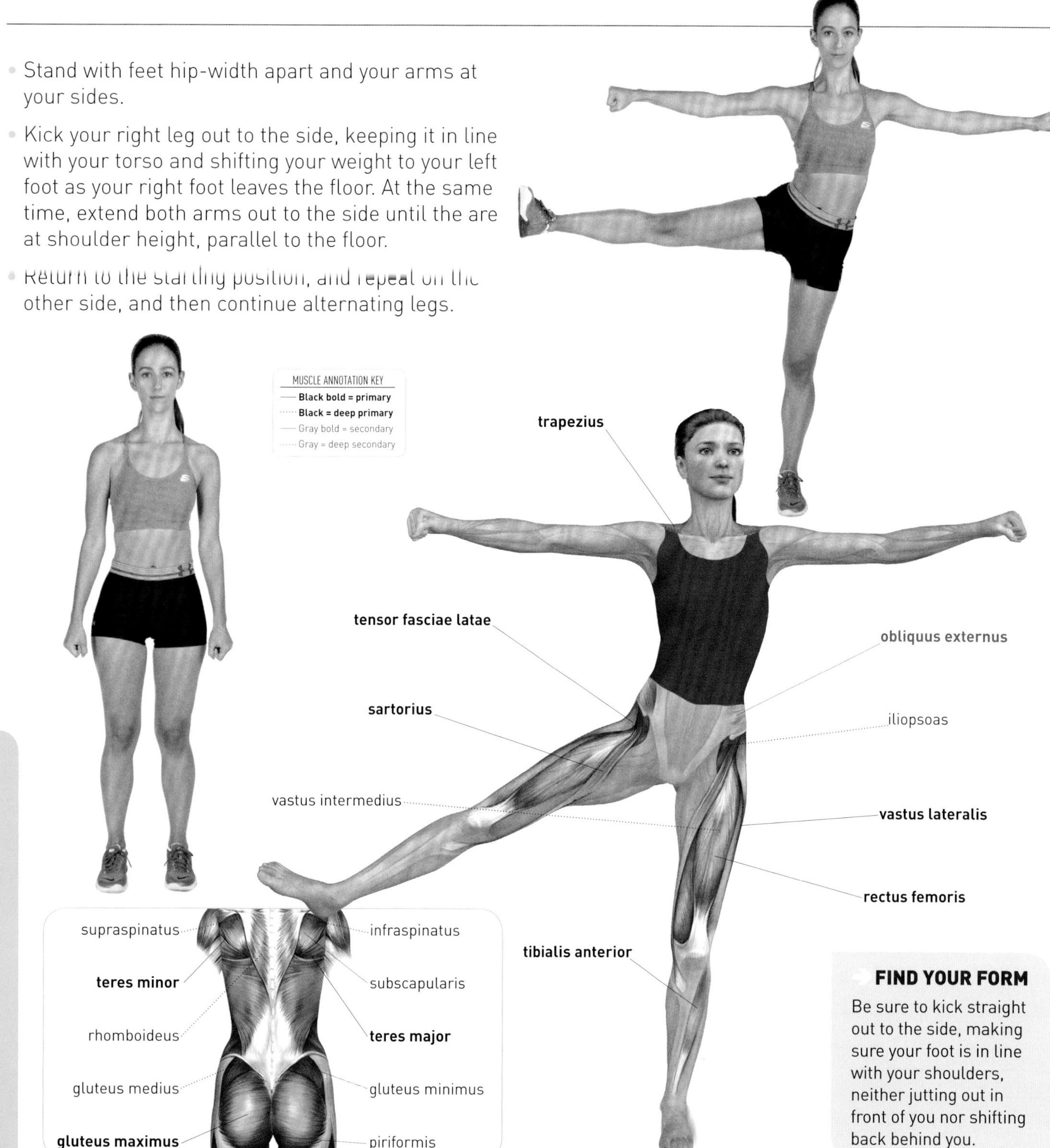

FIND YOUR FORM

Be sure to kick straight out to the side, making sure your foot is in line with your shoulders, neither jutting out in front of you nor shifting back behind you.

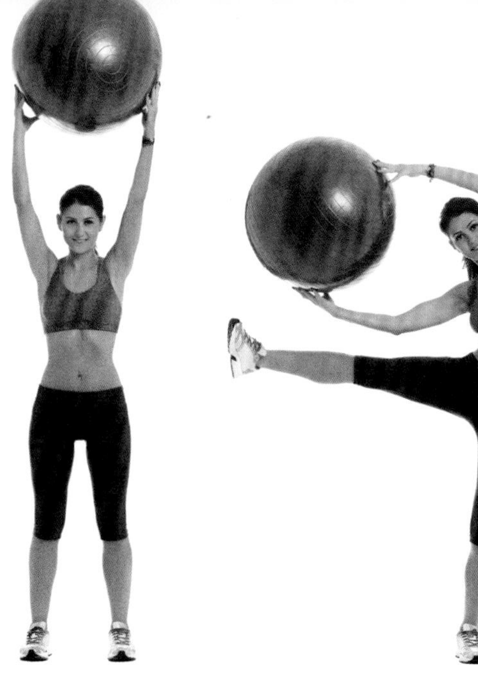

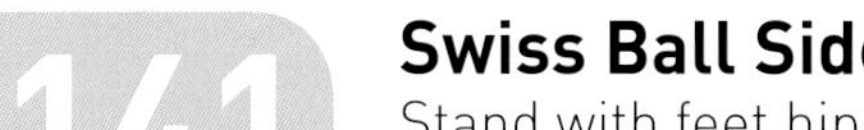

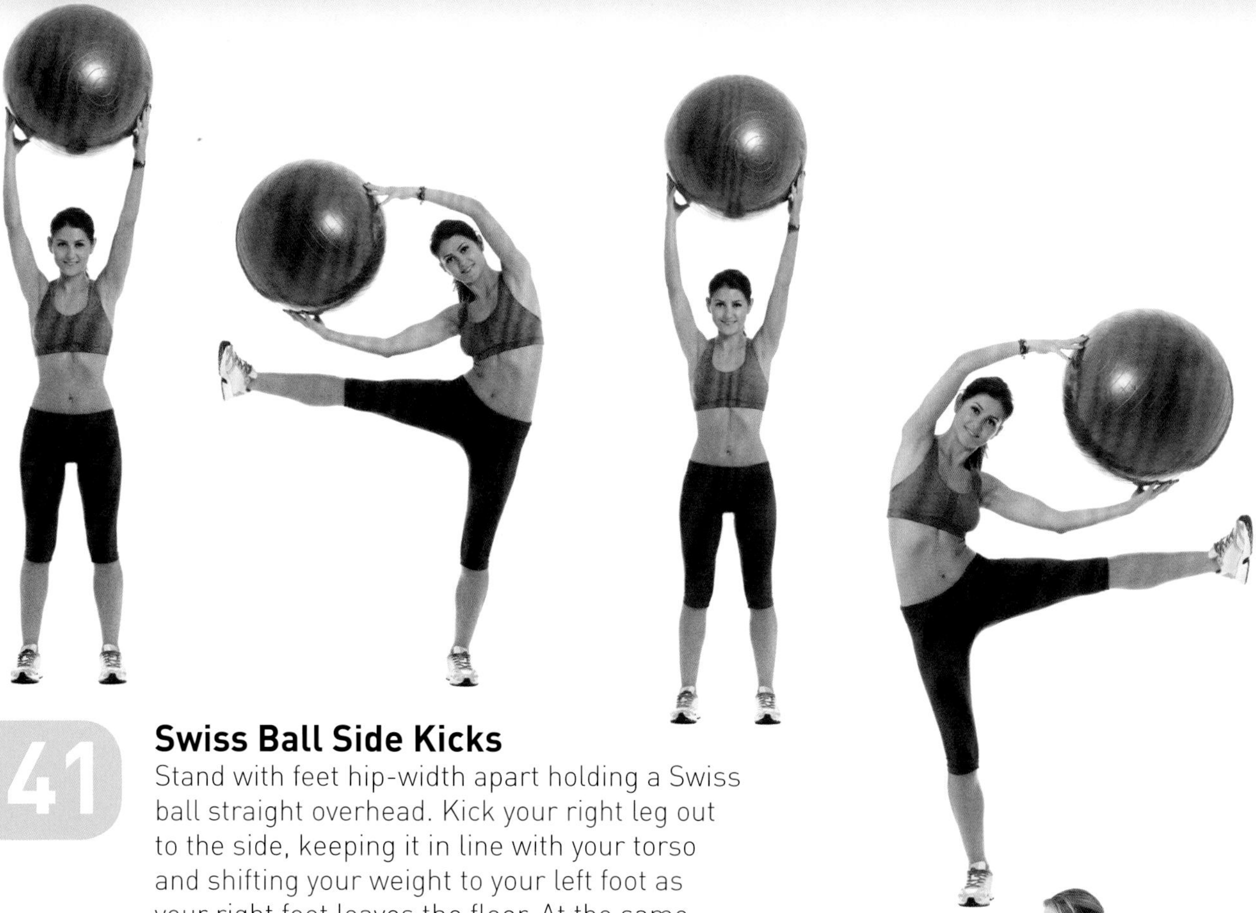

141 Swiss Ball Side Kicks

Stand with feet hip-width apart holding a Swiss ball straight overhead. Kick your right leg out to the side, keeping it in line with your torso and shifting your weight to your left foot as your right foot leaves the floor. At the same time, bend your torso to the right, bringing the ball toward your right foot. Return to the starting position, and repeat on the other side, and then continue alternating legs.

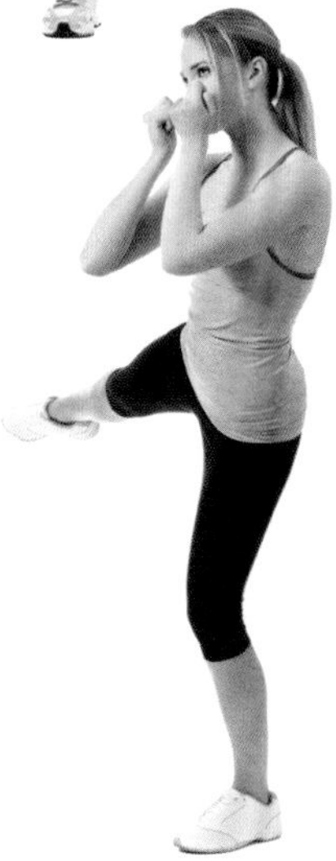

142 Low Round Kick

Assume a boxing stance with your fists up and your left foot forward and your right foot back and to the right. Take a small step with your left foot, pointing your left foot out, and then use your hips to swing your right leg around like a baseball bat, aiming to hit your target at thigh level. Repeat with your left leg and arm to complete one rep.

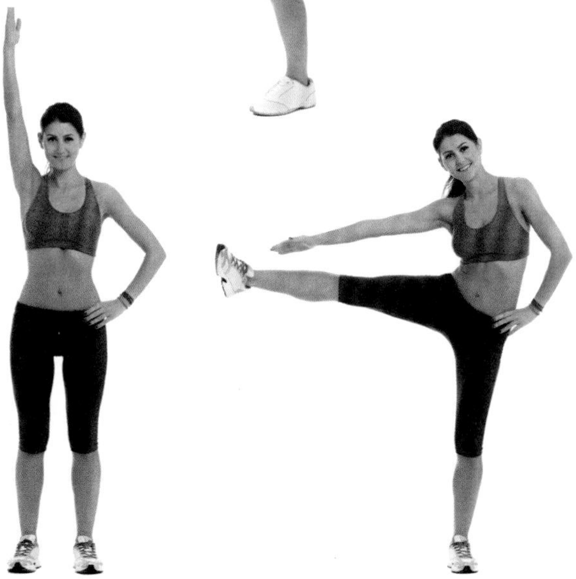

143 Side Kick Reach

Stand with feet hip-width apart. Place your left hand on your hip, and extend your right arm straight up toward the ceiling. Kick your right leg out to the side, keeping it in line with your torso and shifting your weight to your left foot as your right foot leaves the floor. At the same time, reach your right arm toward your right foot. Bring your right foot to the floor as your raise your left arm, and then repeat, kicking with your left leg and reaching with your left hand. Continue alternating legs.

144 Lateral Bounding

Lateral Bounding targets several areas, including the quadriceps, hamstrings, glutes, and calves. Its principal aim is to help you practice lateral movement at speed. Try completing a set of jumps to one side, and then switching. Alternatively, add an extra level of difficulty by performing the routine while holding a medicine ball.

- Start in a quarter-squat position, then bound off your right foot as far and high as possible to your left. Be sure to land on your left foot.
- Next, bound as far and as high as possible back to your right off your left foot. Continue bounding from side to side.

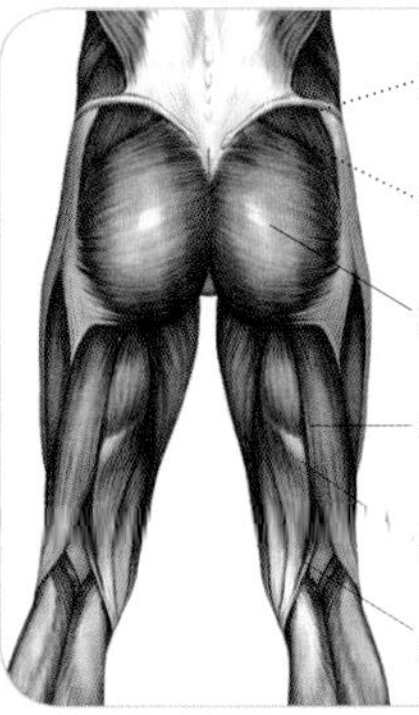

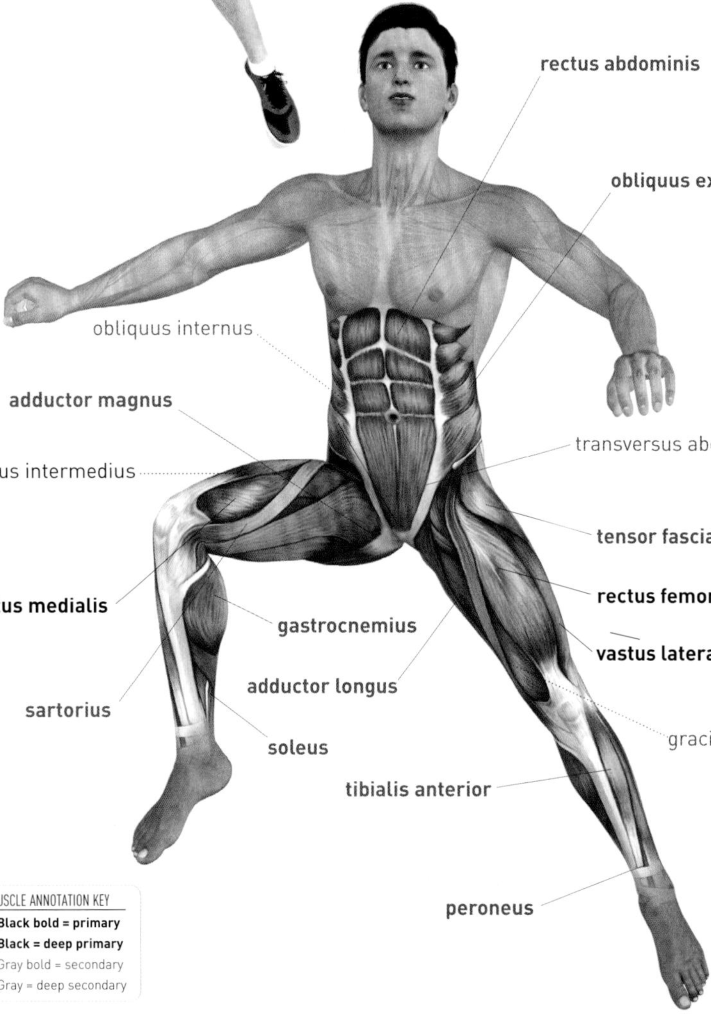

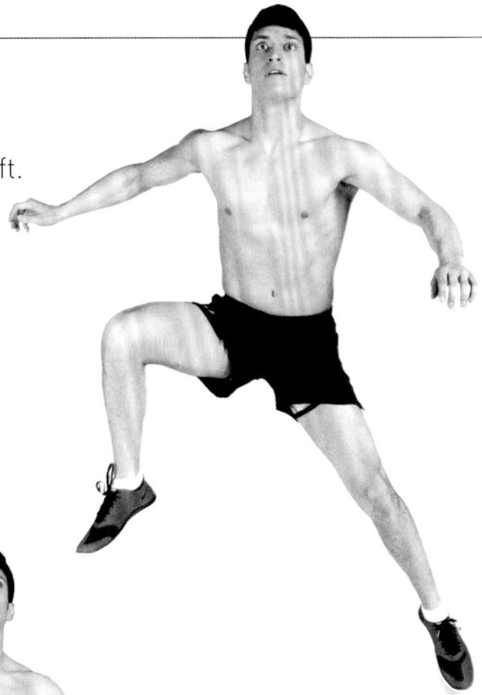

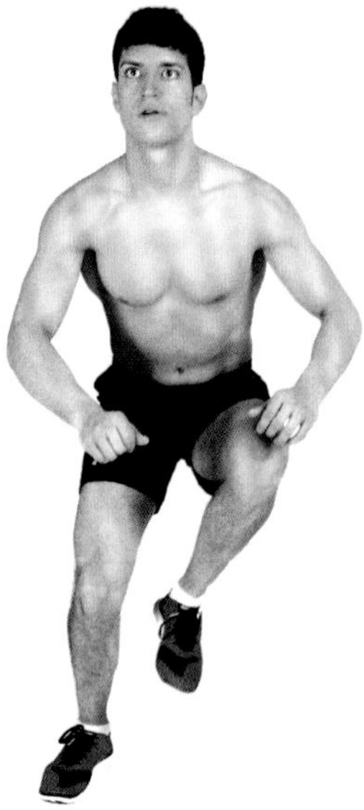

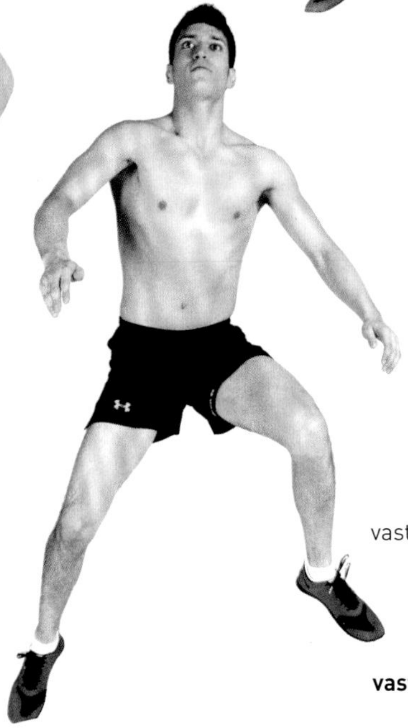

FIND YOUR FORM

To avoid placing too much stress on your knee joint, don't allow your knees to protrude far too far in front of your feet when you decelerate, land, or squat. Be sure to keep a tight core throughout the movement. To prepare for this move, practice your lateral form by working on mastering the Lateral Lunge exercise (#072).

MUSCLE ANNOTATION KEY
- **Black bold = primary**
- Black = deep primary
- Gray bold = secondary
- Gray = deep secondary

145

Lateral Bunny Hops

Stand with your feet together. Jump to the side, keeping your legs as close together as possible. Continue making small jumps side to side for the desired time or reps.

146

Lateral Shuffle

Stand with your legs open, feet placed more than hip-width apart, and bend your knees to assume a half-squat stance. Place your hands on your hips or rest them on your thighs. Stay in the squat position while bringing your left foot to your right, and then your right foot to your left. Hold the squat position while shuffling for the desired reps in each direction.

147

Side-to-Side Hop

Lay a straight-line obstacle, such as a tape measure, yardstick, or a stretched-out resistance band, on the floor. Stand to the right of the line and bend your right knee to stand on your left leg. Hop sideways back and forth, over the line for the desired time or reps, and then switch legs.

148

Side-to-Side Obstacle Springing

Set an agility cone, wire training hurdle, overturned bucket, or other object on the floor. Stand with one foot on either side of it. Spring upward with your knee high and straight. Continue springing upward, back and forth, for the desired time or reps.

149

Slalom Jumps

Stand with your feet together, and bend down to reach your right hand to the floor. In one motion, quickly swing both hands in front of you, elbows bent, and jump to the left, landing softly. Immediately bend your knees to reach your left hand onto the floor, and repeat the movement to the right to return to the starting position. Continue alternating sides.

150

Cone Jumps

Standing to the right of a cone. Jump off both feet to your left to clear the cone, landing on your left foot only. Put your right foot down, and leap off both feet to clear the cone again. Be sure to land on your right foot this time. Only the foot that will be farthest away from the cone should make contact with the floor.

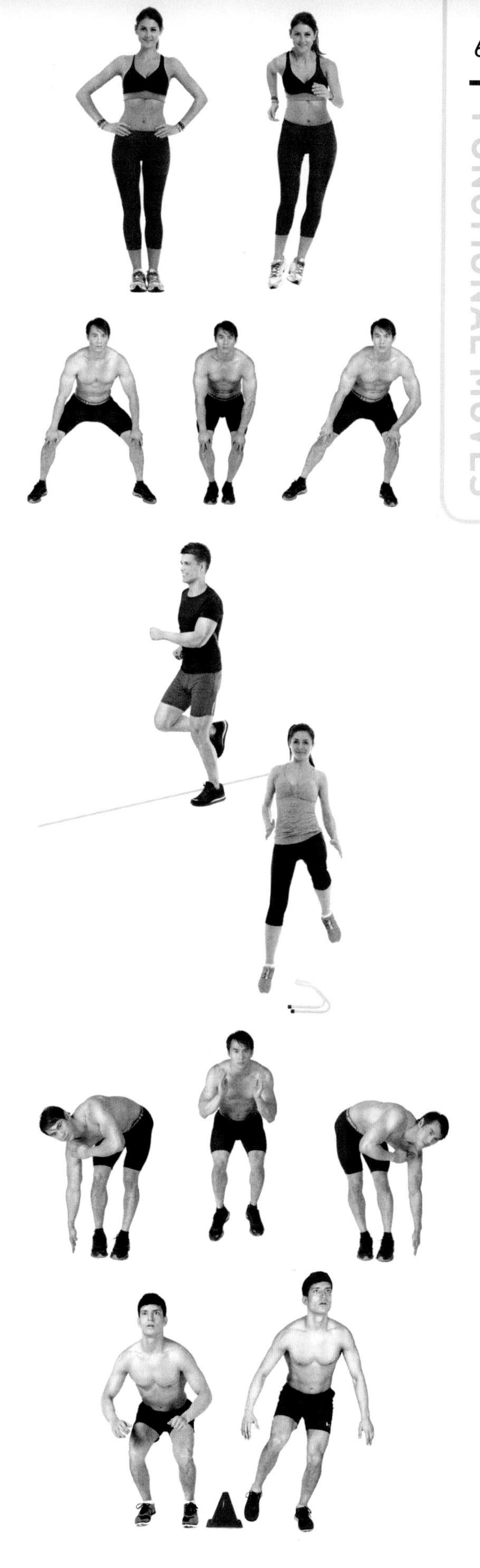

Jumping

Before beginning a high-intensity workout, perform this simple move to warm up the soleus and gastrocnemius muscles of your calves, as well as to get your heart rate going. You can add jumps to just about any exercise, from squats and lunges to push-ups and squat thrusts to add a cardio burst to any workout routine. Once you are strong enough, there are countless variations of jumping exercises—you can take your cure from dance moves like ballet or hip-hop or sport moves like track and field and cheerleading.

- Stand straight with your feet close together, but not touching.
- Jump up slightly, and land without touching your heels to the floor. Continue for the desired time or reps.

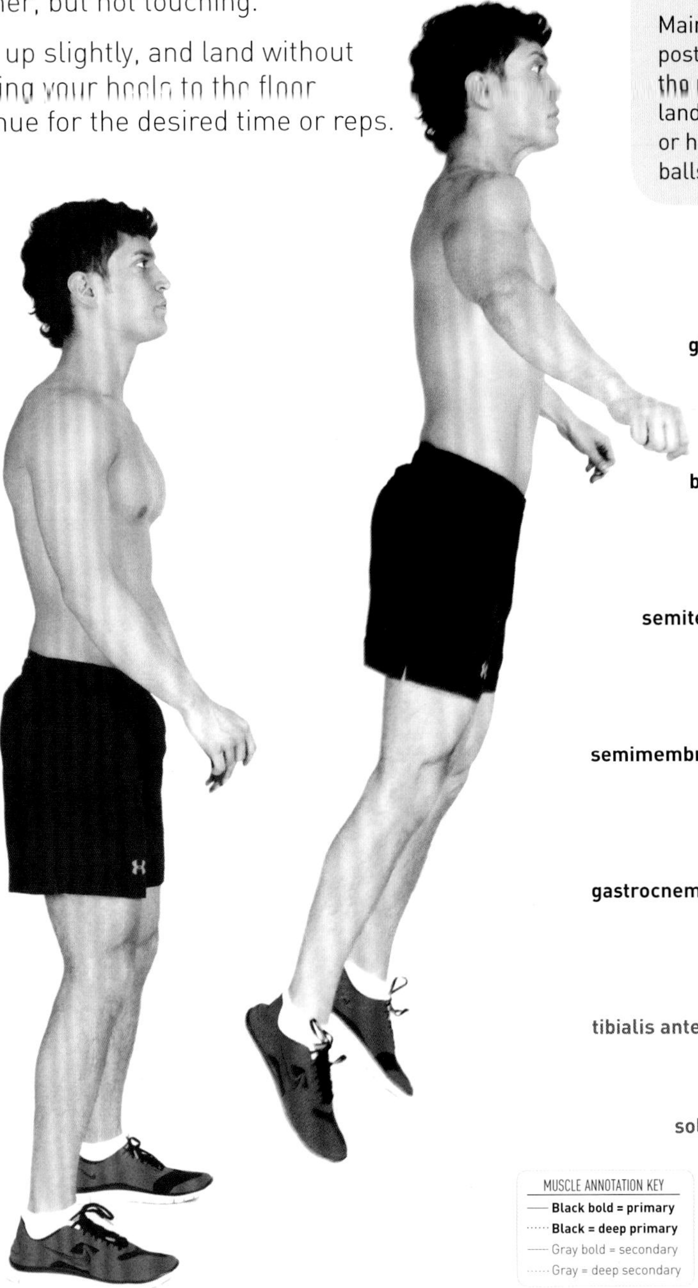

FIND YOUR FORM

Maintain an erect posture throughout the movement. Avoid landing on your toes or heels—land on the balls of your feet.

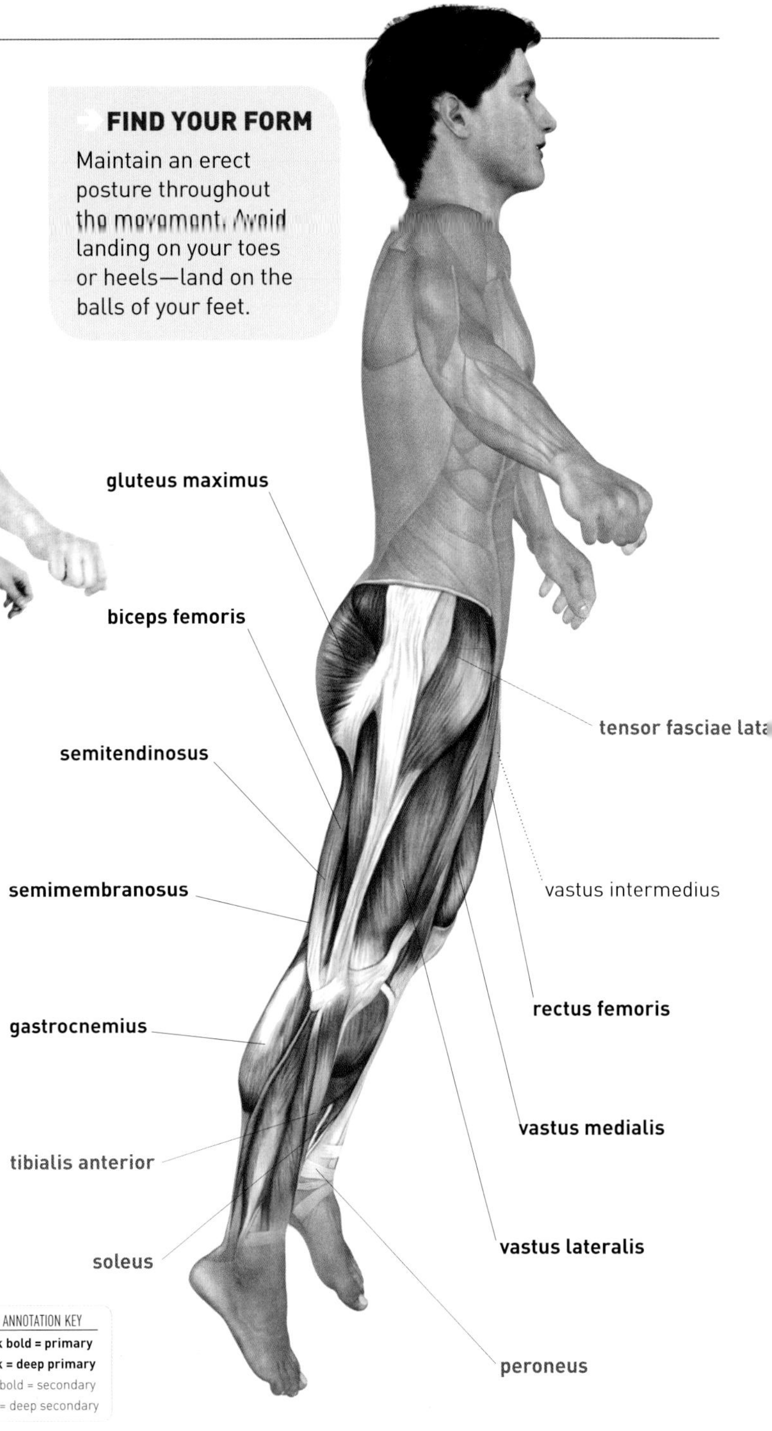

gluteus maximus

biceps femoris

semitendinosus

semimembranosus

gastrocnemius

tibialis anterior

soleus

tensor fasciae lata

vastus intermedius

rectus femoris

vastus medialis

vastus lateralis

peroneus

MUSCLE ANNOTATION KEY
— Black bold = primary
····· Black = deep primary
— Gray bold = secondary
····· Gray = deep secondary

152 **Distance Leap**
Stand straight with your feet close together, but not touching. Jump from your left foot, and land on your right. Then jump from your right foot, and lend on your left. Continue rapidly for the desired time or distance.

153 **Jump to BOSU**
Stand in front of BOSU ball placed dome-side up. Drop down into a quarter-squat, and then push through your heels, swing your arms, and spring up on to dome. Land softly on your heels, and spring backward off the dome.

154 **Cheer Jump**
Stand with your feet together and your hands on your hips. Bend your knees into a half-squat, and then jump upward as high as you can, bending both legs at the knee to bring your feet backward and upward toward your glutes. As your jump, bring your arms over your head into a V position. Continue without pause for the desired amount of time or repetitions.

155 **Depth Jumps**
Face two plyo boxes or platforms placed about 3 feet apart from each other, and then stand on top of the one closest to you. Jump off the box, making sure to land on the balls of your feet between the two boxes. As soon as your feet hit the floor, spring up on to the other box. As soon as you land on the second box, turn around, and repeat in the other direction.

156 **Tuck Jumps**
Stand with your knees slightly bent and your elbows bent to 90 degrees. Bend your knees into a half-squat, and then jump straight upward by bending slightly forward and tucking your knees upward to touch your elbows. Land on the balls of your feet, and continue without pause for the desired amount of time or repetitions.

157 **Stadium Jumps**
Stand at the base of a staircase with steps at least as deep as the length of your feet. Drop down into a quarter-squat, and then push through your heels, swing your arms, and spring up to the first step. Find your balance, and then spring to the next, finding a steady well-balanced rhythm.

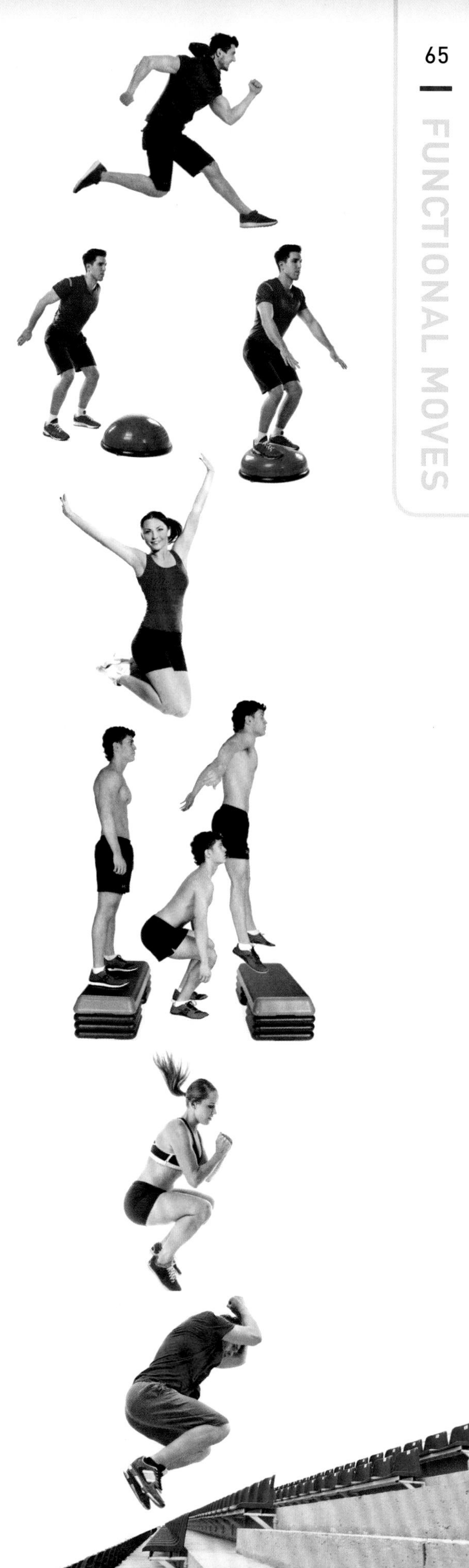

PLYOMETRIC BOXES AND AEROBIC STEPS

A sure way to add intensity to your workout is to work with boxes and steps—just think of the long-standing popularity of step aerobics classes to burn calories and elevate heart rate. I n functional training and boot camp gyms, many lower-body exercise call for you to jump on and off a box or step, which can help you to increase your speed, power, and explosiveness. When choosing a box, look for sturdy construction and a variety of sizes—adjustable models and sets are available that generally range in height from 12 to 30 inches high. Aerobic steps and platforms can vary in height, too. Look for stackable versions that you can adjust, depending on your workout or fitness goals.

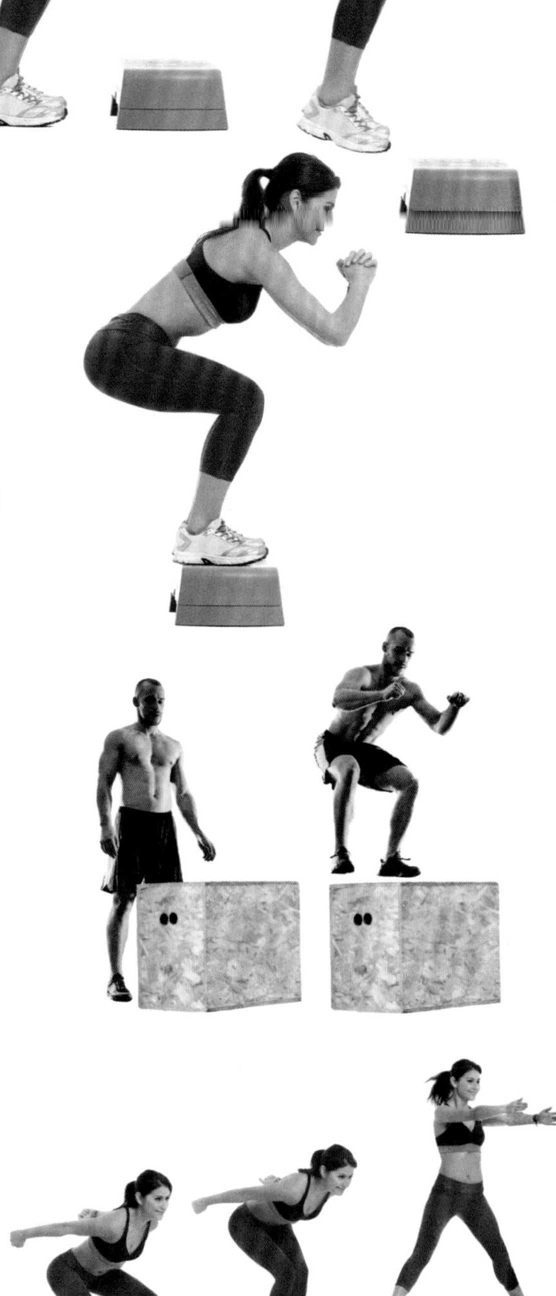

158 Step Jumps

Stand in front of an aerobic step or low box. Bend your knees into a quarter-squat, and then push through your heels, swing your arms forward, and spring up on to the step. Land softly on your heels, and then quickly spring backward off the step. Continue without pause for the desired amount of time or repetitions.

159 Box Jumps

Stand in front of a plyo box or other platform. Bend your knees into a quarter-squat, and then push through your heels, swing your arms, and spring up on to the box. Land softly on your heels, and then step down. Continue for the desired time or reps.

160 Straddle Box Jumps

Stand with your feet on either side of an aerobic step or low box. Bend your knees into a quarter-squat, and then push through your heels, swing your arms forward, and spring upward to land with both feet on the first step. Find your balance, and then jump as high as possible while spreading your legs as wide as you can as you bring your arms forward. Land on the balls of our feet, returning to the starting position with your feet on either side of the step. Continue without pause for the desired amount of time or repetitions.

Skipping Rope

Skipping, or jumping, rope, may be a schoolyard favorite, but many a childhood activity, it is a high-energy exercise that really burns calories. Athletes, such as boxers, and military personnel are known for skipping rope as a training move, and it is an effective exercise to perform as a rest between other exercise sets to recover your heart rate.

- Stand with the jump rope in your hands, letting the rope hang behind your feet.
- Swing the rope around your body and jump over it. Keep your arms as straight as you can during the movement, and land with both feet together on the floor.

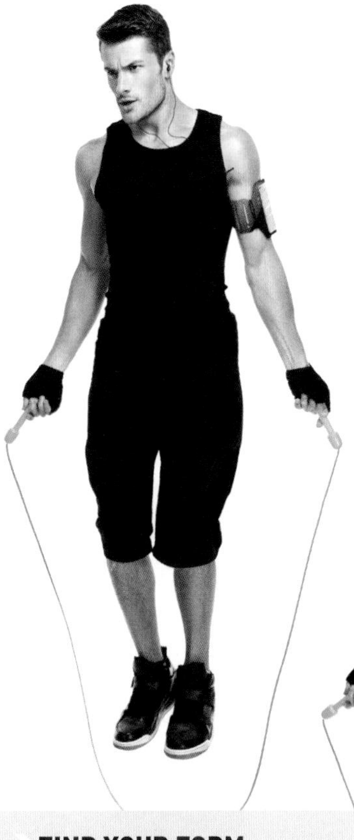

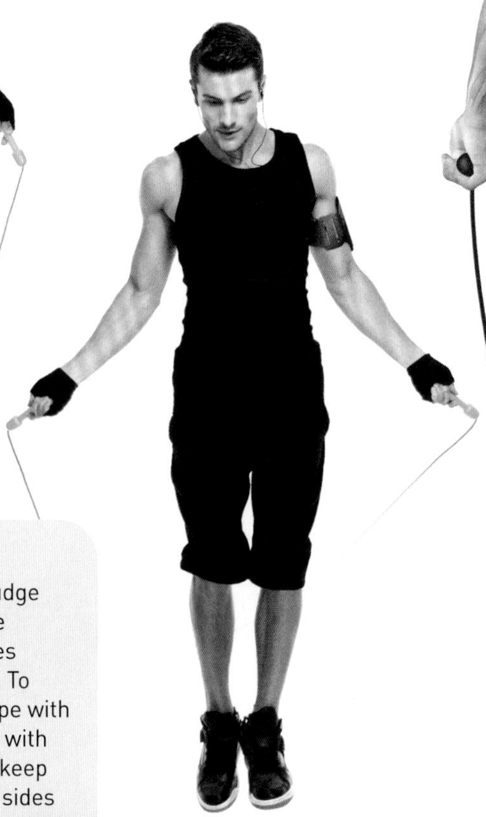

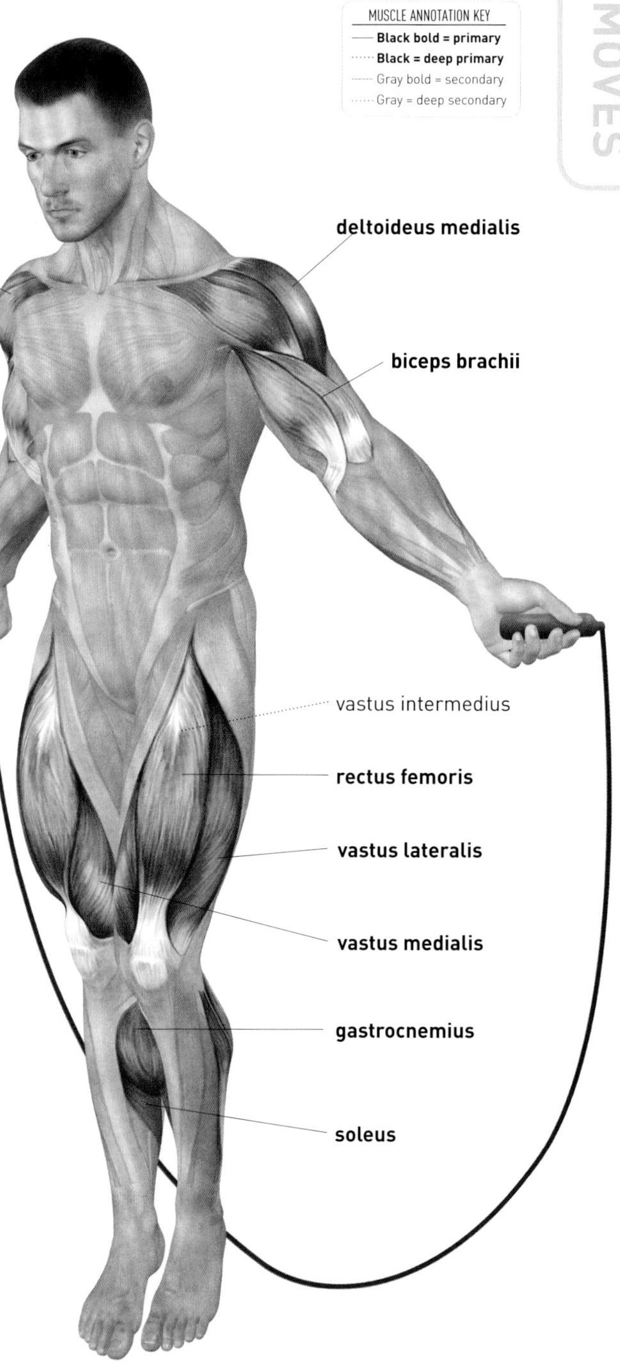

MUSCLE ANNOTATION KEY
Black bold = primary
Black = deep primary
Gray bold = secondary
Gray = deep secondary

deltoideus anterior
deltoideus medialis
biceps brachii
vastus intermedius
rectus femoris
vastus lateralis
vastus medialis
gastrocnemius
soleus

FIND YOUR FORM

Begin with the right rope. To judge the proper length, stand on the middle of the rope—the handles should extend to your armpits. To begin the exercise, hold the rope with your hands at about hip height with your elbows slightly bent, and keep your upper arms close to your sides as you swing the rope with your chest out and shoulders back and down. Keep your jumps small, and make sure to land on the balls of your feet.

162 Star Jump

As many a Navy SEAL candidate or high school cheerleader can attest, the star jump is harder than it looks—you must be able to jump high enough to simultaneously extend your legs and arms outward. To develop leg strength and cardiovascular endurance, as well as improve bone density, you can challenge yourself to perform as many as you can in quick succession, being sure to concentrate on maintaining perfect form.

- Stand with your feet together, and then squat down, keeping your knees in line with your toes.
- In one explosive movement, jump as high as possible while spreading your arms and legs as wide as you can. Your body will make a star shape in the fully extended point of the jump.
- Bend your knees slightly as you land in the standing position. Sink back to a squat, and repeat. Each jump equals one repetition.

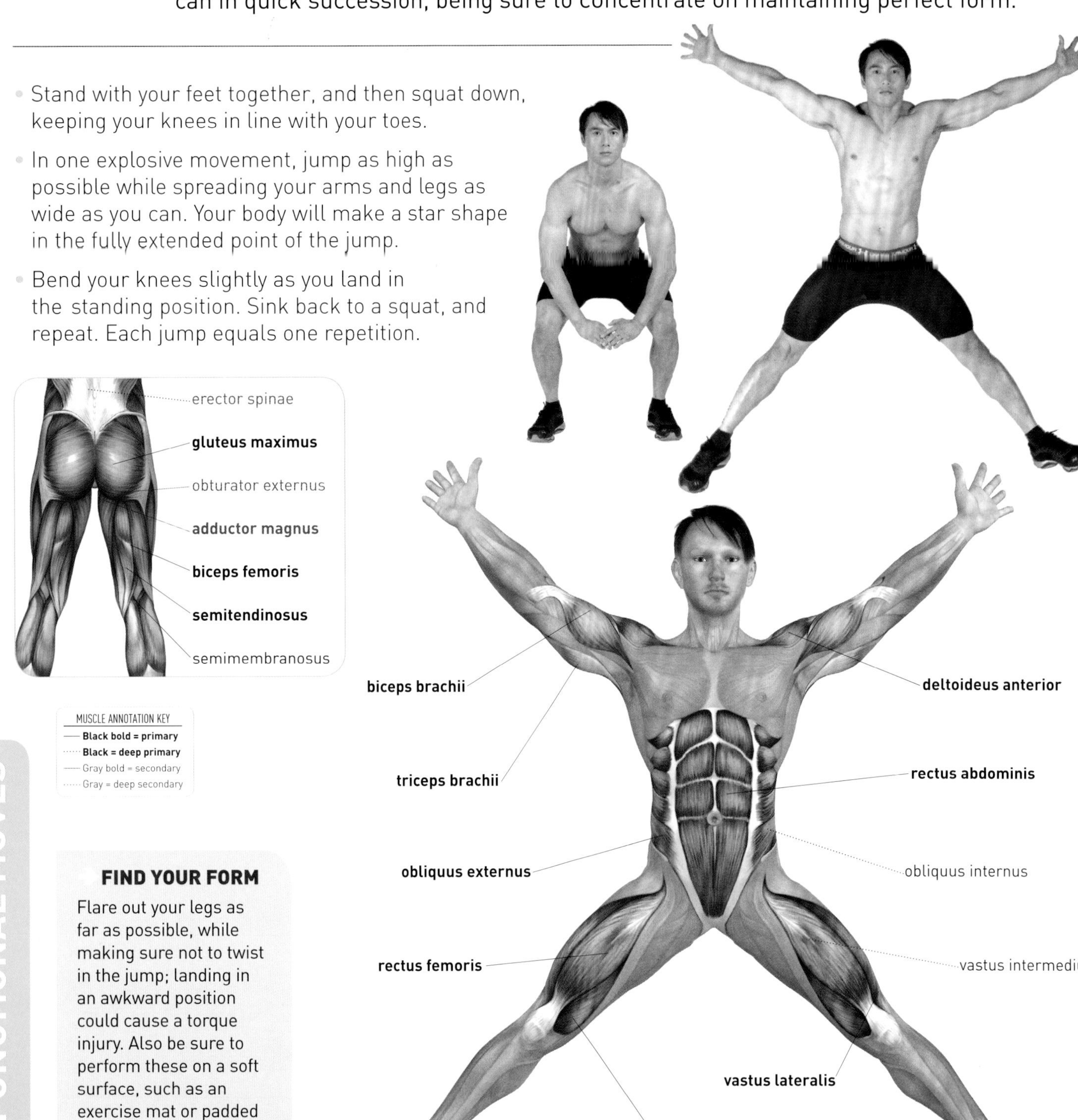

FIND YOUR FORM

Flare out your legs as far as possible, while making sure not to twist in the jump; landing in an awkward position could cause a torque injury. Also be sure to perform these on a soft surface, such as an exercise mat or padded carpeting, to reduce the impact of your landing.

163

Straddle Leap

Stand with your feet together and your arms at your sides. Bend your knees, squatting down completely to the floor with your heels slightly off the floor. Place your hands on the floor for balance, look upward, and then push off the floor to jump straight upward. At the peak of the jump, pop your legs out to the sides, straighten your arms, and reach for your toes. Land softly on the balls of your feet, and continue without pause for the desired amount of time or repetitions.

164

Stag Leap

Stand with your feet together. Bend your knees, and then jump upward as high as you can, bending both legs at the knee and wrapping your back leg around your body, with your knee parallel to the floor. As leap, lift your arms over your head. Land softly on the balls of your feet, and continue without pause for the desired amount of time or repetitions.

165

Jumping Jacks

Stand with your feet together, arms extended with your hands at your sides. Bend your knees slightly, and push through the balls of your feet while straightening your knees to jump upward while spreading your legs a wide as you can. At the same time, raise both arms out and up in a smooth arc. As you return to the floor, bring your feet together and your hands back to your sides. Continue without pause for the desired amount of time or repetitions.

166

Jumping Jack Clap

Perform as your would a Jumping Jack, but at the top of the movement, sharply clap your hands together. Continue without pause for the desired amount of time or repetitions.

167

Scissor-Stance Jacks

Stand with your left foot in front of your right with your knees slightly bent and fists raised in front of you. Bracing your core, kick your right foot in front of you, leg straight, while punching your left fist toward your foot. Quickly return to the starting position, place your right foot in front of your left, and repeat on the other side. Continue alternating without pause for the desired amount of time or repetitions.

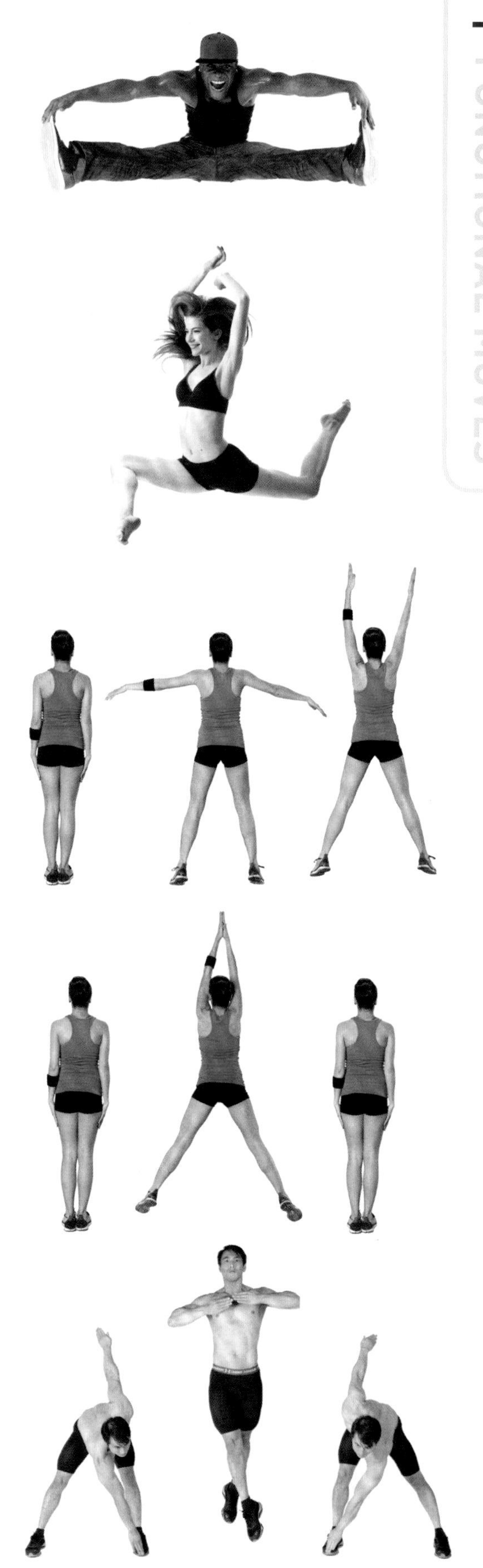

168 Skater

The high-energy Skater targets your inner and outer thighs, including your hip adductor and abductor muscles and iliotibial bands, which all work to keep your knees and hips stable. It is a great exercise for runners, counterbalancing the effects of repetitive flexion and extension and alleviating the resulting strength imbalance between the inner- and outer-thigh muscles and the quadriceps and hamstrings.

- Stand with your legs spaced wider than shoulder-width apart and your toes pointing forward.
- Slide to your side into a side lunge as you bend forward slightly, with your hands placed on your thigh, and then move in the opposite direction.
- Slide back and forth for the desired time or repetitions.

FIND YOUR FORM

Push through your heels to drive the exercise, moving with control and keeping a steady, quick pace. Avoid hyperextending your knee past your toes.

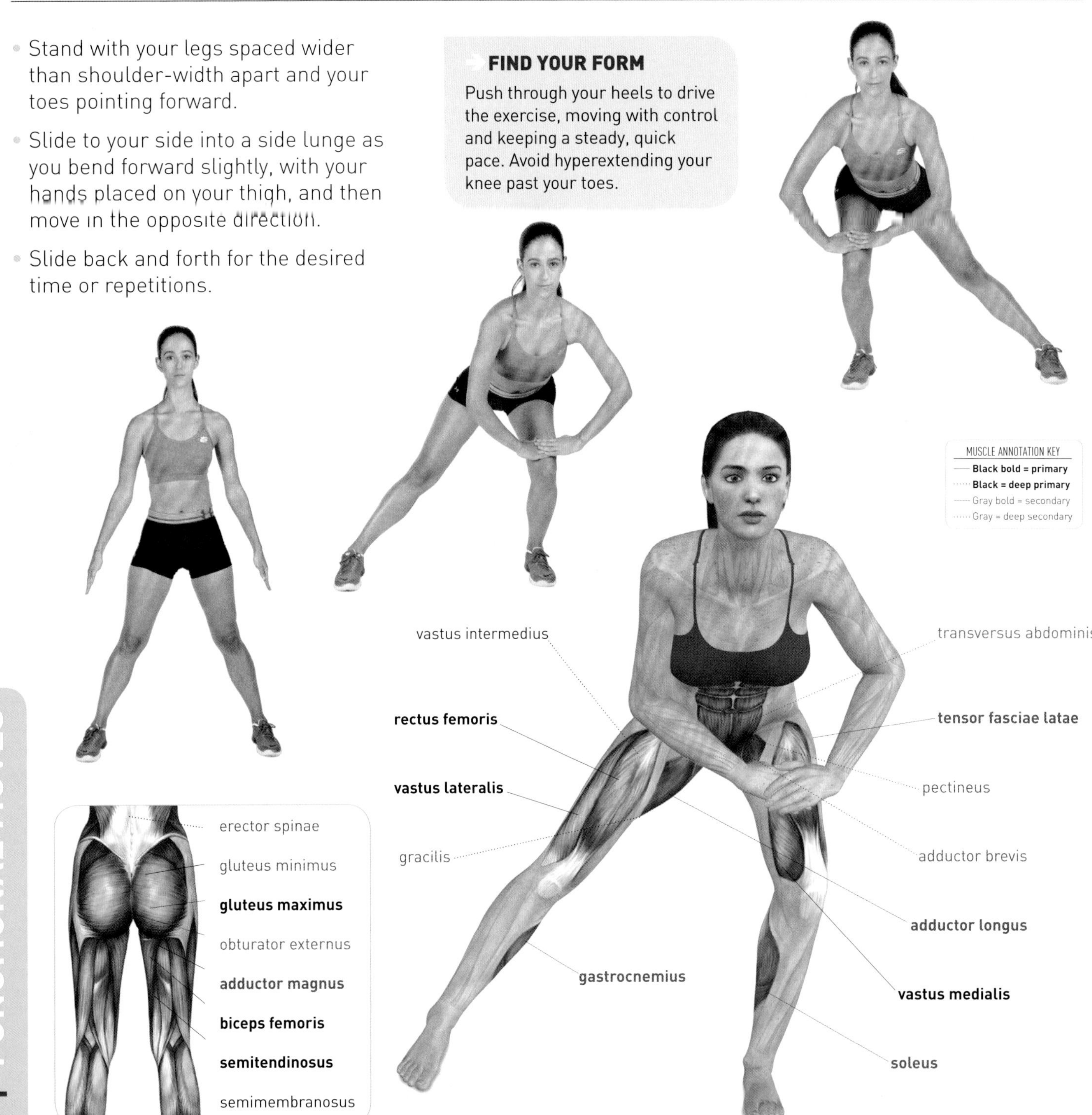

169 **Dumbbell Skater**

Grasp a dumbbell in each hand, and perform the Skater (#XX) while curling the dumbbells upward as you move from side to side.

170 **Straight-Leg Skater**

Stand straight, and place your left leg slightly behind your right. Keeping your legs and back straight, jump to your left as far as possible while swinging your arms toward the left. Land in a standing position with your right leg slightly behind your left. Continue jumping side-to-side, crossing one leg behind the other. Switching back and forth equals one repetition.

171 **Speed Skater**

Stand in a half-squat position, and place your left leg slightly behind your right. Jump to your left as far as possible while swinging your arms toward the left. Land in a half-squat position with your right leg slightly behind your left. Immediately jump back toward the right as far as possible, as if you were skating in long strides. Continue to alternate sides for the desired amount of time or repetitions.

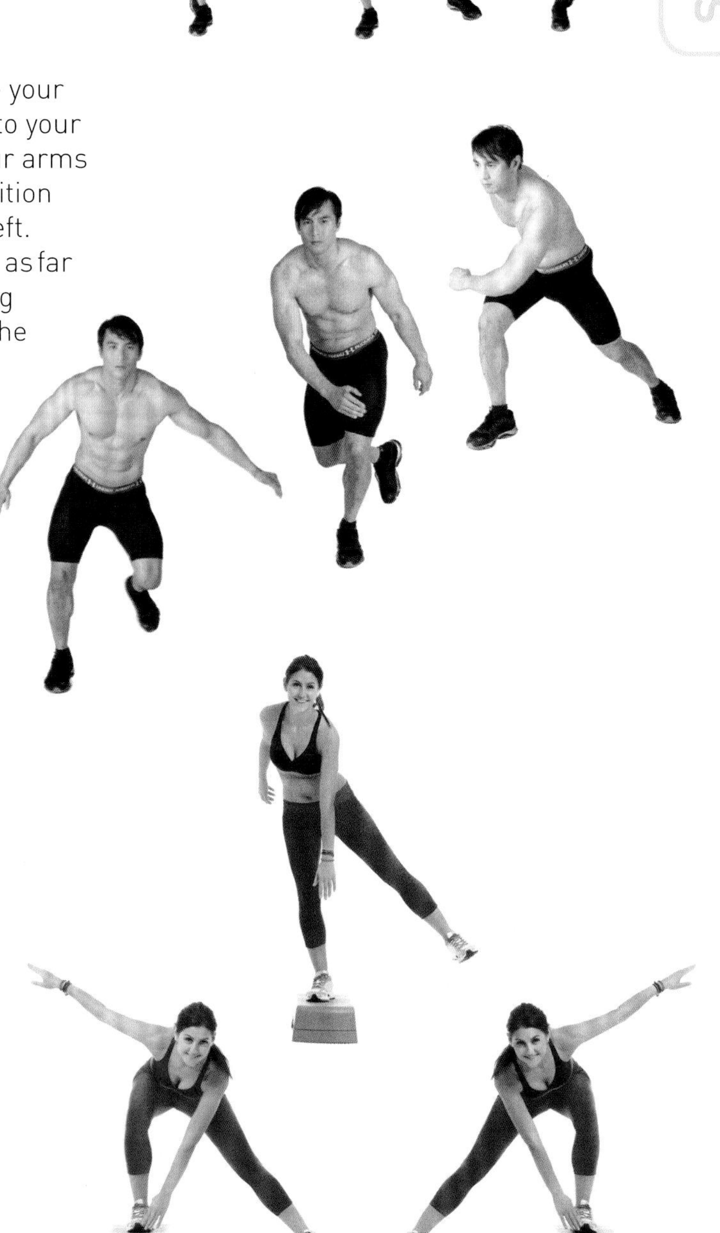

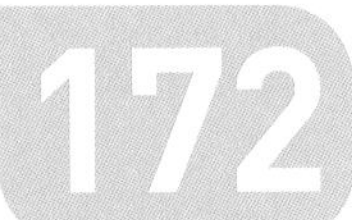

172 **Step Skater**

Stand with your right foot on an aerobic step with your left foot planted at least a foot from the step. Extend your arms out at shoulder height. Bend forward at the hip, reaching down to touch your right foot with your left hand. Rise back up, placing both feet on the step, and then drop your right foot to the floor. Bring your right hand to your left foot. Bring both feet back to the step, and then repeat all steps, continuing to alternate sides for the desired amount of time or repetitions.

Swimming

A functional move that is also a Pilates staple, the swimming exercise can strengthen your core muscles while improving your coordination and endurance. As your strength improves, keep increasing the speed and tempo of your strokes.

- Lie prone on the floor with your legs hip-width apart. Stretch your arms beside your ears on the floor. Engage your pelvic floor, and draw your navel into your spine.
- Extend through your upper back as you lift your left arm and right leg simultaneously. Lift your head and shoulders off the floor.
- Lower your arm and leg to the starting position, maintaining a stretch in your limbs throughout.
- Extend your right arm and left leg off the floor, lengthening and lifting your head and shoulders. Continue to alternate arms and legs.

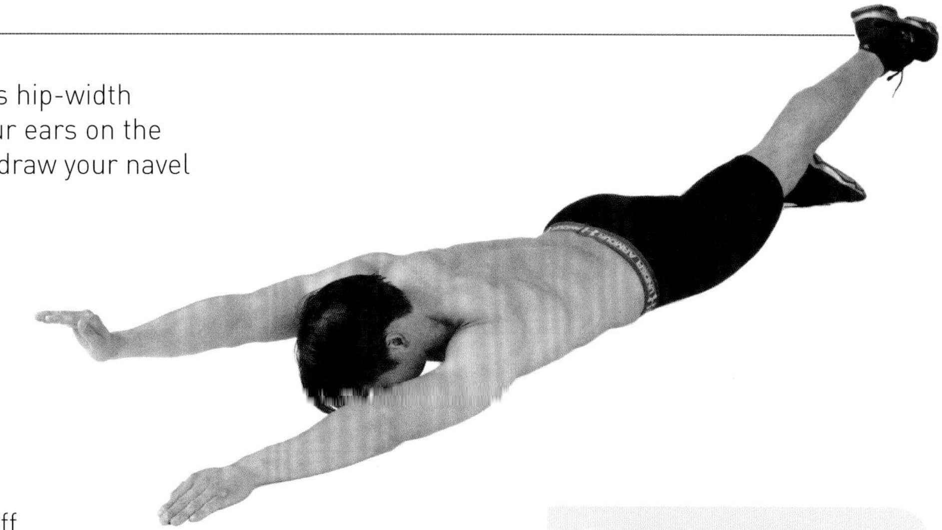

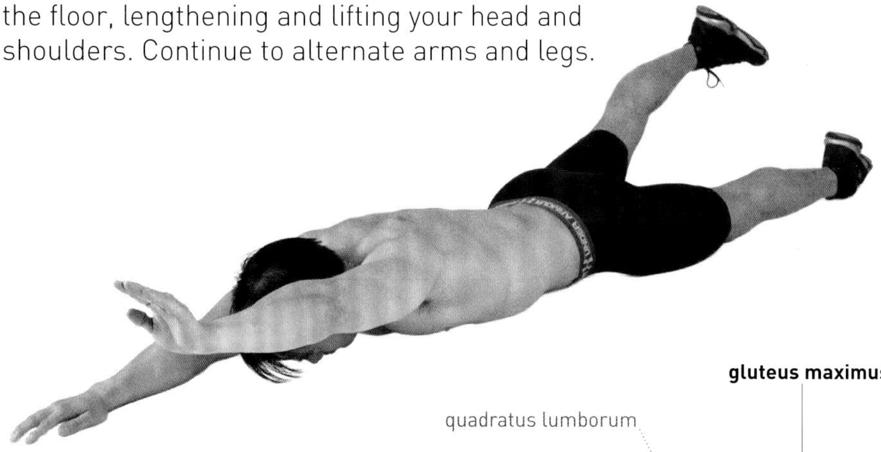

FIND YOUR FORM

Extend your limbs as long as possible in opposite directions. Tightly squeeze your glutes, and draw your navel into your spine throughout the exercise.

MUSCLE ANNOTATION KEY
- **Black bold = primary**
- Black = deep primary
- Gray bold = secondary
- Gray = deep secondary

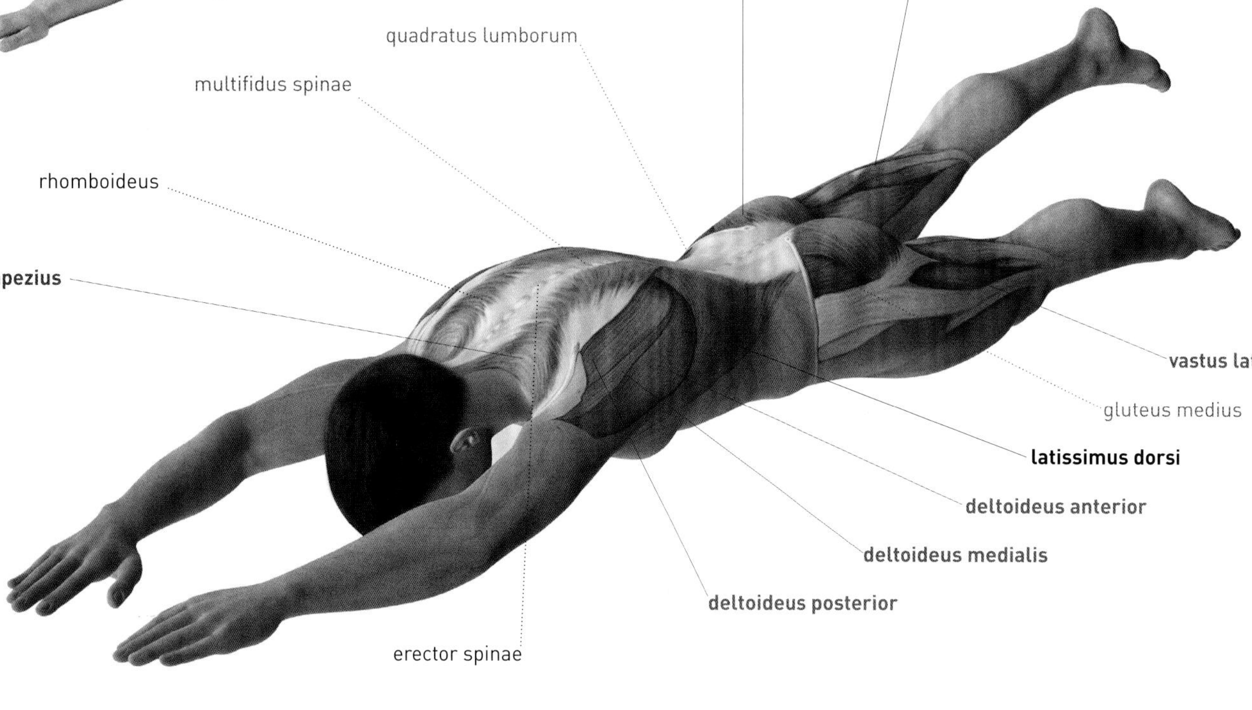

biceps femoris
gluteus maximus
quadratus lumborum
multifidus spinae
rhomboideus
trapezius
vastus lateralis
gluteus medius
latissimus dorsi
deltoideus anterior
deltoideus medialis
deltoideus posterior
erector spinae

174 Arm Hauler

Lie facedown with your arms spread wide, keeping them level with your shoulders. Lift your head, keeping your chin up while arching your lower back. Bring your arms off the floor and reach behind you as far as your can. Without letting your hands touch the floor, bring your arms forward to touch your fingertips together. Draw your arms back to the start, and continue for the desired repetitions.

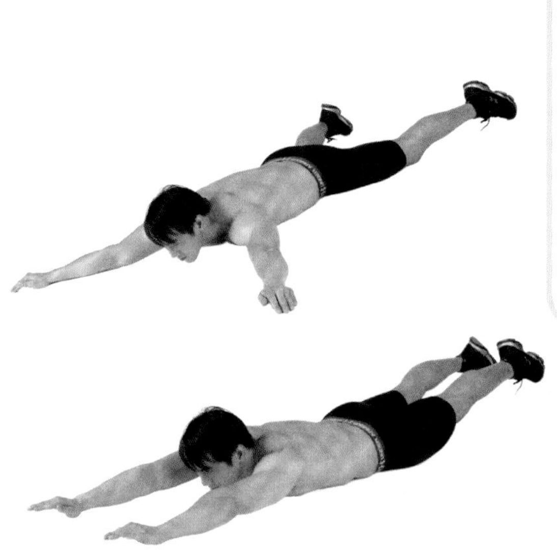

Facedown Snow Angel

Lie facedown on the floor with your legs hip-width apart. Lift your arms and legs at the same time, and move them as if you were making snow angels.

Superman

Lie prone on the floor with your legs hip-width apart. Lift both arms and legs simultaneously, continuing to draw your navel into your spine.

Heel Beats

Work your hamstrings, glutes, inner thighs, lower back, and lower abs all while lying prone on your mat. This Pilates staple will also boost your coordination and endurance.

- Lie facedown with your arms lifted off the floor by your hips, palms up. Draw your shoulders down away from your ears. Turn your legs out from the top of your hips and pull your inner thighs together.
- Lengthen your legs and lift them off the mat, tightening your thigh muscles, and then press your heels together, and then separate them in a rapid but controlled motion.

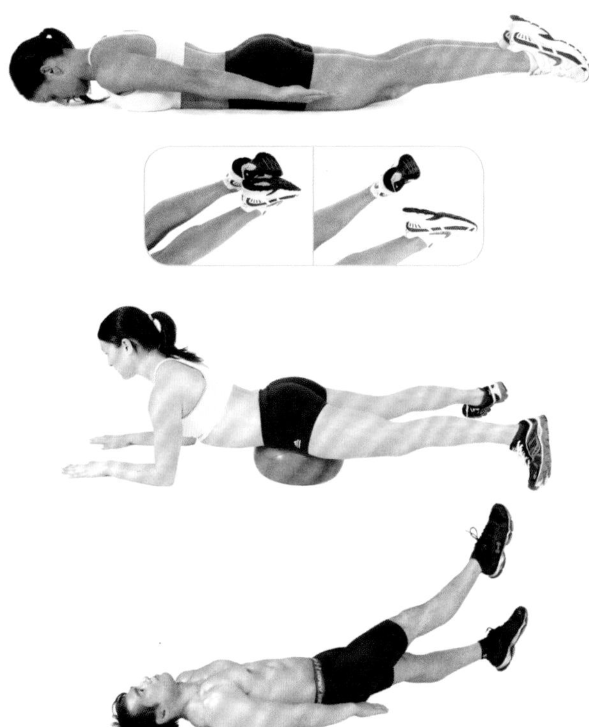

Swiss Ball Heel Beats

Lie facedown with your forearms on the floor. Rest your hips on top of a small Swiss ball. Extend your legs behind you. Press your heels together, and then separate them in a rapid but controlled motion.

Supine Flutter Kicks

Lie on your back with your arms stretched along the sides of your body. Keeping your heels a few inches off the floor, kick up and down, alternating legs.

Bear Crawl

The Bear Crawl is a favorite of Navy SEALS and other military special forces, helping to train recruits for real-world movements. Crawling exercises can be tough, but they are great for increasing agility, cardiovascular health, and upper-body strength. They are anaerobic exercises, meaning that they trigger lactic acid formation, which promotes strength, speed, and power.

- Place both hands and feet on the floor.
- Walk your left arm and right leg forward, and then your right arm and left leg.
- Keep moving forward and backward in this position, keeping your weight evenly distributed between your arms and legs.

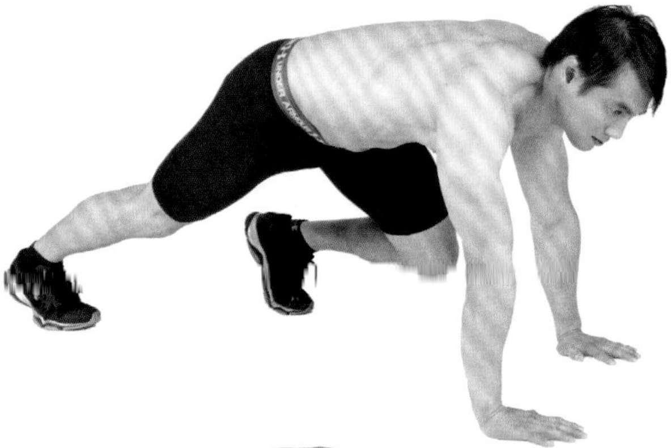

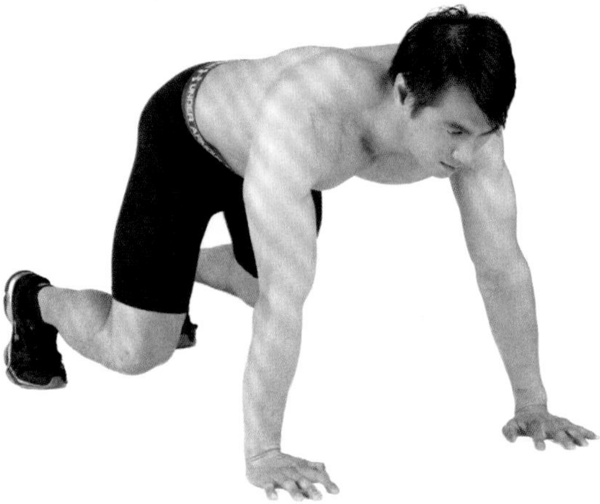

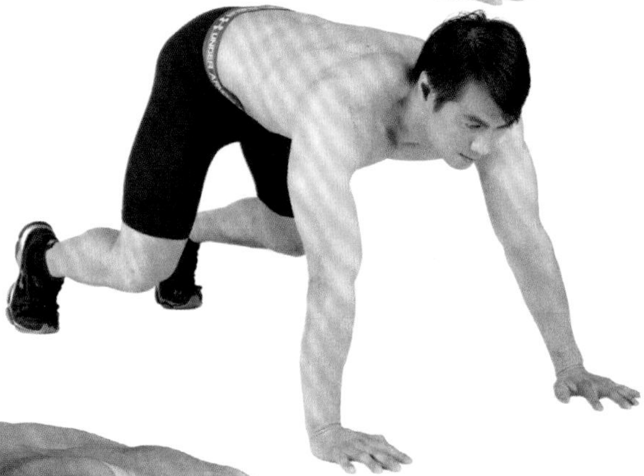

FIND YOUR FORM

Move as steadily and as smoothly as possible, being careful to distribute your weight and not placing all of your weight on your arms and shoulders, which can stress your rotator cuffs. Avoid touching your knees to the floor.

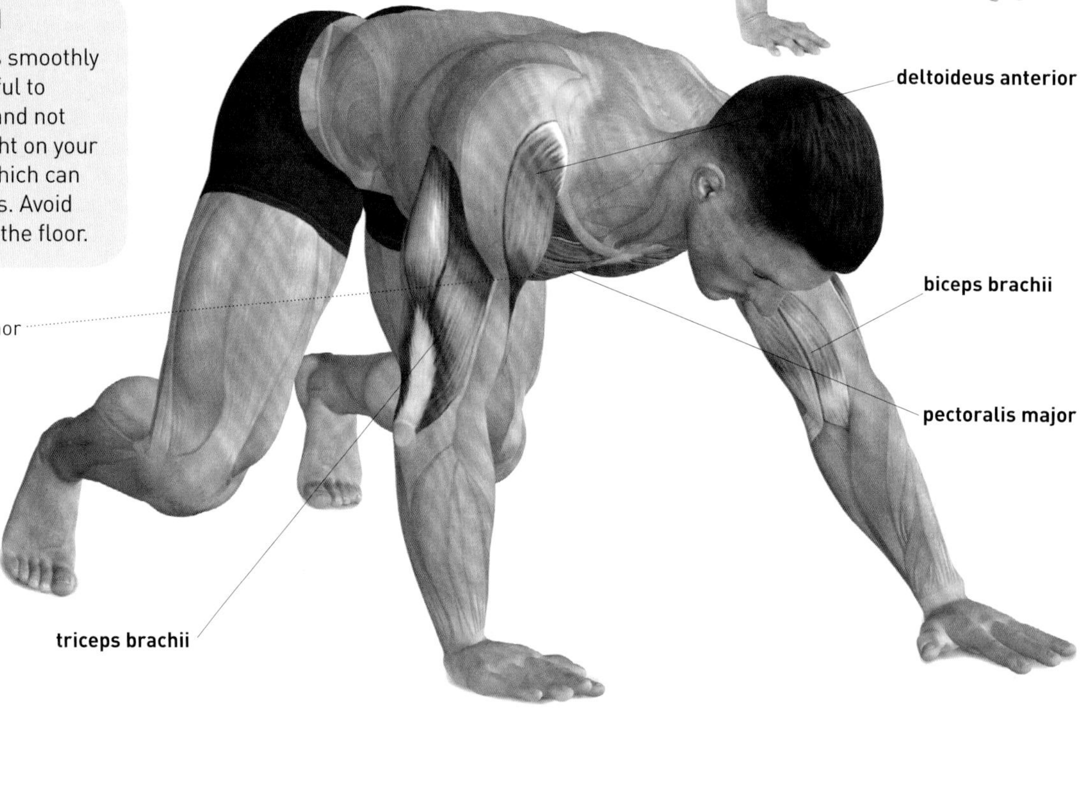

deltoideus anterior

biceps brachii

pectoralis minor

pectoralis major

triceps brachii

MUSCLE ANNOTATION KEY
- Black bold = primary
- Black = deep primary
- Gray bold = secondary
- Gray = deep secondary

181 **Alligator Crawl**

Start in the drop position, with your hands directly below your shoulders. Lower into a half push-up with your back straight. Keeping your body low to the floor, bring your right knee to your right elbow while walking your left hand forward. Reverse this movement by walking your right hand forward and bringing your left knee to your left elbow. Continue moving forward, reversing your hand and knee positions for the desired time.

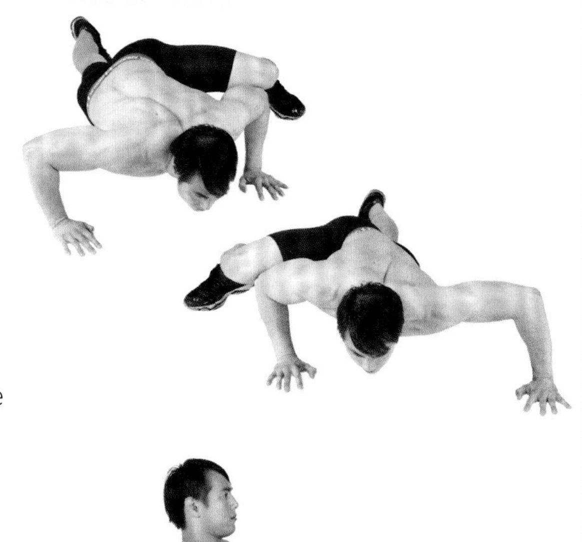

182 **Crab Crawl**

Begin with both hands and feet on the floor. Lift your body slightly so that your butt is just above the floor. Walk your right foot forward. Walk your left foot forward. Continue moving forward, taking several steps with each leg. Next, walk each leg back. Alternate moving backward and forward for the desired time.

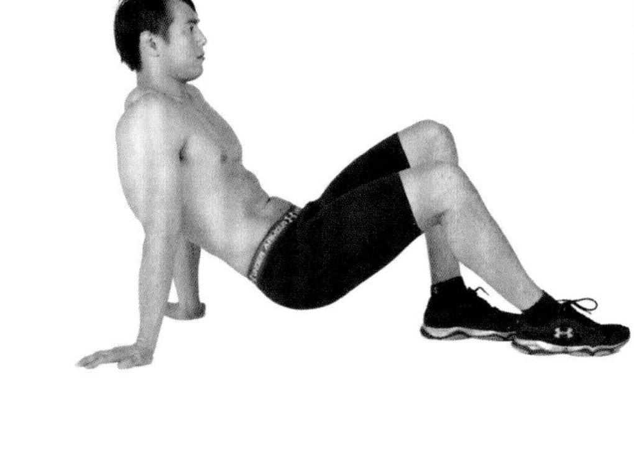

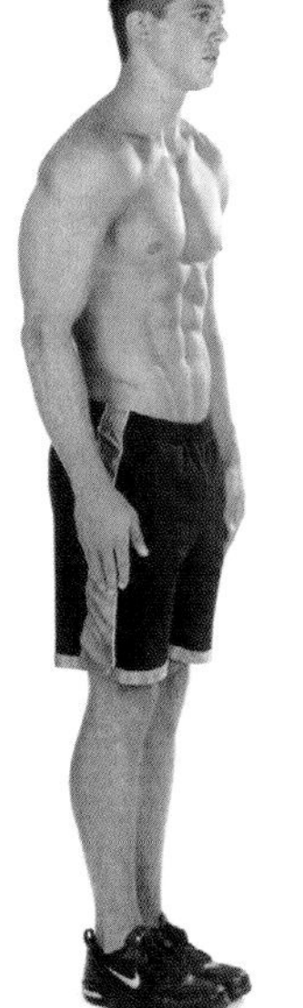

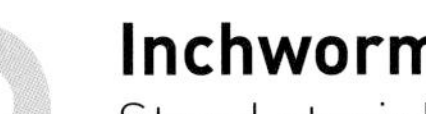

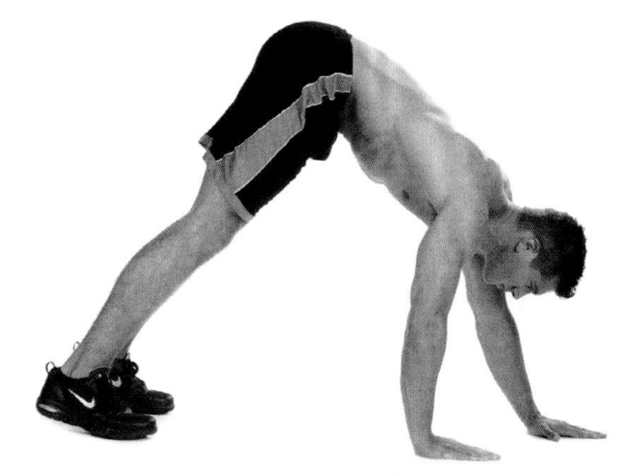

183 **Inchworm**

Stand straight, arms at your sides. Bend forward from the waist, and place your hands on the floor in front of you, at a distance slightly wider than your feet. Keep your knees as straight as possible. Shift your weight to your hands, and slowly "walk" them forward, while keeping your knees straight, your hips up, and your spine straight. Return by walking back toward the starting position and pushing your hips upward, folding your torso at the hips. This exercise is also called the Hand Walk-Out.

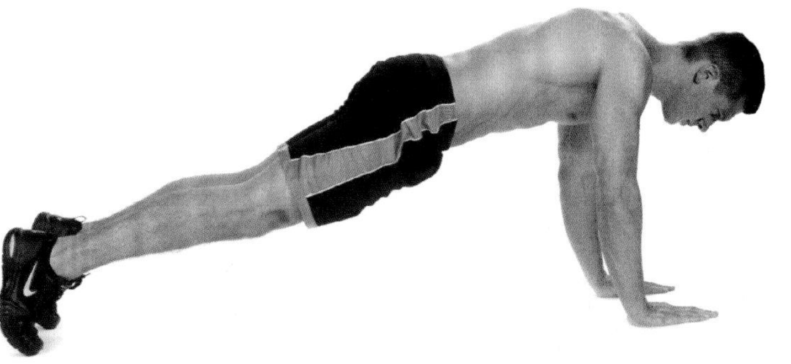

184 Mountain Climber

A favorite of military special forces, the mountain climber exercise is a high-intensity move that gets your heart rate going while it challenges the muscles of your legs and core. This compound exercise helps to develop muscular endurance in your arms, as well as hone your balance, agility, proprioception, and coordination. Keep a steady pace by moving to a 1-2 count.

- With your hands shoulder-width apart, place your palms on the floor, keeping your feet together and back straight. Push your body up until your arms are straight. This starting position is the high plank, or drop position.
- Bring your right knee in toward your chest, and rest the ball of the foot on the floor for count 1.
- Jump, and bring your left knee to your chest for count 2. Continue alternating your feet as fast as you can safely go for the desired time or repetitions, keeping pace by counting 1-2, 1-2.

FIND YOUR FORM

Perform this exercise on a stable, nonslippery surface. Avoid exercise mats for his one—a surface like a hardwood floor will offer traction, but not shift under your feet or impede your movements.

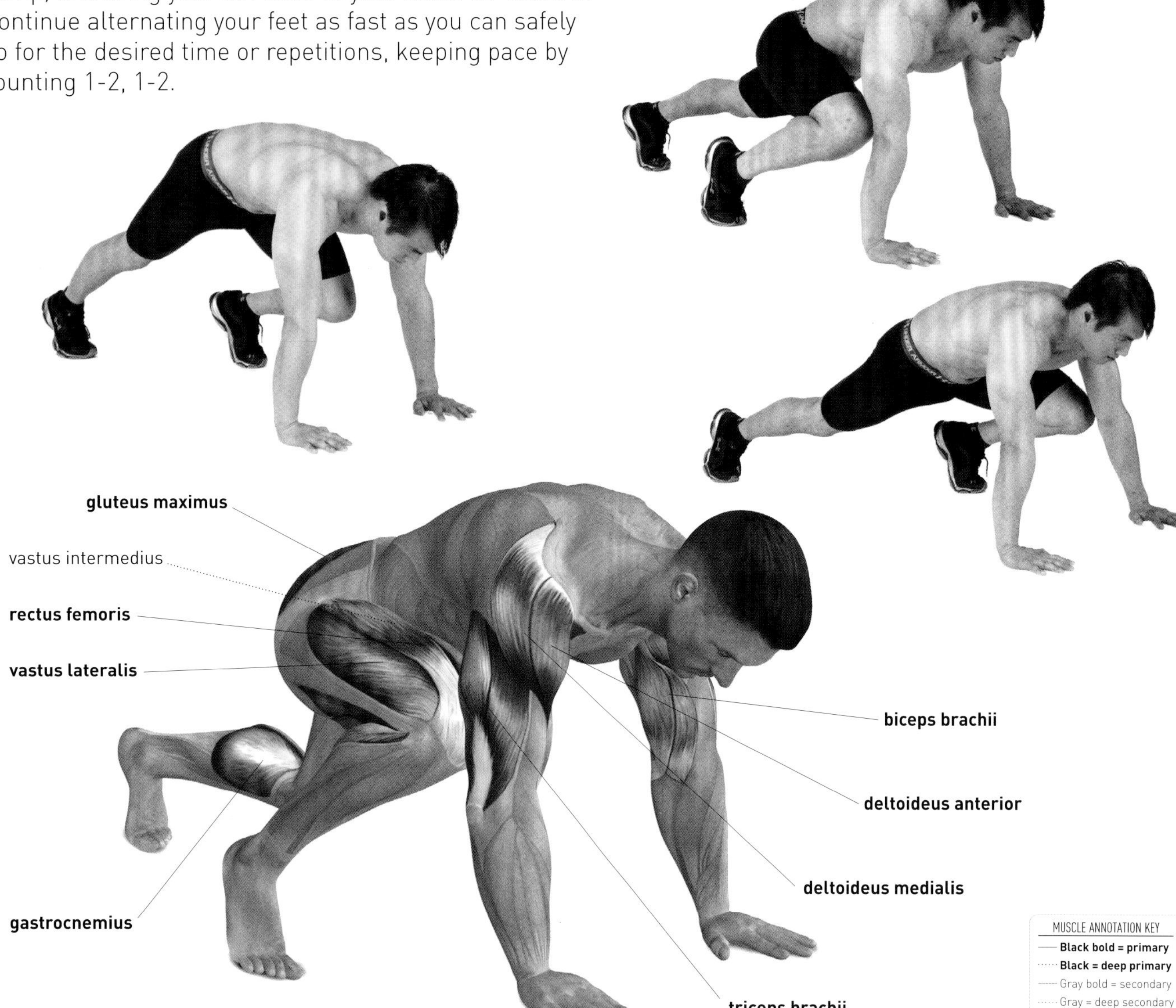

185 Cross-Body Mountain Climber
Assume the drop position with your body straight and core tight. Pick up one foot, and bring your knee toward the opposite shoulder. Return to the starting position, and then quickly alternate legs.

186 BOSU Mountain Climber
Place a BOSU ball dome-side down, and then get into a high plank position with your shoulders directly over your wrists. Keeping your hips in place and your core tight, bring one knee toward your chest, and then quickly alternate legs.

187 Spider Mountain Climber
Assume a low plank position with your shoulders over your elbows. Bend one leg and bring your knee as close to your same-side shoulder as you can. Take it back down and repeat, on the other side.

188 Sliding Mountain Climber
Place a sliding disc, paper plate, or small towel under each foot. Assume the high plank position with your hands just wider than shoulder-width apart. Bring one knee toward your chest, pulling the sliding disc, and then quickly alternate legs.

189 Swiss Ball Mountain Climber
Place your hands on a stability ball, and then extend your legs behind you in the high plank position. Raise one foot, and slowly bring your knee toward your chest, then lower it. Repeat with the other leg, and continue alternating legs as you try to keep the ball in place.

190 Fire Hydrant Mountain Climber
Assume a low plank position with your shoulders over your elbows. and then drive your knee forward, out, and up, aiming to get your thigh parallel to the floor and your knee as far forward as possible.

191 Suspended Mountain Climber
Start in the high plank position facing away from the anchor point with your hands under your shoulders, your feet in the foot cradles, and one leg pulled up to your chest. Alternate pulling your knees toward your chest.

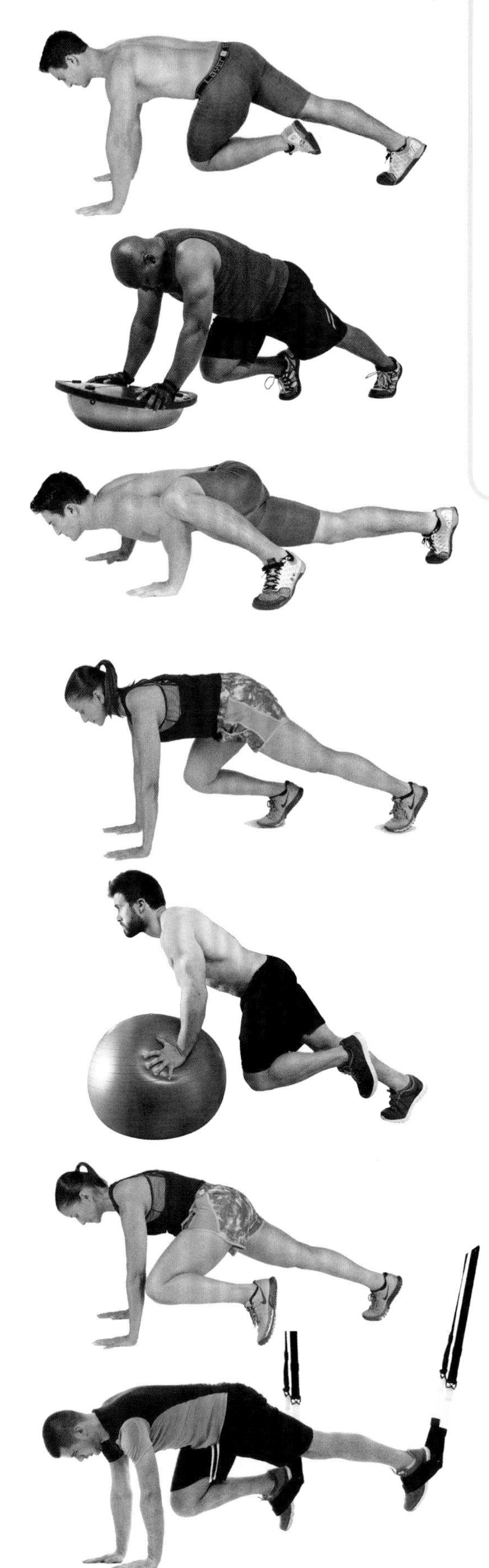

192 Mountain Climber with Hands on Desk or Bench

Assume the drop position with your hands on top of a bench and your feet planted firmly on the floor. Keep your arms fully extended and directly beneath your shoulders. Brace your core, and drive one knee to the mid-line of your body. Reverse the motion, and step your foot back to the starting position.

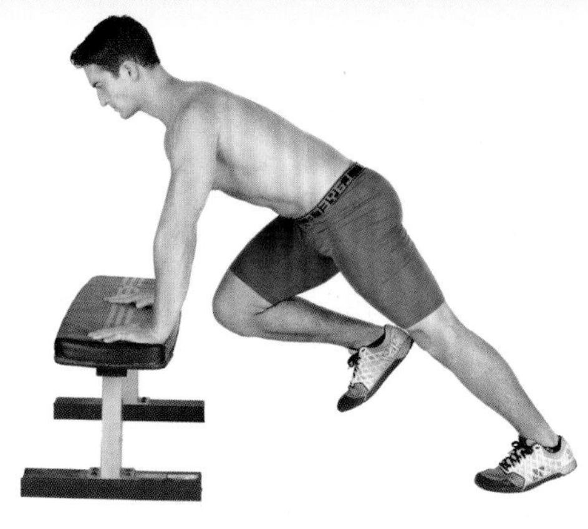

193 Resistance Band Mountain Climber

Loop or tie a resistance band loosely around your ankles. Assume the drop position, and then perform as your would a Mountain Climber (#184).

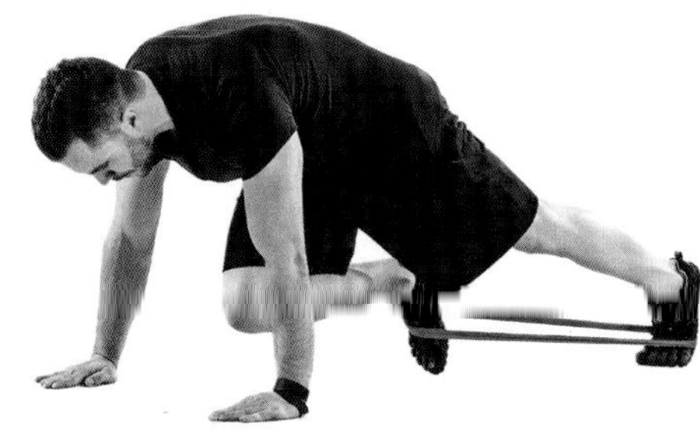

194 Slalom Skier

Assume the drop position. Jump both feet together to the left so that both feet land outside your left arm. Tuck your knees toward your chest while you jump. Jump your feet back to the leaning rest position, and then jump both feet back across your body to the right, landing with both feet outside your right arm and both knees bent toward your chest. Immediately jump back to the left, and continue alternating sides. Both left and right equal one repetition.

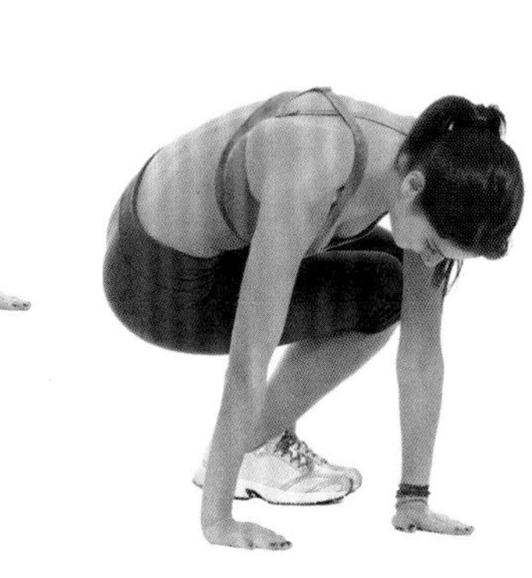

195 Plank Bunny Hop

Lay a straight-line obstacle, such as a tape measure, yardstick, or a stretch-out resistance band, on the floor. Assume the drop position with one hand on each side of the line and both feet to the left of it. Jump both feet forward do that your calves are parallel to the floor, forming a right angle with your thighs. In one explosive movement, jump both feet to the right, lifting your body as far as you can. Land both on the balls of your feet, and then immediately jump to the other side. Continue jumping back and forth over the line without pause for the desired amount of time or repetitions.

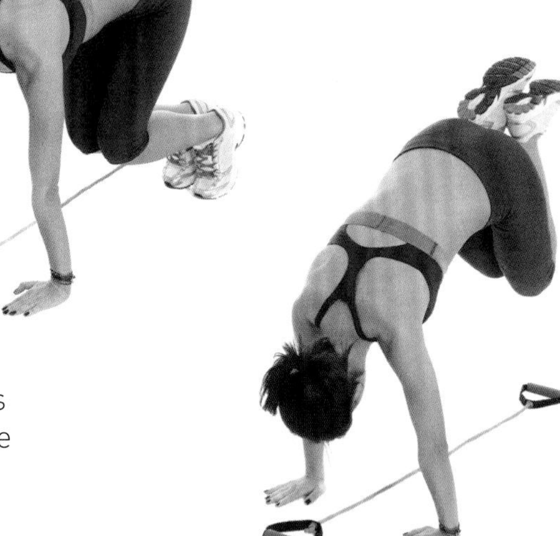

196 Diagonal Reach

As simple as it may look, the Diagonal Reach trains multiple muscles at once—especially your abdominals and obliques. This exercise, along with the Medicine Ball Over-the-Shoulder Throw is a multipurpose move that helps you to develop balance, coordination, and power while stabilizing and strengthening your core.

- Stand with your feet hip-width apart and your arms at your sides.
- Raise both arms upward and to the right to form a diagonal line. Follow your hands with your gaze. Return to starting position.
- Repeat to the left side.

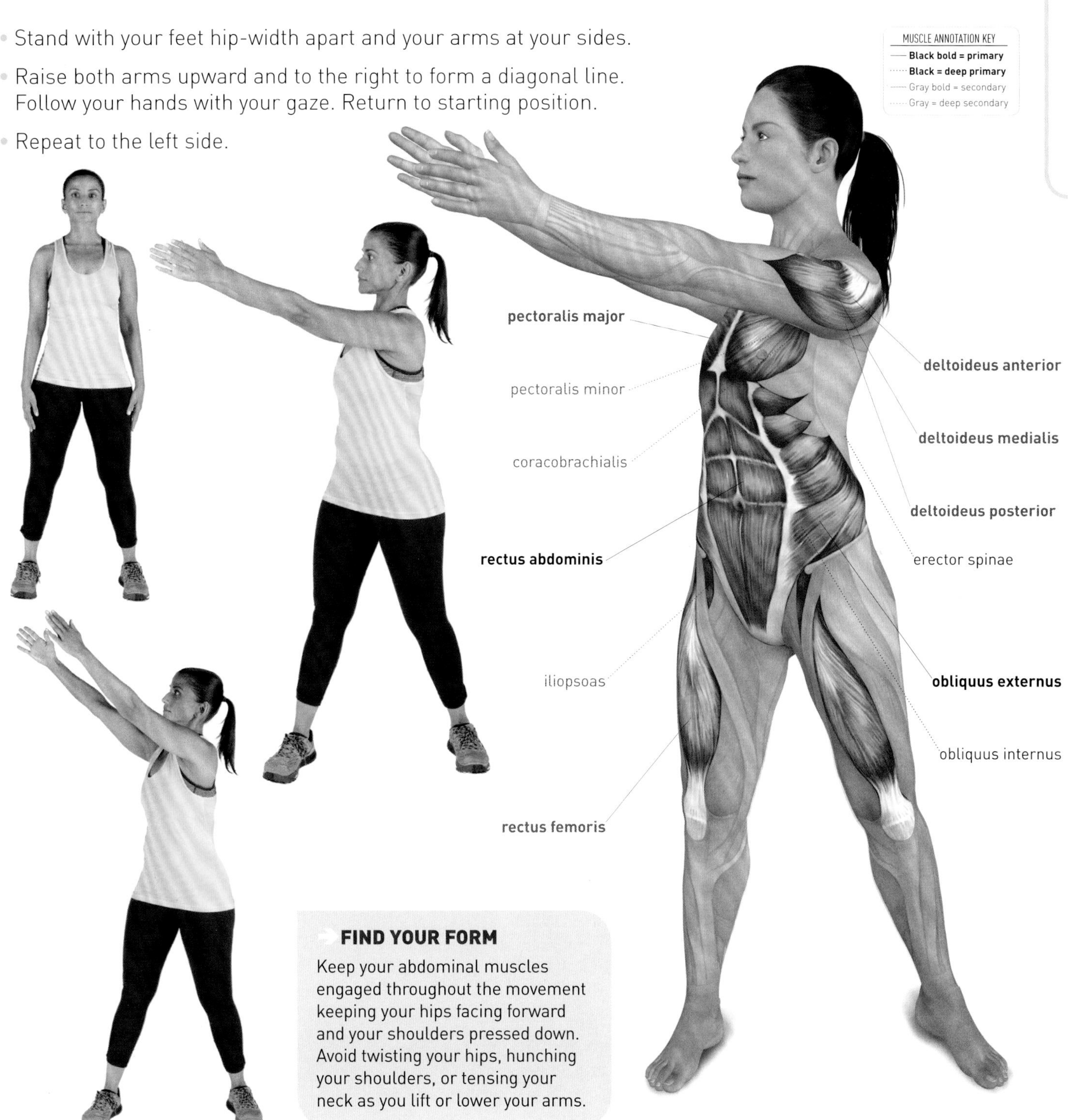

FIND YOUR FORM

Keep your abdominal muscles engaged throughout the movement keeping your hips facing forward and your shoulders pressed down. Avoid twisting your hips, hunching your shoulders, or tensing your neck as you lift or lower your arms.

197 Over-the-Shoulder Throw

Working with a medicine ball during the Over-the-Shoulder Throw adds resistance and force to the Diagonal Reach movement, and like that exercise, it has multiple benefits—helping you to improve your balance and coordination while stabilizing and strengthening your core. You can perform it with a partner, taking turns to throw the ball to each other, or you can perform it facing a wall.

- Stand with your feet hip-width apart holding a medicine ball in your hands, held low at waist height. Extend your arms forward, and rotate your core, moving your extended arms slightly upward and to the side so that the medicine ball follows your body's twist.
- Twist your torso in the other direction as you raise your arms in an arc. At the top of the arc, with your torso twisted, release the ball to your partner.
- Lower your arms and return your torso to center, and then retrieve the ball. Perform the desired repetitions, and then switch sides.

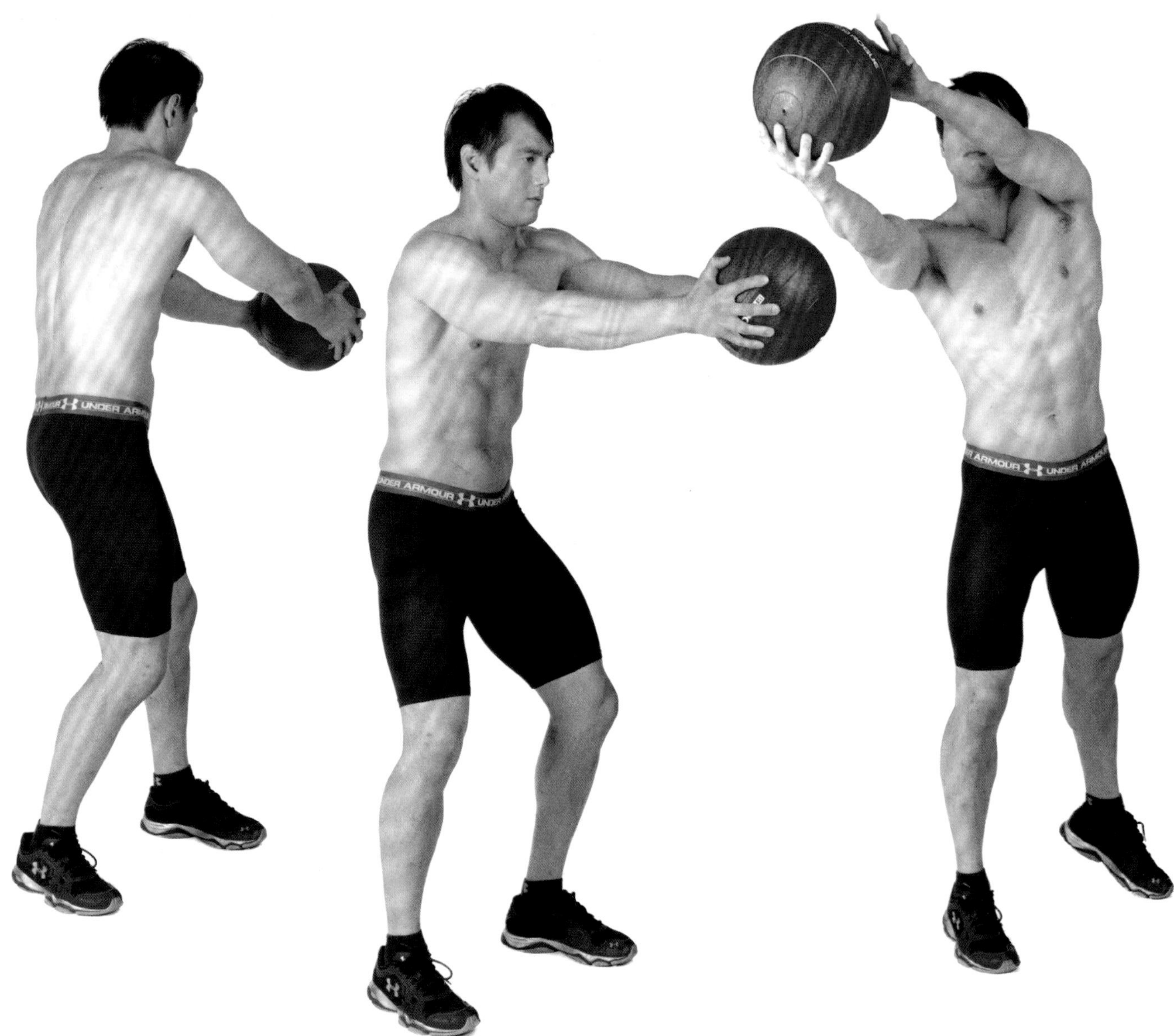

198 Figure 8

The Figure 8 exercise is both a core stabilizer and a core strengthener. It is great for anyone who wants to build rotational power, such a baseball pitcher or golfer. You can experiment with form and speed when performing this move—the bigger your make the 8s, the more of a challenge it will be. Try upping your speed, too, while still keeping good form.

- Stand with your feet hip-width apart and your arms at your sides.
- Raise both arms upward and to the right to form a diagonal line. Follow your hands with your gaze. Return to starting position.
- Repeat to the left side.

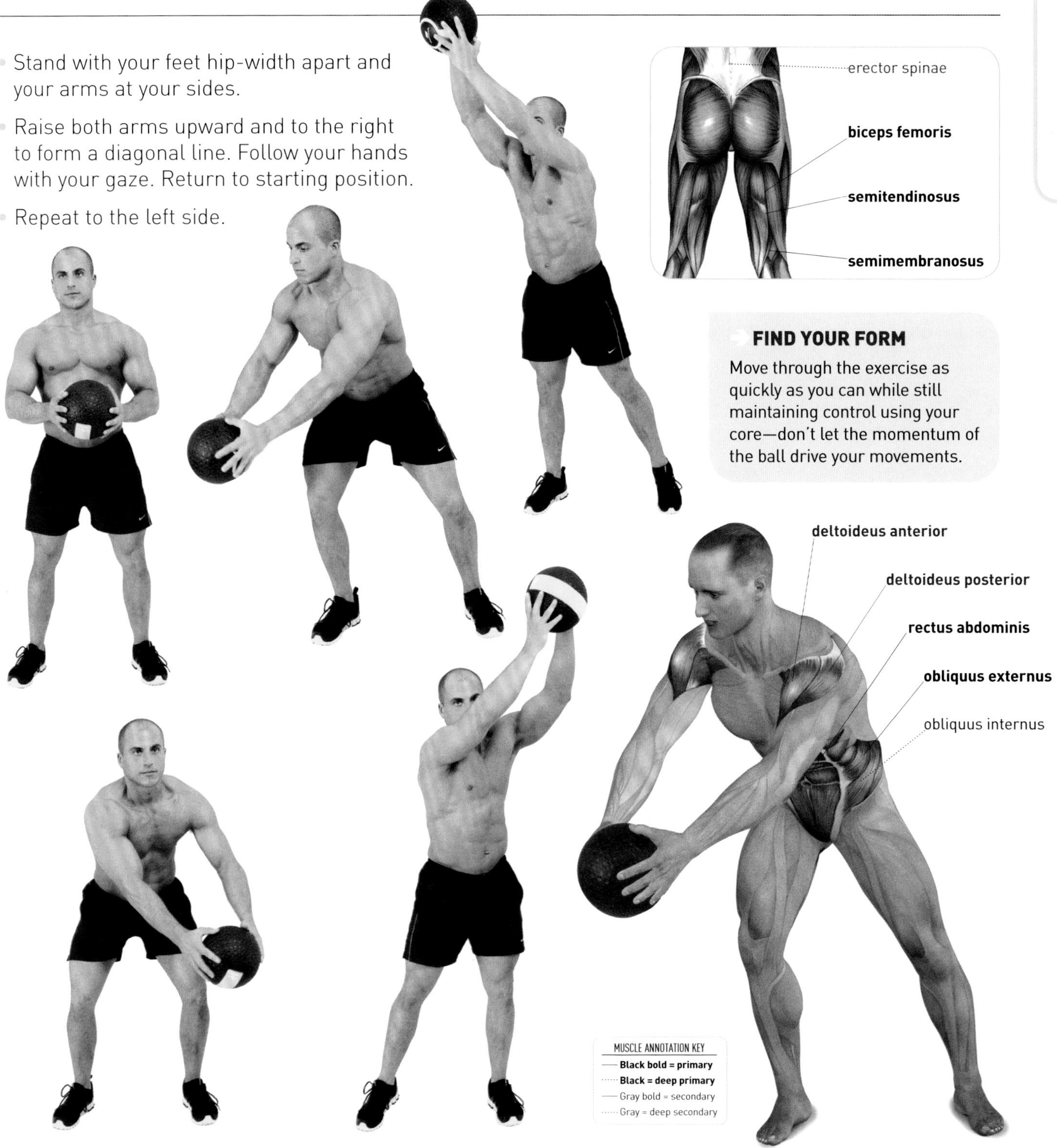

FIND YOUR FORM

Move through the exercise as quickly as you can while still maintaining control using your core—don't let the momentum of the ball drive your movements.

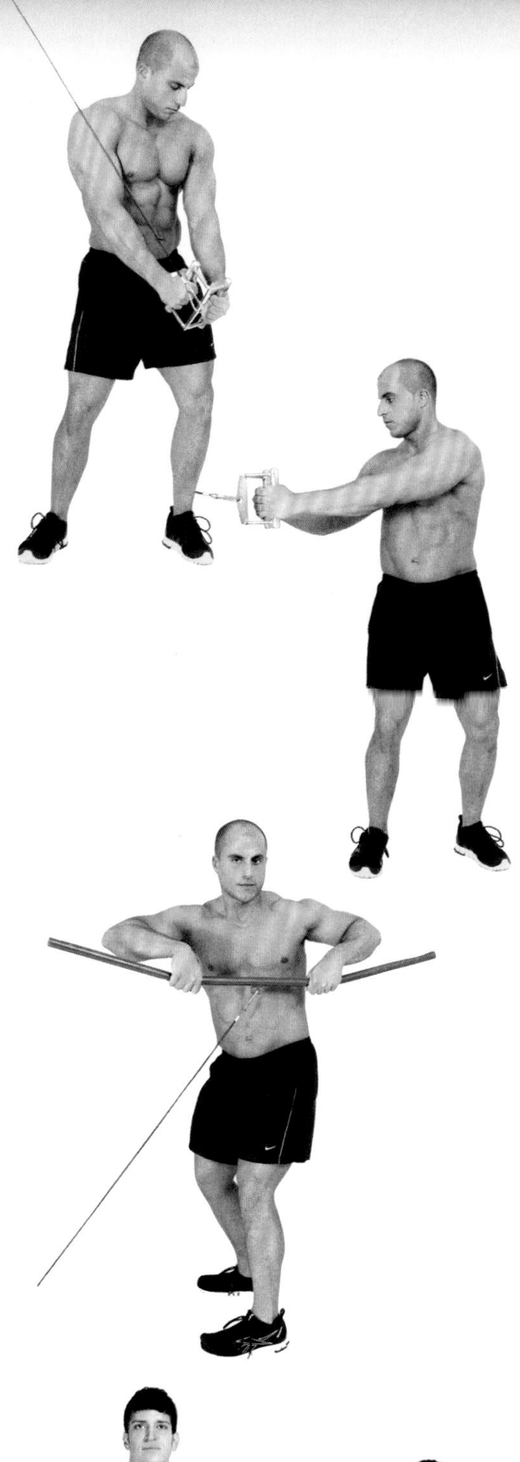

199 Cable Woodchop

Stand with your feet slightly wider than hip-distance apart, with a cable weight machine to your right. Grasp the handle of the cable in both hands. With your legs slightly bent, smoothly rotate your core and raise your arms diagonally to the upper right, toward the cable machine. In a controlled chopping motion, bring your arms diagonally back to the starting position and then down to the other side, rotating your core away from the machine. Complete the desired number of repetitions, and then repeat in the opposite direction.

200 Waist-Height Woodchop

Perform a Cable Woodchop (#199), only bringing the cable to shoulder height. This offers you a chance to focus on your form without straining your arm muscles.

201 Twisting Lift

Stand with your planted hip-distance apart or slightly wider facing a cable machine with a lat bar attached to the cables. Take hold of the lat bar with both hands. In a smooth movement, pull the bar toward your body as you bend your elbows to bring the bar in toward your chest. Your elbows should be almost at shoulder height. Using your hips as a hinge, turn to the right side, keeping your arms stationary and allowing your left knee to bend slightly. Gradually twist back to face the machine. Straighten your arms, releasing the cable to return to starting position. Complete the desired number of repetitions, and then repeat in the opposite direction.

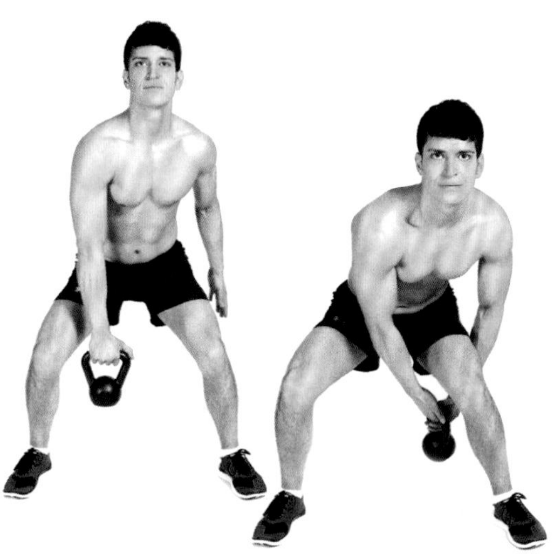

202 Kettlebell Figure 8

Assume a wide stance and hold a kettlebell in your right hand, between your legs, close to your right thigh. Bend forward slightly, keeping your back flat and pushing out your buttocks. Bring the kettlebell toward your left leg and receive it in your left hand, which should come from behind the left leg. Repeat the movement with the left hand, switching the kettlebell from in front of the left leg to the right hand behind the right leg. This forms a figure 8 around your static legs. Continue passing the kettlebell between your legs to form the 8s for the desired time or repetitions.

203 Hand-Clap Figure 8

Perform as you would a Kettlebell Figure 8 (#202), but rather than moving a kettlebell from hand to hand, clap your hands between your legs.

204 Big Circles with Medicine Ball

Stand with your feet hip-width apart or slightly wider, holding a medicine ball above your head, with your arms straight. Swing your arms downward and to the side, keeping your arms straight all through the movement. Continue swinging the ball to the opposite side and up in a continual 360-degree circular motion. Complete the desired number of circles, and then repeat in the opposite direction.

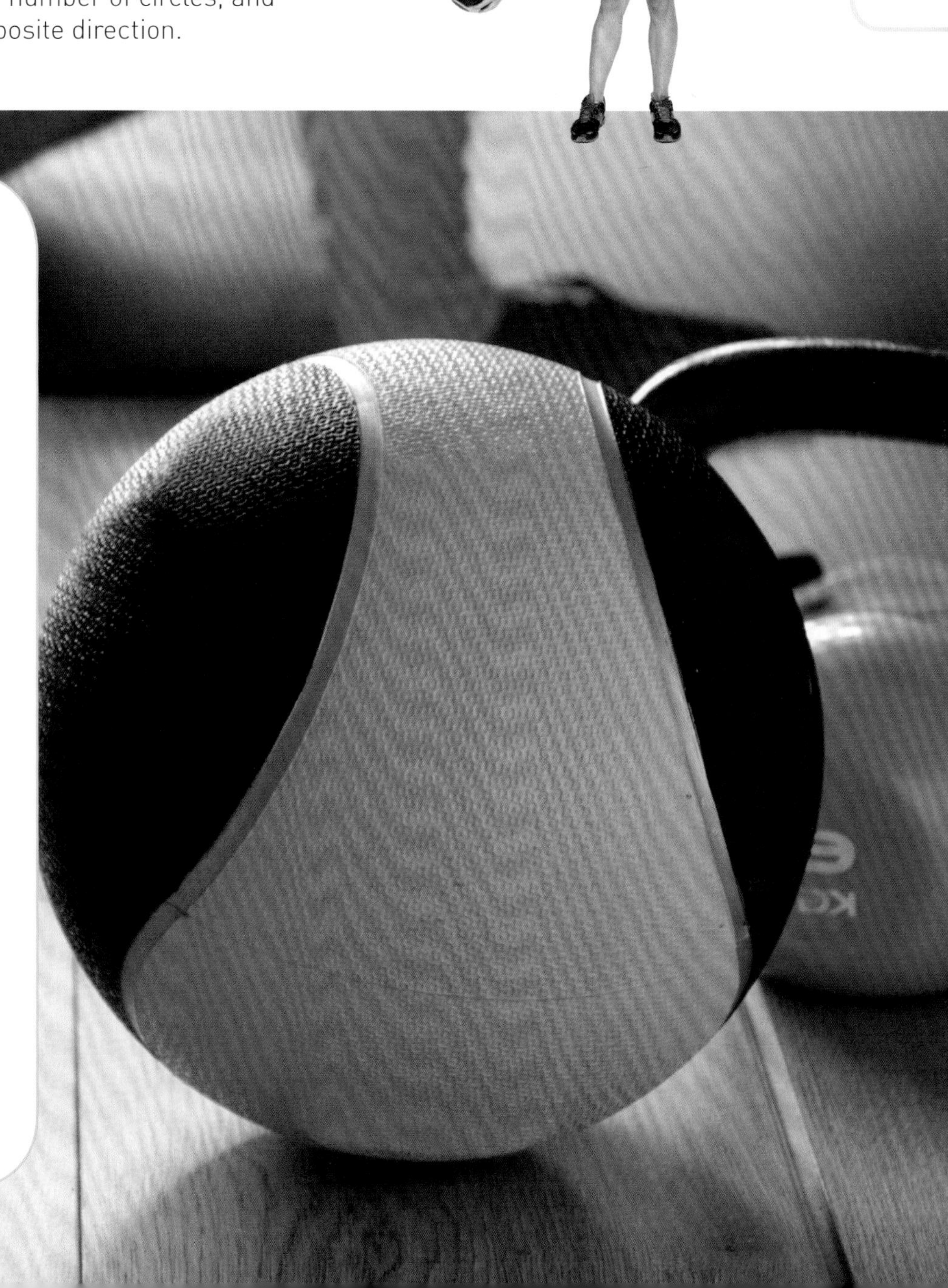

WHY USE A MEDICINE BALL?

A medicine ball is a useful piece of fitness equipment—you can hold it or lift it as you would a dumbbell to add resistance to an exercise, and you can toss it, slam it, or pass it to add explosive power to a move. It also allows you to work in all three planes of motion — frontal (forward and back), sagittal (side to side), and transverse (up and down), and it is great for working on strength, stability, balance, and coordination. Medicine balls come in a wide variety of sizes and weights, from small 2-pound versions to enormous 150 pounders. You can also choose from hard versions to softer bouncing balls, as well as ones with handles or ropes and water-filled varieties. For the most stable grip, be sure to hold a medicine ball with your hands open, fingers spread wide.

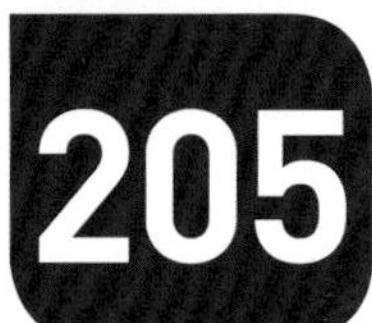

Medicine Ball Throw

The Medicine Ball Throw takes a real-world movement—throwing—and adds the explosive power of a medicine ball to provide rotational drive that can help you build stamina and core stability. You can perform it alone or try it with an exercise buddy, going through the same motions as you toss the ball back and forth between you.

- Hold a weighted medicine ball in front of your chest, taking a few steps forward to get ready.
- Prepare to throw the ball by positioning your left foot behind you, heel off the floor. Keeping your torso stable, raise the ball until it is positioned above your right shoulder.
- Bend the knee of your back foot to lift it off the floor as you throw the ball forward.
- Retrieve the ball, and then repeat on the opposite side. Continue for the desired time and repetitions.

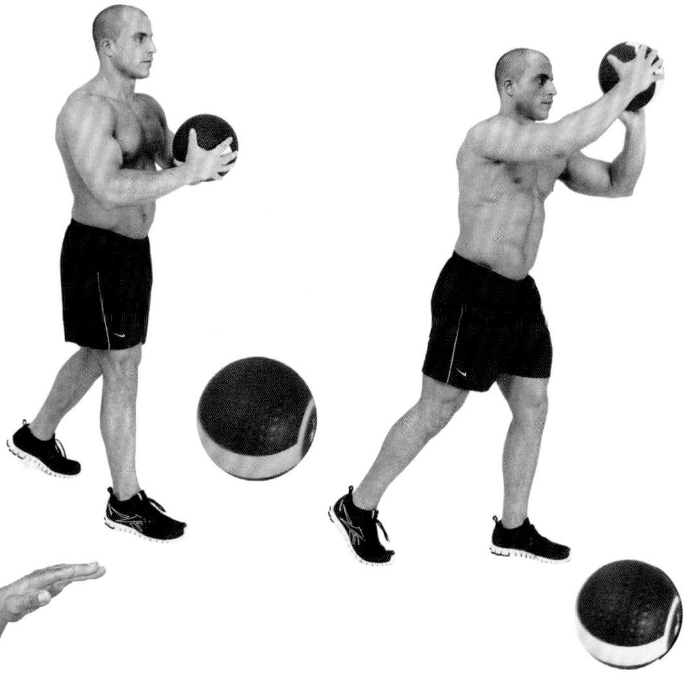

MUSCLE ANNOTATION KEY
Black bold = primary
Black = deep primary
Gray bold = secondary
Gray = deep secondary

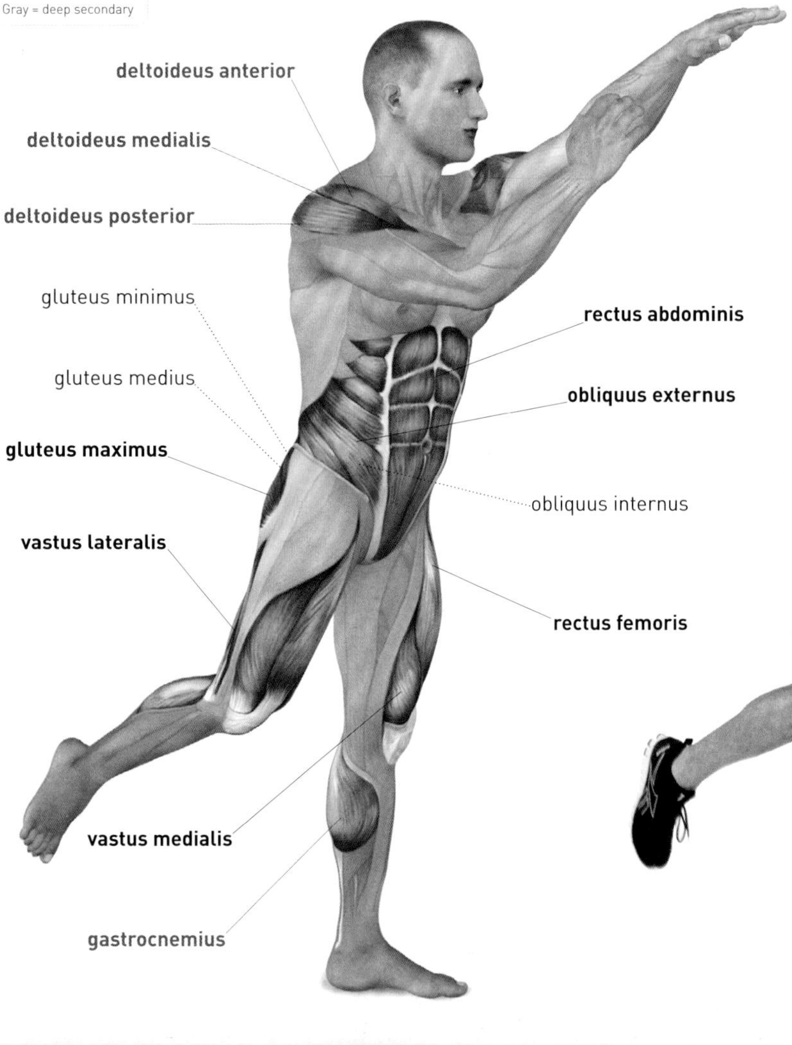

deltoideus anterior
deltoideus medialis
deltoideus posterior
gluteus minimus
gluteus medius
gluteus maximus
vastus lateralis
vastus medialis
gastrocnemius
rectus abdominis
obliquus externus
obliquus internus
rectus femoris

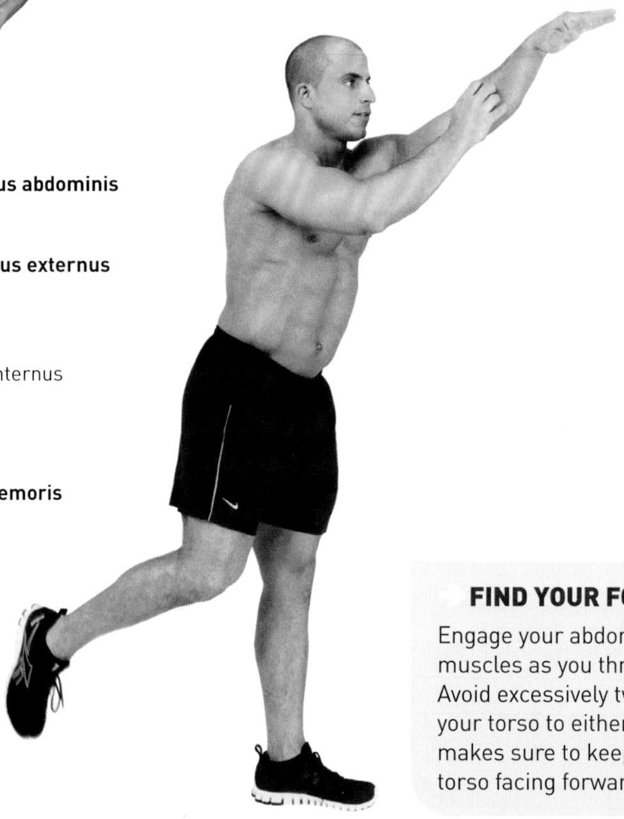

FIND YOUR FORM

Engage your abdominal muscles as you throw. Avoid excessively twisting your torso to either side—makes sure to keep your torso facing forward.

206

Medicine Ball Throw and Catch

Begin in a standing position, holding a medicine ball behind your head. Raise the ball over your head and forward in a sweeping throwing motion, and then release the ball to your partner. Receive the returned ball, and repeat with each partner alternating throwing and catching.

207

Medicine Ball Slam

Stand upright, holding a medicine ball behind your head with elbows bent. Swing the ball over your head, and slam it straight down with force, squatting as you do so. Catch the ball in the squat position. Stand up, and repeat.

208

Wall Ball

Holding a medicine ball below your chin, face a wall at arms length, and stand with your legs and feet parallel and shoulder-width apart, and your knees bent very slightly. Tuck your pelvis slightly forward, lift your chest, and press your shoulders down and back. Lower into a squat, and then forcefully stand up, throwing the medicine ball upward at an overhead target on the wall. Continue squatting and throwing for the desired time.

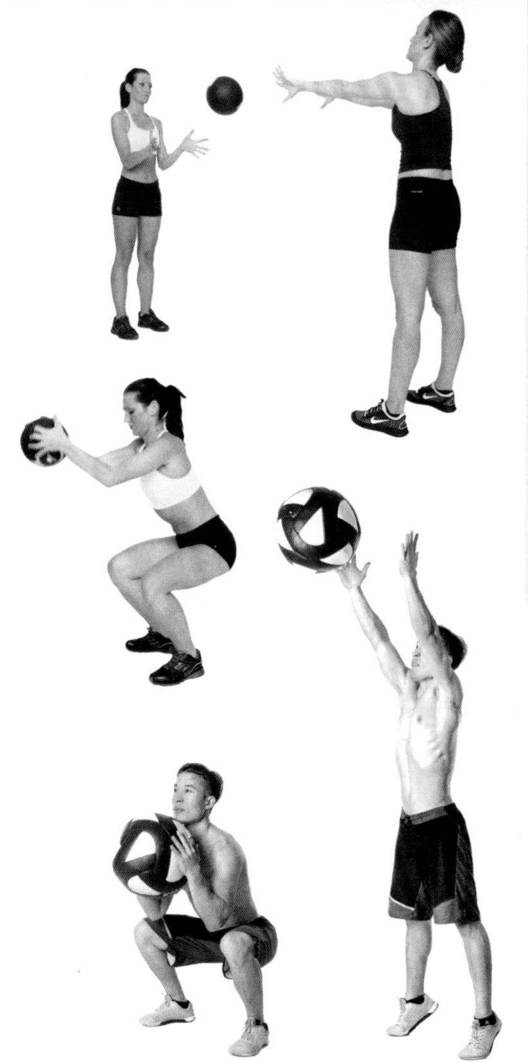

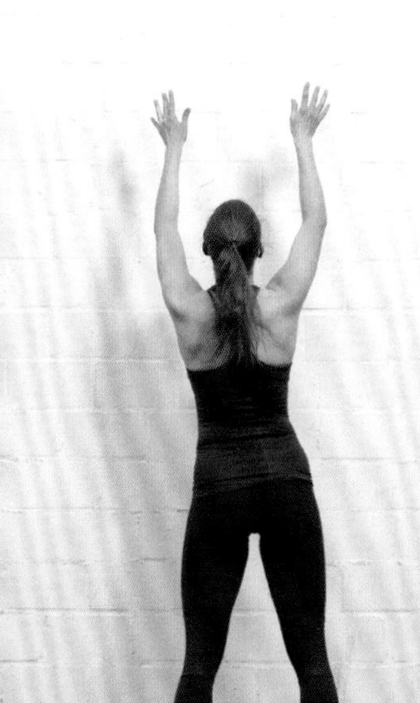

HIGH-INTENSITY FUNCTIONAL TRAINING

Wall Balls, Box Jumps, Kettlebells Swings . . . high-intensity exercises like these have taken gyms by storm as functional training and boot camp–style programs have risen in popularity. The most well-known of these may be CrossFit®, a branded fitness regimen created by Greg Glassman, which according to the company, is a strength and conditioning program consisting of "constantly varied functional movements executed at high intensity across broad time and modal domains." CrossFit gyms and others with similar programs use a range of fitness techniques and equipment, including weights (like barbells, dumbbells, kettlebells, and medicine balls), gymnastics rings, pull-up bars, jump ropes, plyo boxes, and resistance bands. The regimen changes regularly, with workouts of the day (WODs) a feature. Wall Balls are often included because this grueling exercise works so many muscles—including your abs, glutes, quads, hamstrings, calves, lower back, chest, deltoids, biceps and triceps—and increases your overall power and explosive strength.

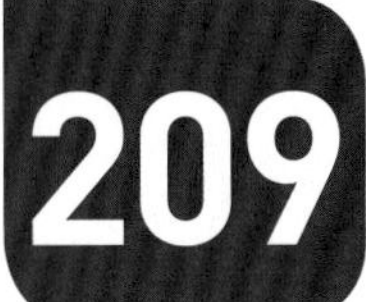

Power Punch

You don't have to step into the ring to reap the benefits of boxing—which is a great way to incinerate calories, build strength, and boost stamina. To get the most out of this high-intensity, high-energy kind of workout, you need to get to know the basic fighting stance and the basic punches: the jab, cross, uppercut, and hook. Exercises, like the Power Punch lays the groundwork so that you can go on to practicing combo moves. You can perform punching exercises alone,in other words, shadowboxing, or you can work with punching bags or a sparring partner.

- Stand with your feet shoulder-width apart and one leg placed slightly in front of the other, placing most of your weight on your back leg. Keep your elbows in, and raise your fists up. This is the basic fighting stance.
- Transferring your weight to your front leg, punch straight in front of you with the fist closest to your body as you turn your torso in to lend power to the punch.
- Punch for the desired time or repetitions, and then reverse sides, switching both arms and legs.

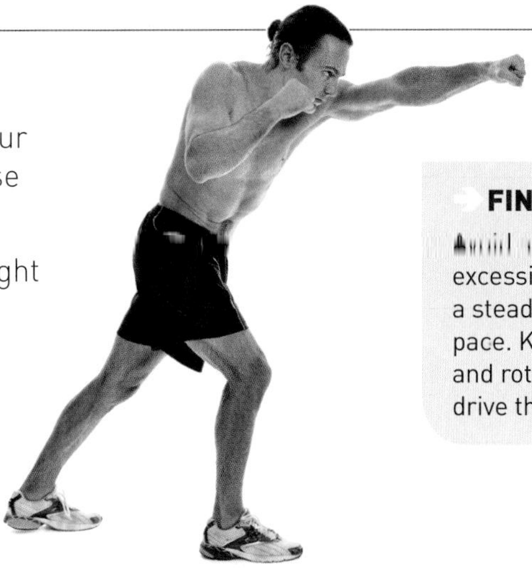

FIND YOUR FORM

Avoid sloppy form or excessive speed—maintain a steady, even, but modest pace. Keep your fist ups, and rotate your torso to drive the movement.

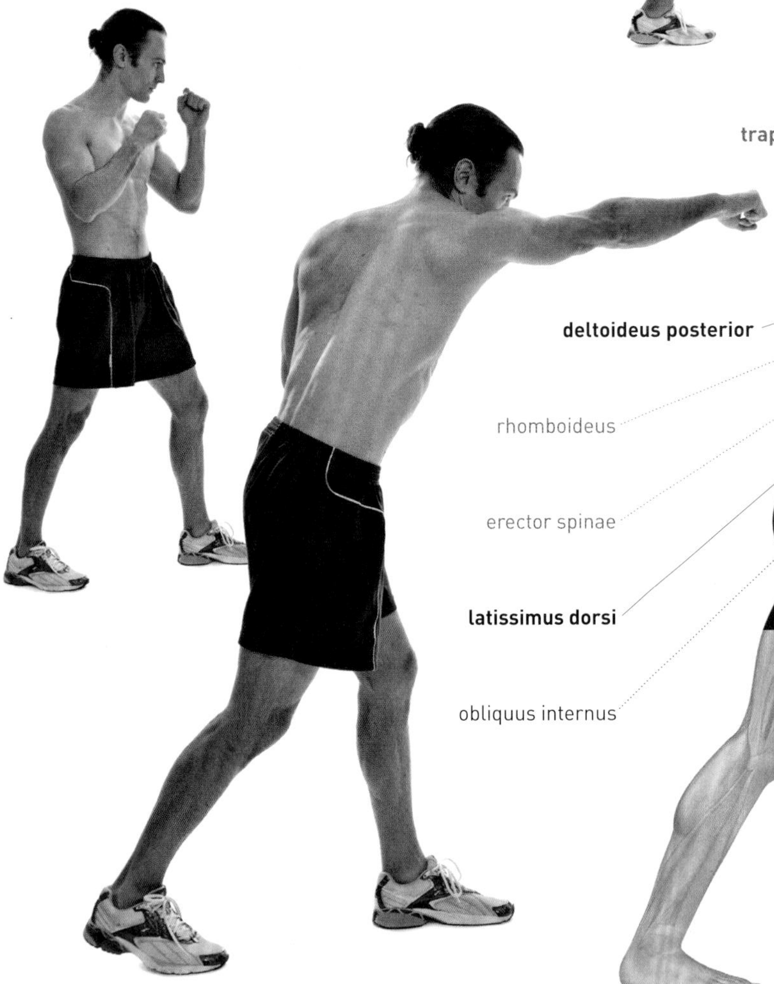

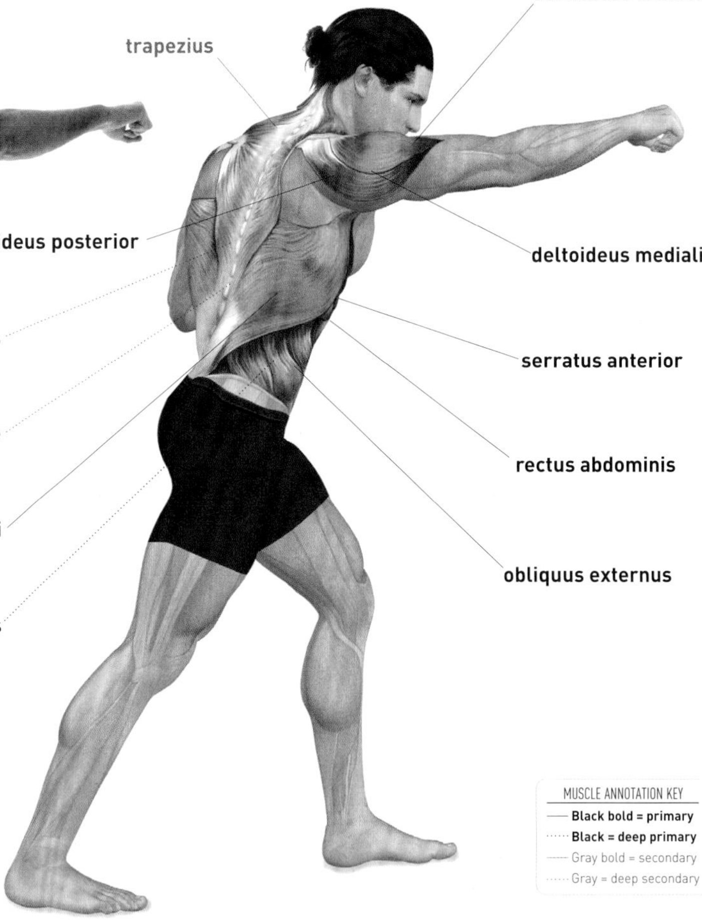

deltoideus anterior
trapezius
deltoideus posterior
deltoideus medialis
rhomboideus
serratus anterior
erector spinae
rectus abdominis
latissimus dorsi
obliquus externus
obliquus internus

MUSCLE ANNOTATION KEY
Black bold = primary
Black = deep primary
Gray bold = secondary
Gray = deep secondary

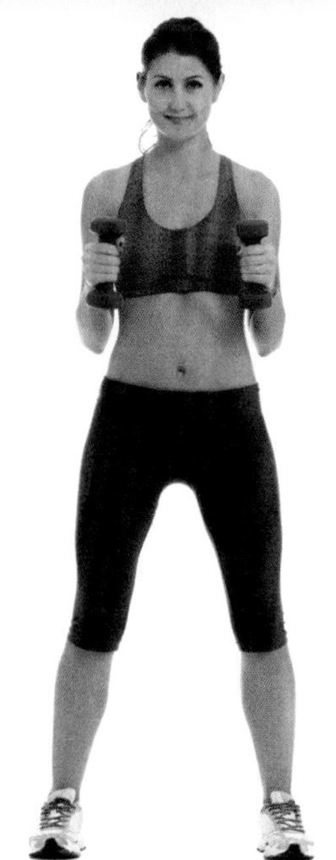

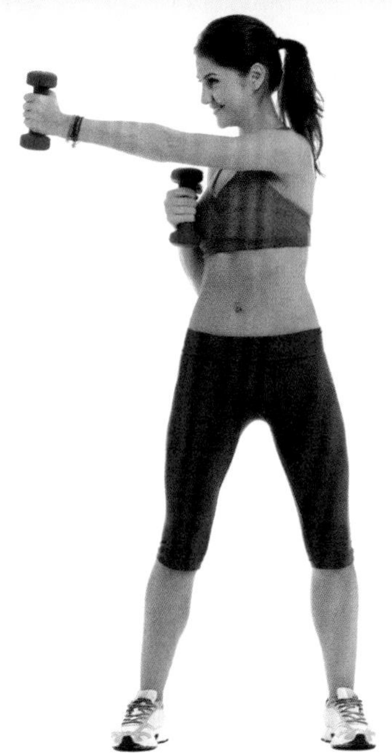

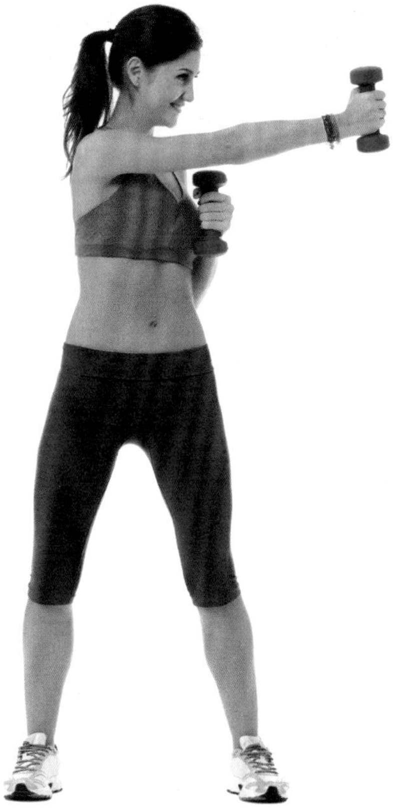

210 Dumbbell Cross Jab

Stand with your feet a bit wider than hip-width apart and your knees very slightly bent. Hold a dumbbell in each hand at chest height with your elbows bent and palms facing each other. Extend your left arm across your body until the weight is in line with your right shoulder. As you return to start, repeat with the right arm. That's one rep. Punch for the desired time or reps, continuing to alternate arms.

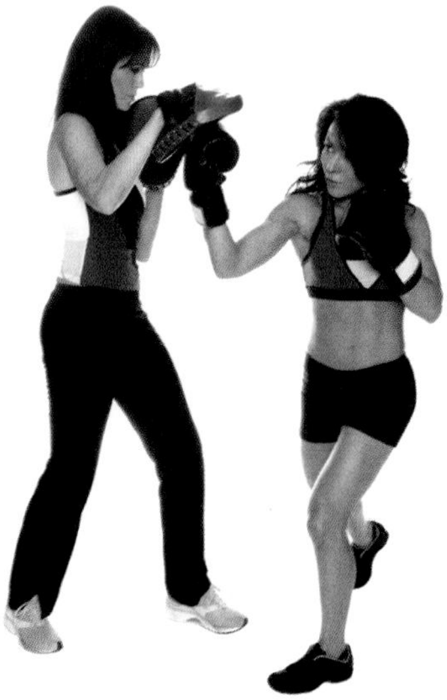

211 Uppercut

Stand with your feet shoulder-width apart and one leg placed slightly in front of the other, placing most of your weight on your back leg. Keep your elbows in, and raise your fists up. Keeping your elbows in, raise your fists and punch upward toward the sky as you rotate your torso and transfer most of your weight to your front foot. Punch for the desired time or reps, and then reverse sides, switching both arms and legs.

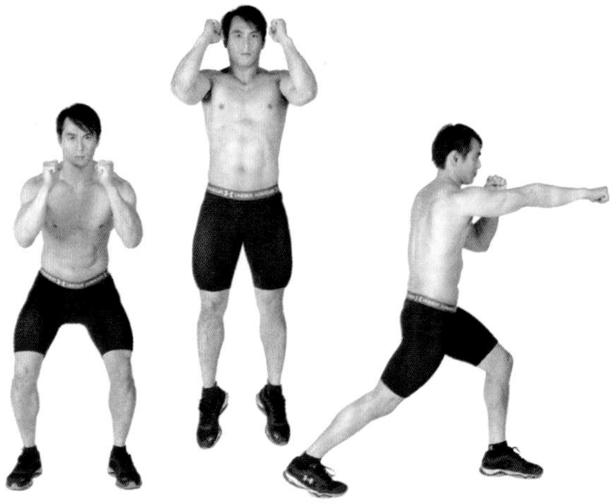

212 Jump Cross

Stand with your feet hip-width apart, your knees bent and your fists raised to shoulder height. Jump upward, raising your arms overhead. As you land, pivot to the left, and punch your right fist straight out in front of you. Quickly return to the starting position, and repeat on the other side, pivoting to the right and punching with your left fist. Continue alternating sides for the desired time or reps.

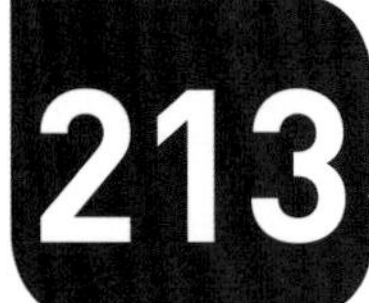

Battle Rope Side-to-Side Swings

The rising popularity of rope training comes as no surprise. Working with these simple tools provides you with powerful strength training and high-energy cardio and helps you to build speed and agility. Battle rope exercises particularly target your core and upper body, with a strong contribution from your lower-body muscles. Moves like the Battle Rope Side-to-Side Swings also call for your obliques to kick in. Whatever moves you choose, battle ropes offer an efficient way to build lean muscle (without heavy weights), while incinerating calories and upping your heart rate.

- Stand with your knee slightly bent, and take a battle rope in each hand. Bring your hands together, keeping the ropes around waist height.
- Brace your core. And in one motion, forcefully swing the ropes to the left. Reverse the motion, bringing the ropes to the right.
- Continue swinging the ropes from side to side while maintaining a strong, tight, and braced stance.

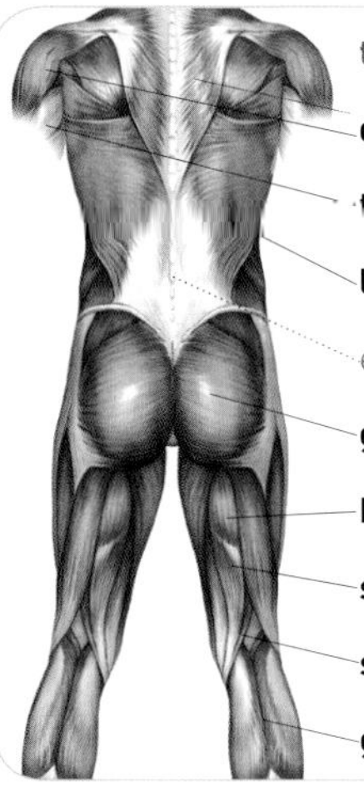

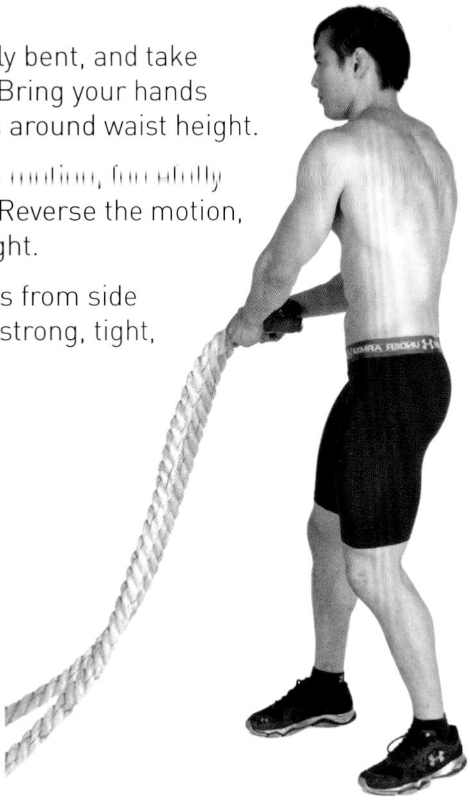

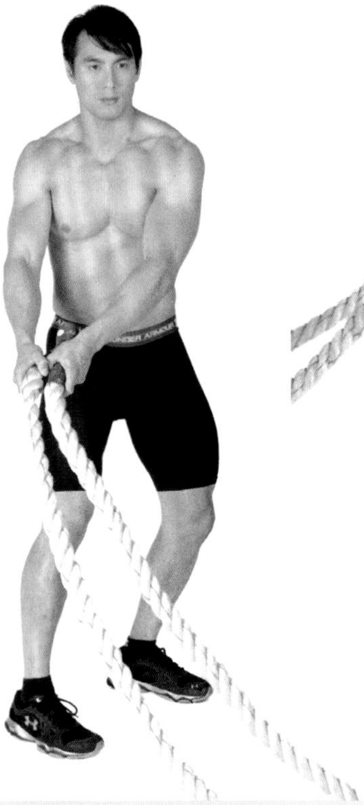

trapezius
deltoideus posterior
triceps brachii
latissimus dorsi
erector spinae
gluteus maximus
biceps femoris
semitendinosus
semimembranosus
gastrocnemius

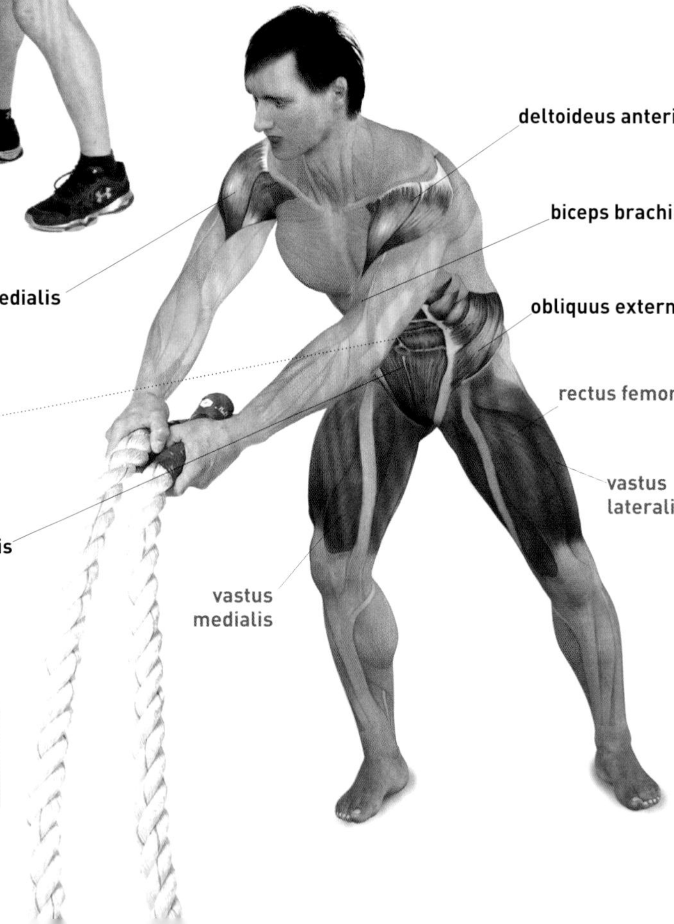

deltoideus anterior
biceps brachii
deltoideus medialis
obliquus externus
rectus femoris
obliquus internus
vastus lateralis
rectus abdominis
vastus medialis

FIND YOUR FORM

When working with ropes, don't be afraid to mix things up—vary your stance, your grip, and your movements to avoid the drudgery of repetitive, old-school cardio.

MUSCLE ANNOTATION KEY
Black bold = primary
Black = deep primary
Gray bold = secondary
Gray = deep secondary

214 Battle Rope Alternating Waves

Stand with your knees slightly bent, holding the ends of the rope at arm's length in front of your hips with your hands shoulder-width apart. Tuck your elbows into your sides, and brace your core, and then begin alternately raising and lowering each arm explosively. Keep alternating arms for the desired time.

215 Full-Squat Alternating Wave

Holding a battle rope in each hand, bend your knees and drive your hips back while you brace your core to assume a full squat position. Bring the left rope up as you move the right rope down, and then immediately bring the right rope up and the left rope down. Keep repeating this alternating motion while remaining in the squat position for the desired time.

216 Jump Squat and Slam

Holding a battle rope in each hand, bend your knees, and then drive your hips back while you brace your core to assume a full squat position. Explosively jump as high as you can, and when you land, immediately squat down, and jump again. Continue squatting and jumping for the desired time, and then finish by slamming the rope down. Keep repeating this motion for the desired time.

217 Snakes

Stand with your knee slightly bent, and take a battle rope in each hand. Bring your hands together, keeping the ropes around waist height. Brace your core, and then move the rope in and out, close to the floor to create two symmetrical zigzags.

218 External-Rotation Spirals

Stand with your knee slightly bent, and take a battle rope in each hand, starting with your hands at your sides. Move each arm outward (never inward) to create two symmetrical spirals.

219 Claps

Stand with your knee slightly bent, and take a battle rope in each hand. Bring your hands together, keeping the ropes around waist height. Brace your core, and then move your arms in and out as if your were clapping your hands together.

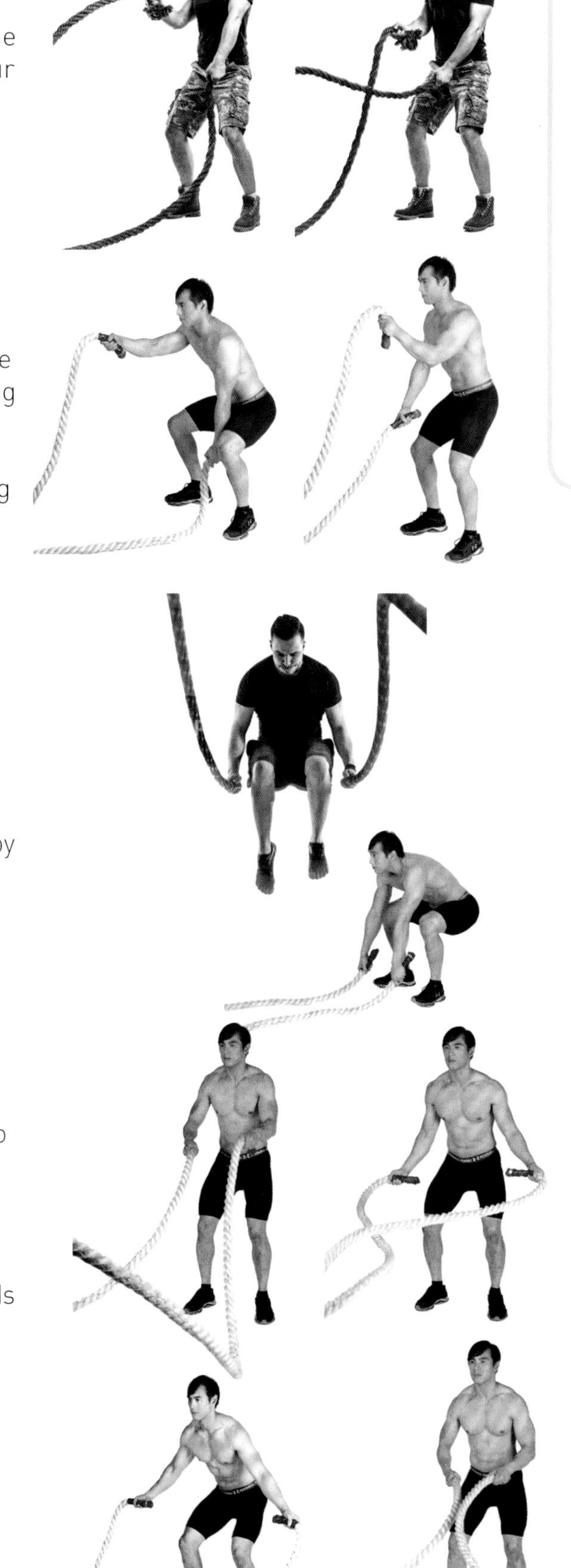

220 Crossover Slam

Stand with your knees slightly bent, and take the ends of a battle rope in each hand. Bring your hands together, and then move the ends of the ropes in an arc above your head, lifting them to your left, and then slamming them down hard to your right, while keeping both feet flat on the floor. Repeat in the opposite direction. Keep alternating sides for the desired time or repetitions.

221 Battle Jacks

Stand with your knees slightly bent, and take the ends of a battle rope in each hand, starting with your hands at your sides. Forcefully push off the floor into a small jump, and extend your legs to each side to land with your feet spread wide. At the same time, bring the ropes up above your head. Jump again, bringing your feet together, and moving your arms back down toward your hips. Repeat the movement, mimicking a traditional Jumping Jack.

222 Double-Arm Wave

Stand with your knees slightly bent, holding the ends of the rope at arm's length in front of your hips with your hands shoulder-width apart. Tuck your elbows into your sides, brace your core, and then pump your arms up and down together, creating waves in the ropes. Continue for the desired time or repetitions.

223 Double-Arm Slam

Stand with your knees slightly bent, and take the ends of a battle rope in each hand. Lift both ends of the rope overhead, as high as you can, and then slam the rope down to the floor with as much force as you can generate. Continue lifting and slamming, going as fast as possible.

224 Double-Arm Slam Jump

Stand with your knees slightly bent, and take the ends of a battle rope in each hand. Brace your core, and then in an explosive movement, bring the ropes upward to shoulder level as you perform a small jump in the air. At the top of the movement, immediately come down into a squatting position, and slam the ropes downward to the floor. Repeat the movement, being sure to maintain the rope's pattern. Continue for the desired time or repetitions.

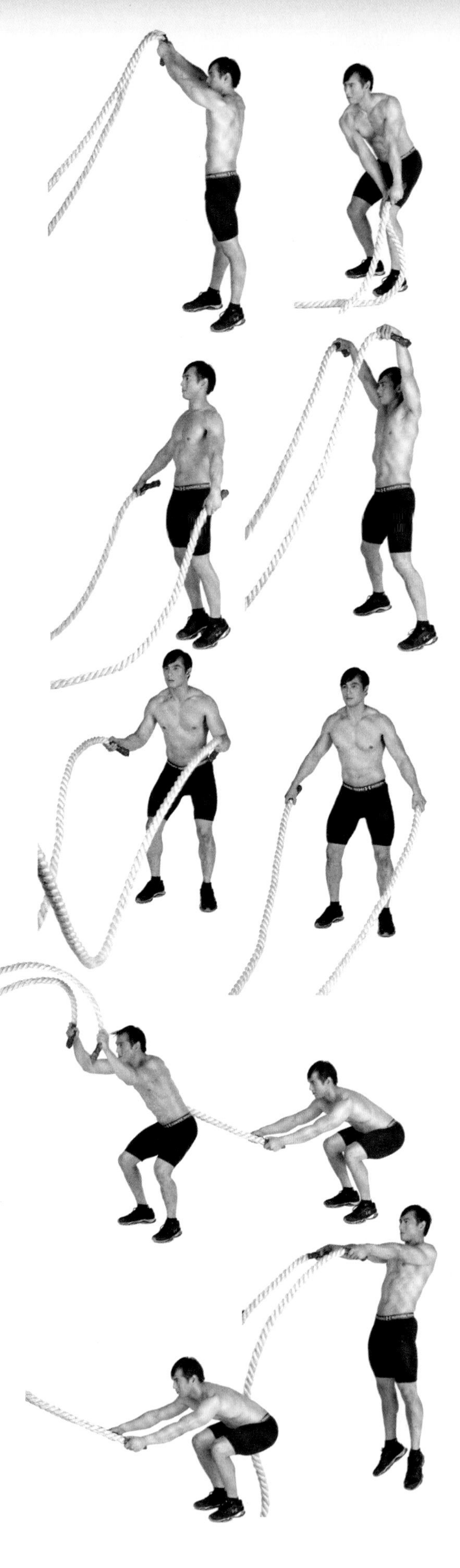

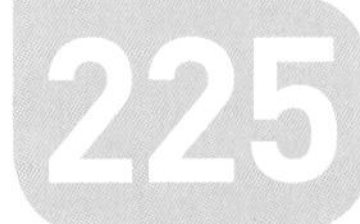

Grappler Throes

Stand with your knee slightly bent, and take a battle rope in each hand, grasping it so that the ends are sticking out from between your thumb and index fingers. Bring the ends down next to your right hip.. Keeping both feet grounded, pivot your torso from to the left. During the pivot, flip the ropes over your hip as if you were throwing a grappling opponent to the ground. Pivot back to the other side, switching back and forth for the desired time.

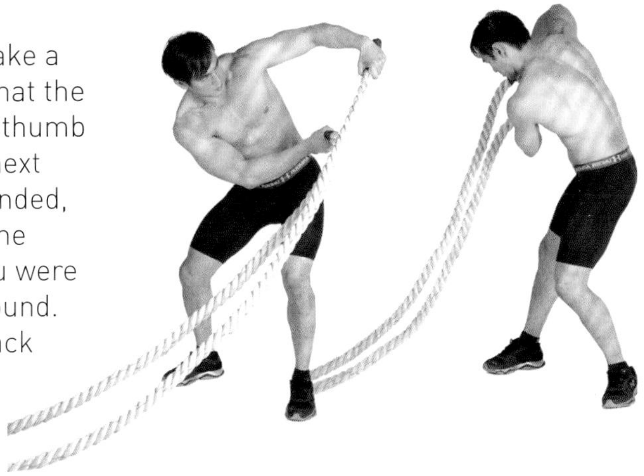

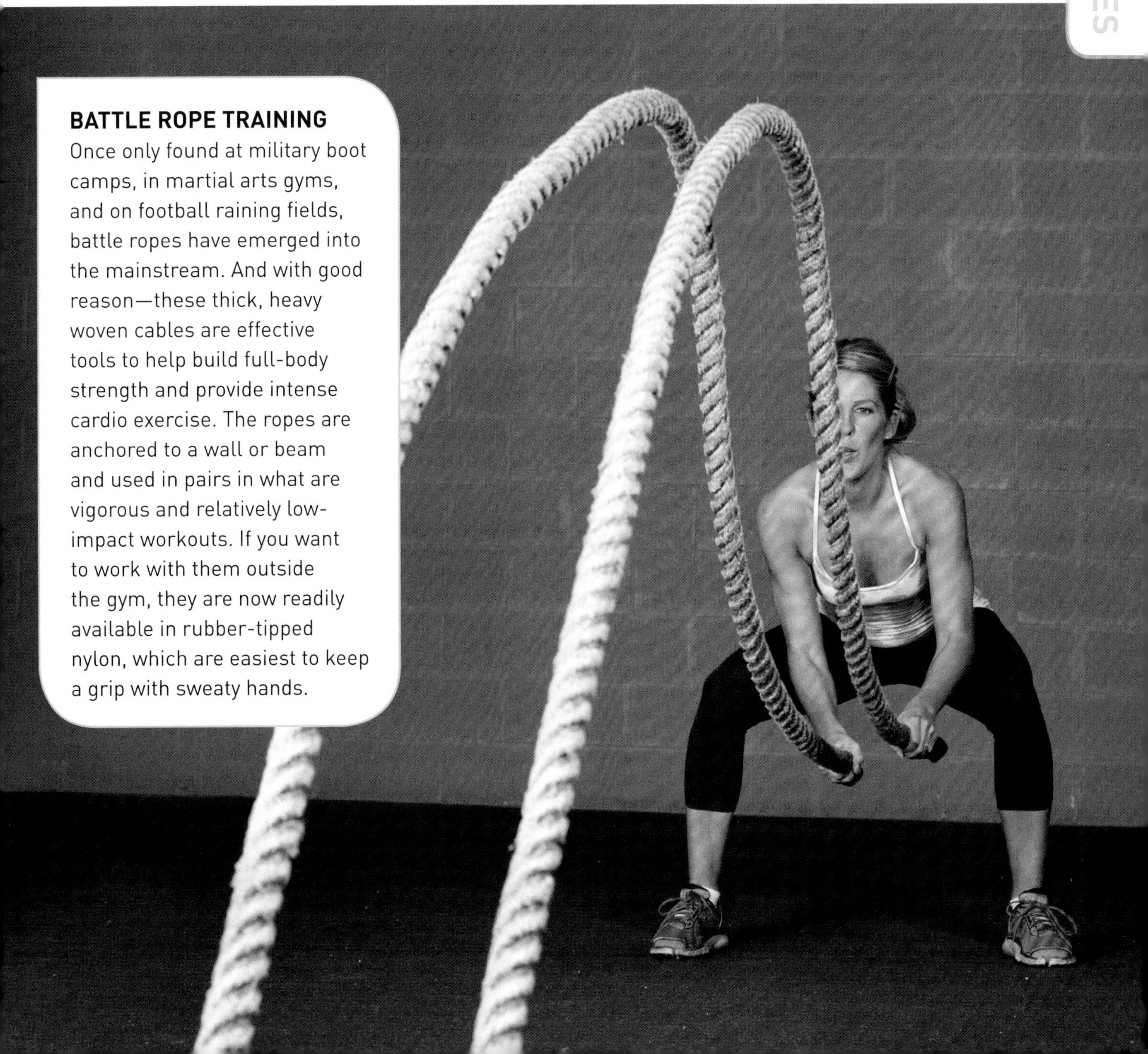

BATTLE ROPE TRAINING

Once only found at military boot camps, in martial arts gyms, and on football raining fields, battle ropes have emerged into the mainstream. And with good reason—these thick, heavy woven cables are effective tools to help build full-body strength and provide intense cardio exercise. The ropes are anchored to a wall or beam and used in pairs in what are vigorous and relatively low-impact workouts. If you want to work with them outside the gym, they are now readily available in rubber-tipped nylon, which are easiest to keep a grip with sweaty hands.

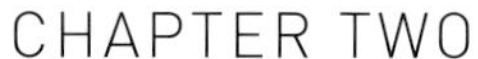

CHAPTER TWO

Power Exercises

Traditional exercises, like the push-up, pull-up, or crunch, have earned their places in both military boot camps and boot camp–style gym classes because they are so versatile—while you're working to pump up your muscles, you can also pump up your power and endurance. You can perform these classic exercises at high intensity and high volume to really get your heart rate up and challenge your stamina and endurance. You can also combine them with other power moves or functional exercises—the high-intensity Burpee and its many variants, for example, mixes a squat thrust with a variety of aerobic and strength moves, like jumps, push-ups, and pull-ups.

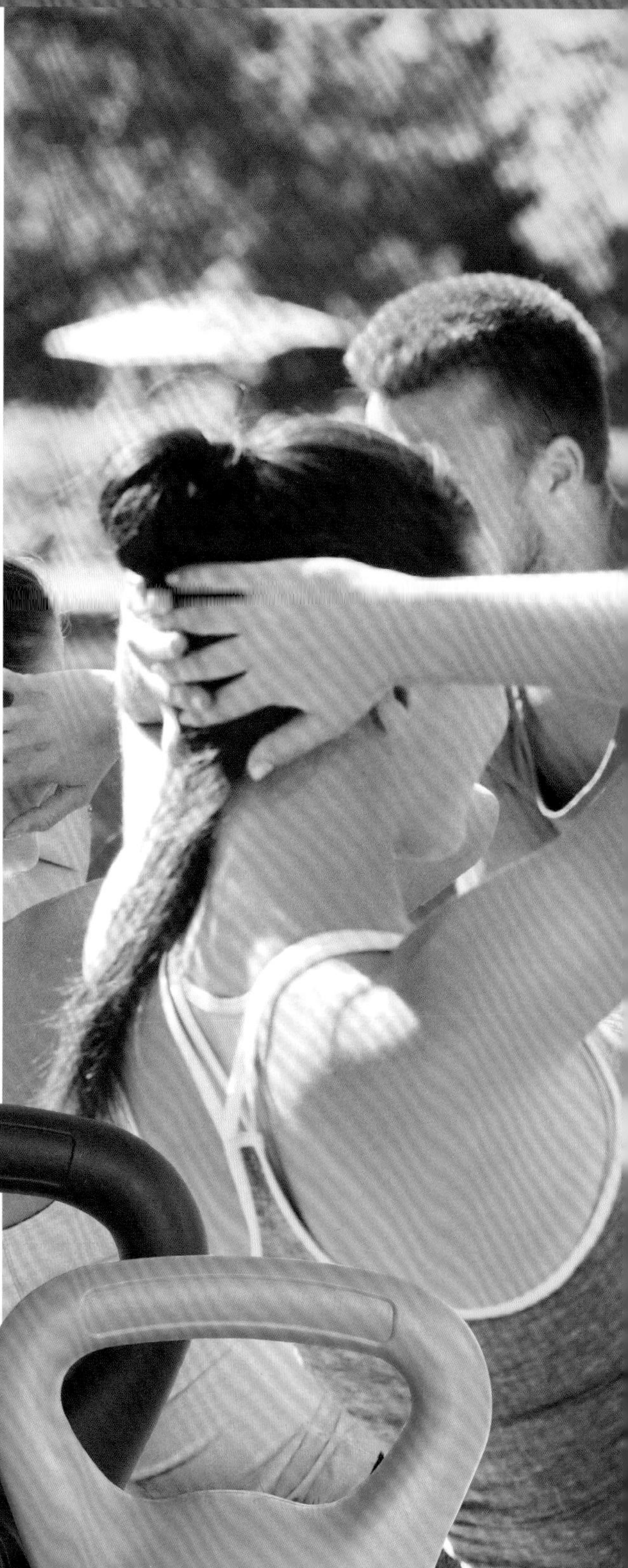

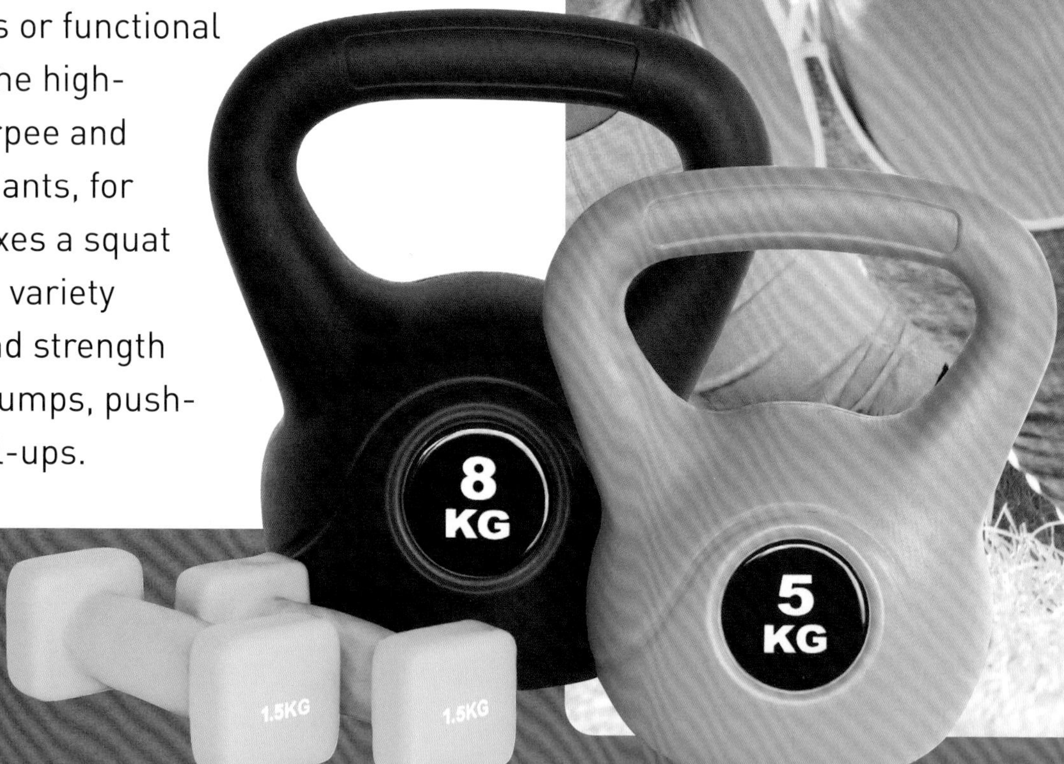

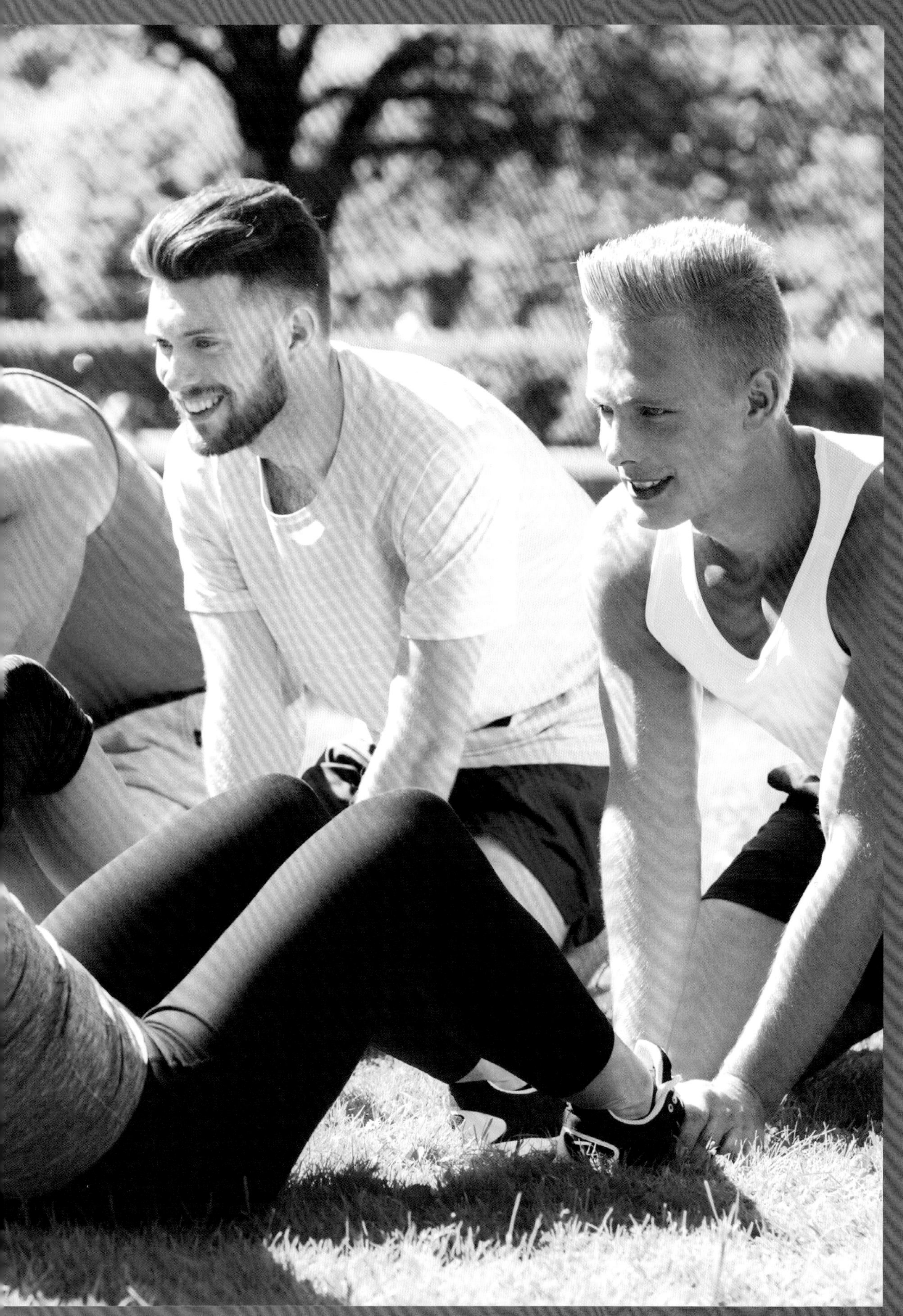

Power Exercises

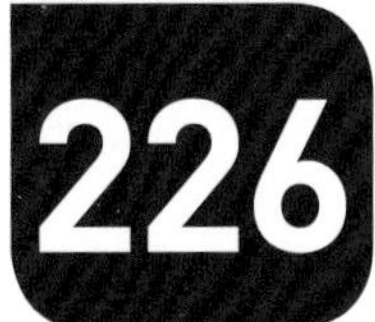

226 Basic Push-Up

From boot camps to school gyms, anywhere you find serious exercisers, you'll find the push-up. This classic move is used to assess fitness levels, and it is a fundamental component of military basic training. It can be a basic strength exercise, but it also serves as the foundation of many high-energy moves and can be combined with other exercises to amp up its intensity. Its "drop" starting position—legs extended and arms straight—is the launching point for numerous power exercises. Push-ups target the pectorals, triceps, and anterior deltoids, while also benefiting the midsection.

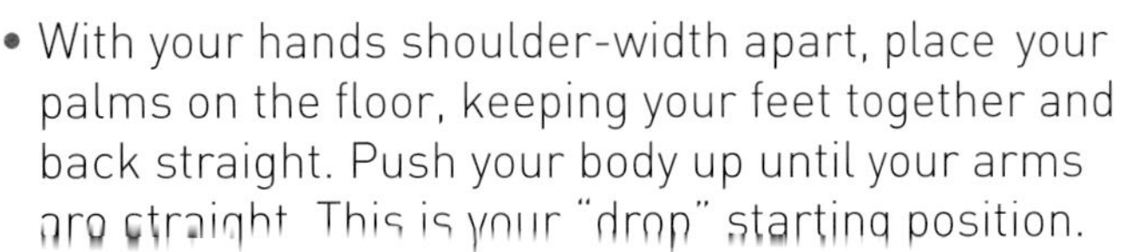

- With your hands shoulder-width apart, place your palms on the floor, keeping your feet together and back straight. Push your body up until your arms are straight. This is your "drop" starting position.
- Bend your arms, and lower your torso until your chest touches the floor. Straighten your arms to rise back up to the starting position to complete the repetition. Perform for the desired sets and reps.

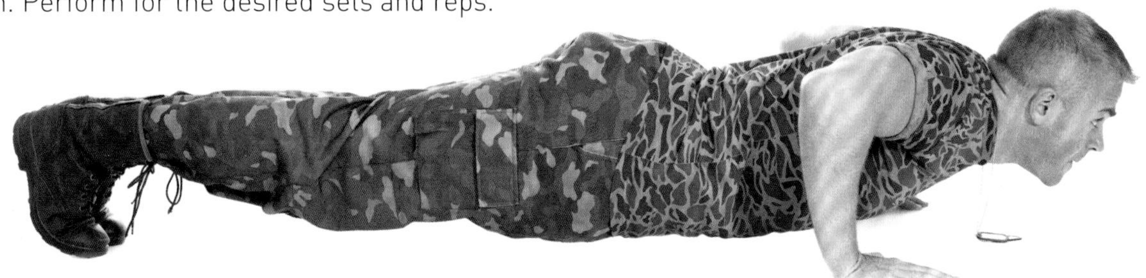

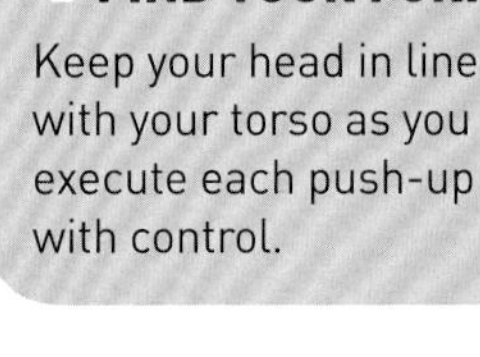

FIND YOUR FORM

Keep your head in line with your torso as you execute each push-up with control.

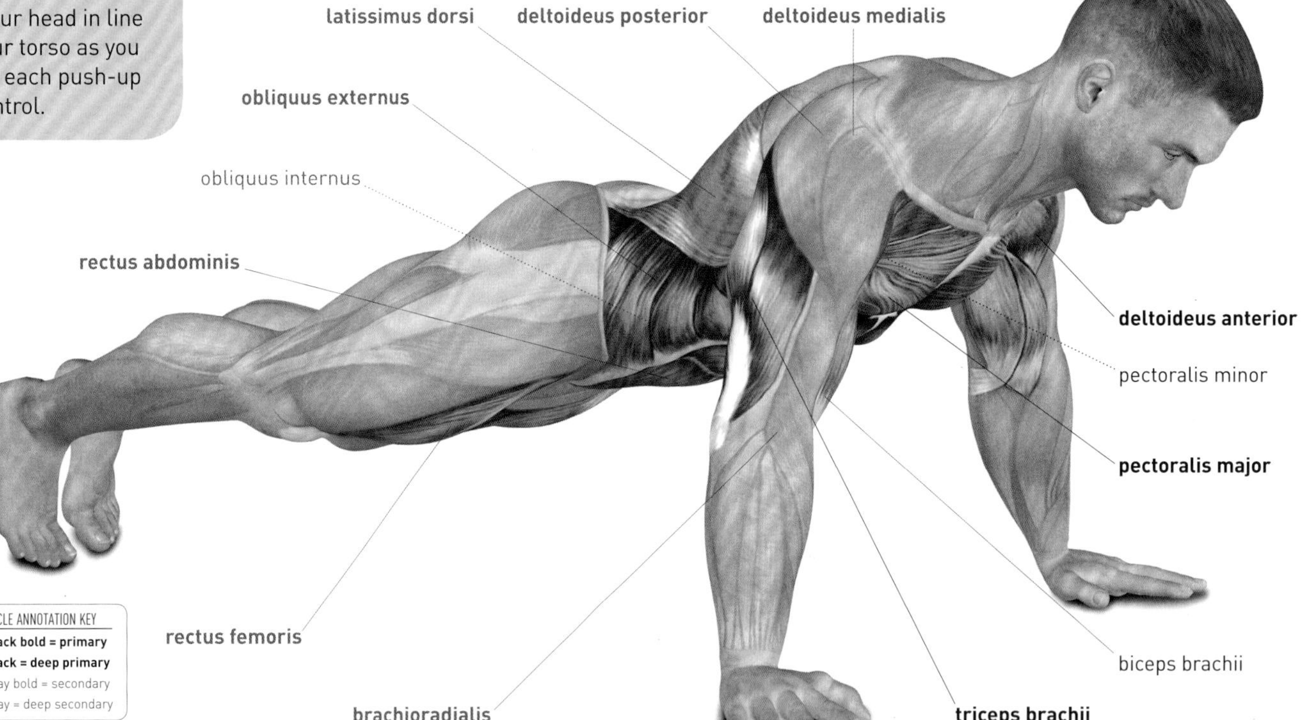

MUSCLE ANNOTATION KEY
— **Black bold = primary**
····· Black = deep primary
— Gray bold = secondary
····· Gray = deep secondary

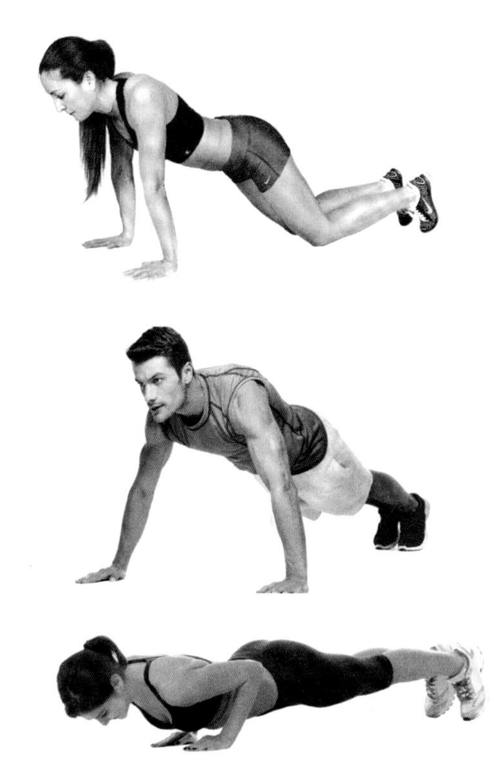

227 Knee Push-Up

Begin on your hands and knees, and then walk your hands forward, dropping your hips so that your body forms a straight line from shoulders to knees. Perform as you would a Basic Push-Up (#226). This easier version shortens the lever, reducing your lifting load by about half.

228 Wide Push-Up

Assume the drop position, with your hands spaced wider than shoulder width. This hand position will take your shoulder and chest muscles through a different range of movement than a Basic Push-Up (#226), isolating the lateral part of the pectoralis major.

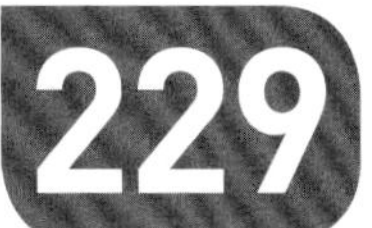

229 Triceps Push-Up

Assume the drop position, with your hands placed close together, and perform as you would a Basic Push-Up (#226). This hand position shifts the emphasis from the pectorals to the deltoids and triceps.

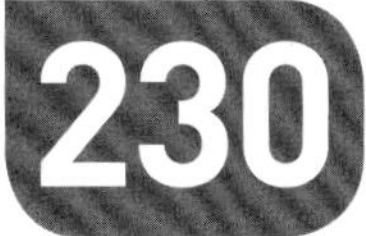

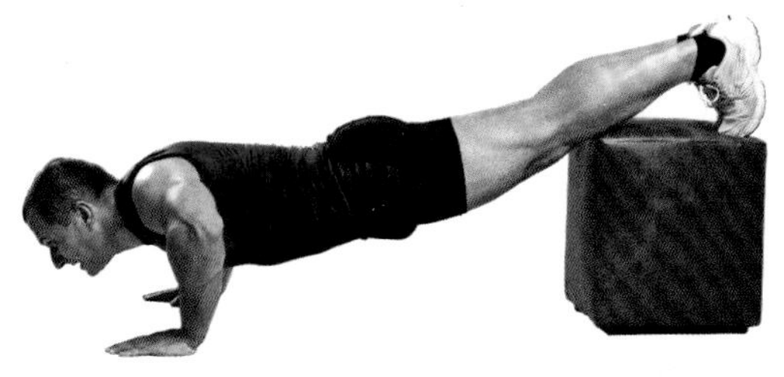

230 Decline Push-Up

Begin on your hands and knees, with your hands about shoulder-width apart, and then prop your feet on an elevated surface. With your back flat, bend your elbows to touch your chest to the floor, and then extend your arms back to the upright position. The decline angle applies greater pressure to the upper chest and front deltoids and isometrically contracts the core muscles.

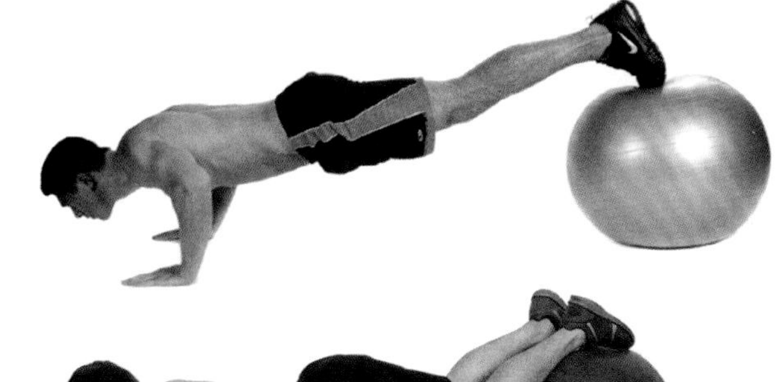

231 Swiss Ball Decline Push-Up

Begin on your hands and knees, with your hands about shoulder-width apart. Prop your toes on a Swiss ball, and perform as you would a Decline Push-Up (#230).

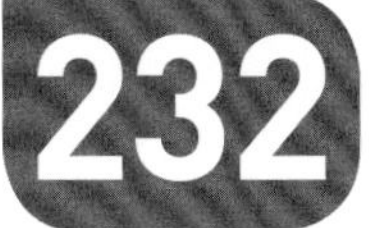

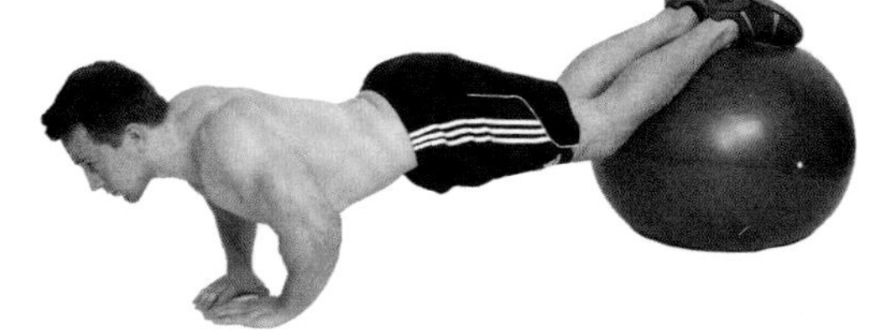

232 Diamond Decline Push-Up

With your hands placed together so that your thumbs and index fingers touch, rest the tops of your feet on an elevated surface, and perform as you would a Decline Push-Up (#230).

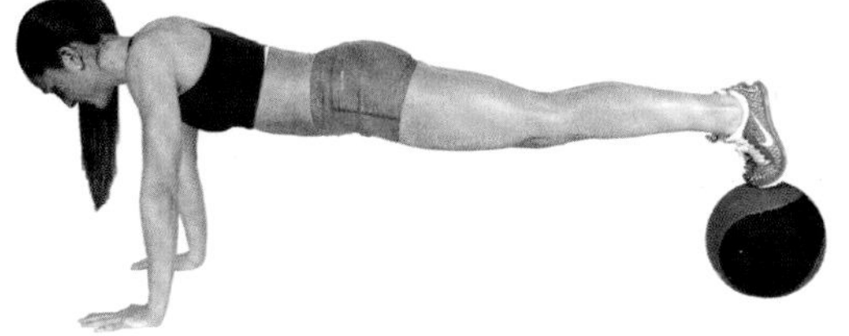

233 Medicine Ball Decline Push-Up

Begin on your hands and knees,with your hands about shoulder-width apart. Balance your toes on a medicine ball, and perform as you would a Decline Push-Up (#230).

234 Incline Push-Up

Assume the drop position with your hands your hands placed slightly wider than shoulder width on an elevated surface. Keeping your body straight, bend your arms, and lower your torso until your chest touches the surface. Pause, and then push back to the starting position. The incline angle places more emphasis on the lower chest and triceps.

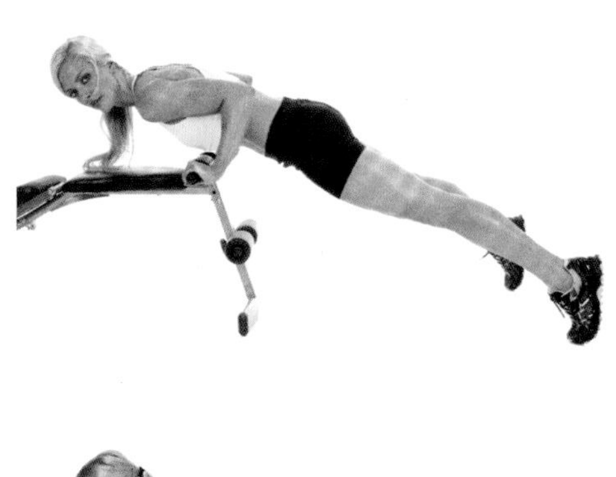

235 Medicine Ball Knee Push-Up

Begin on your hands and knees, and place your hands on a medicine ball. Perform as you would an Incline Push-Up (#234). Performing on the slightly unstable surface calls for increased contributions from the rotator cuff and shoulder stabilizers, which can help you to improve shoulder function.

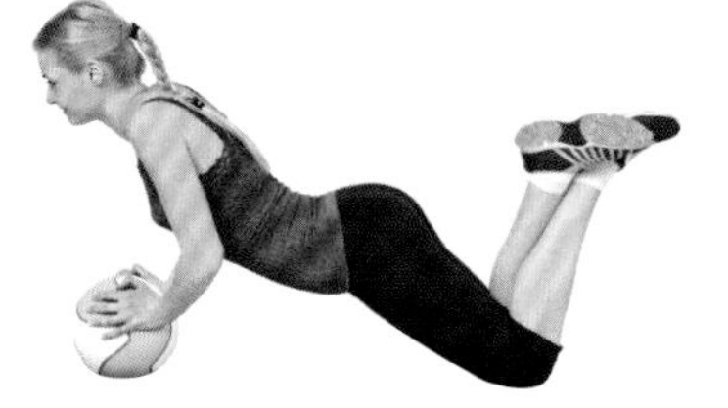

236 Medicine Ball Push-Up

Assume the drop position, with your hands on a medicine ball, and perform as you would an Incline Push-Up (#234).

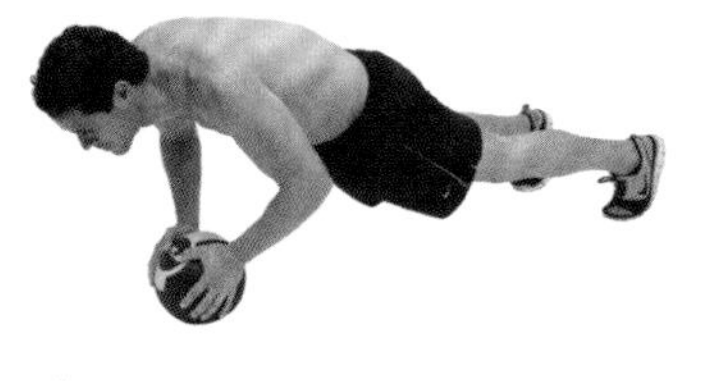

237 Swiss Ball Incline Push-Up

To add an element of instability, assume the drop position, with your hands on a Swiss ball, and perform as you would an Incline Push-Up (#234).

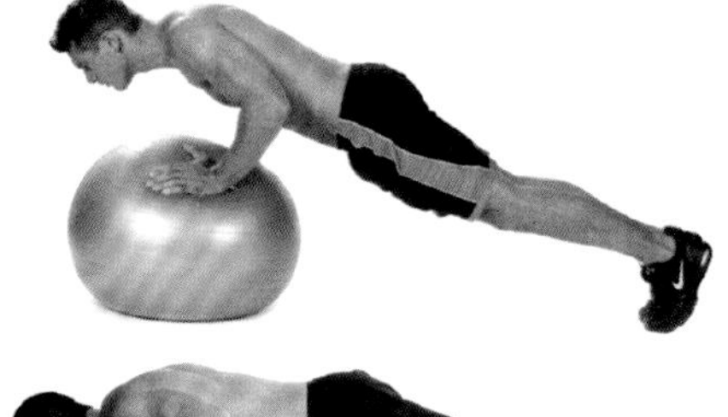

238 Foam Roller Push-Up

To add an element of instability, assume the drop position, with your hands on a foam roller, and perform as you would an Incline Push-Up (#234).

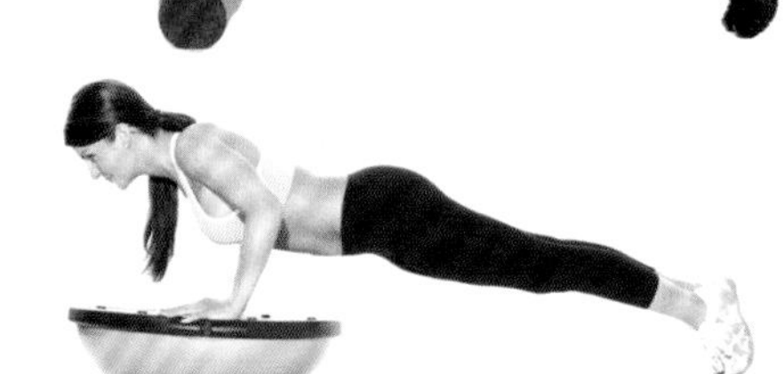

239 BOSU Push-Up

To add an element of instability, assume the drop position, with your hands on the flat side of a BOSU ball, and perform as you would an Incline Push-Up (#234).

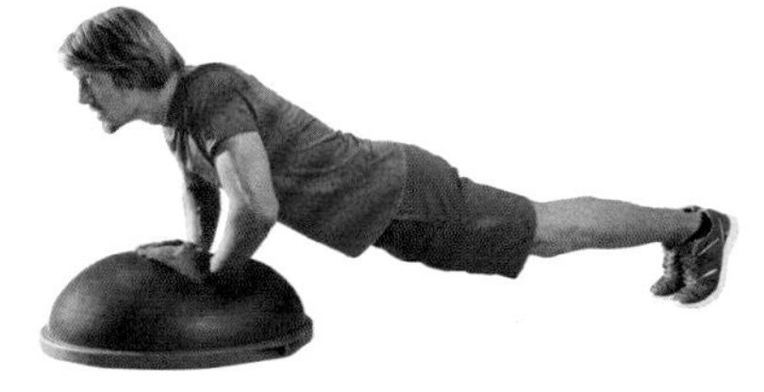

240 BOSU Diamond Push-Up

Place both hands on the rounded side of a BOSU ball, positioning them close together so that your thumbs and index fingers touch. Perform as you would an Incline Push-Up (#234).

241 Balance Board Push-Up

To add an element of instability, assume the drop position, with your hands on the flat side of a balance board, and perform as you would an Incline Push-Up (#234).

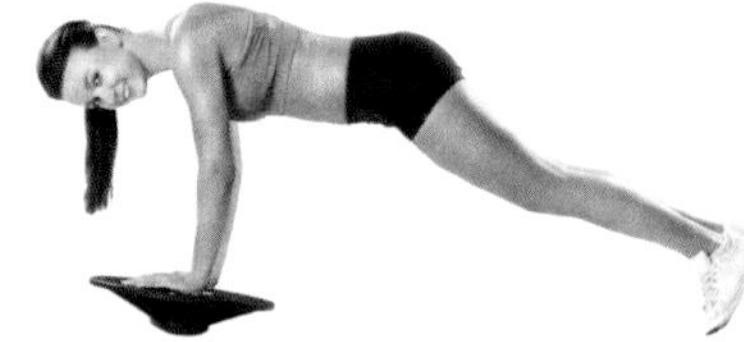

242 Pilates Magic Circle Push-Up

Place the ring on the floor with the bottom pad down. Rest your sternum on the pad and your hands on the floor. Push down on the pad with your sternum until you can squeeze your upper arms against your ribcage, and then, step both feet back to come into the drop position. Perform as you would a Basic Push-Up (#226).

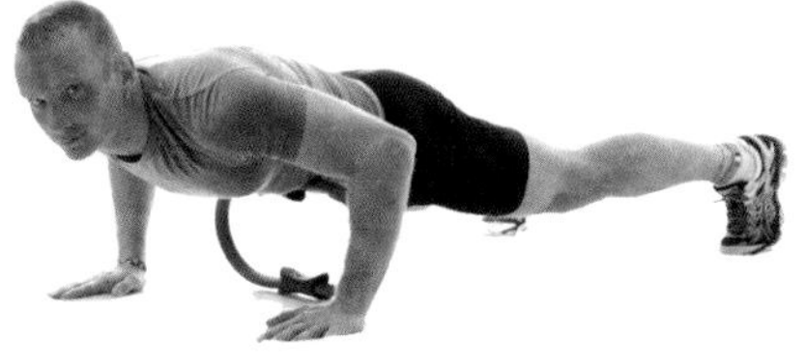

243 Knuckle Push-Up

Clench your fists by wrapping your thumbs around the outside of your curled index and middle fingers, and assume the drop position. Perform as you would a basic push-up. This version is a great option for those with wrist issues, and it also allows for a slightly deeper range of motion.

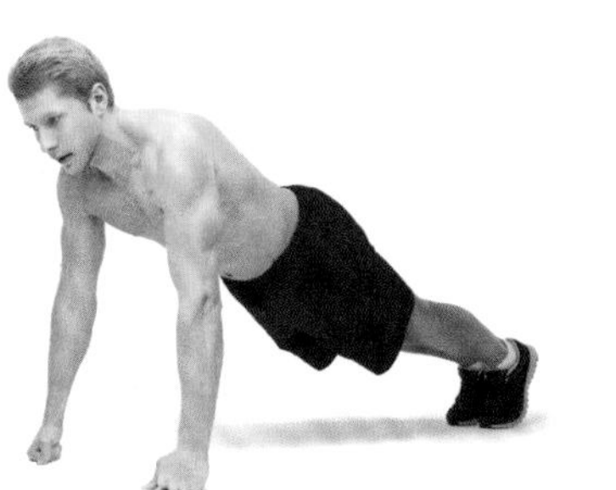

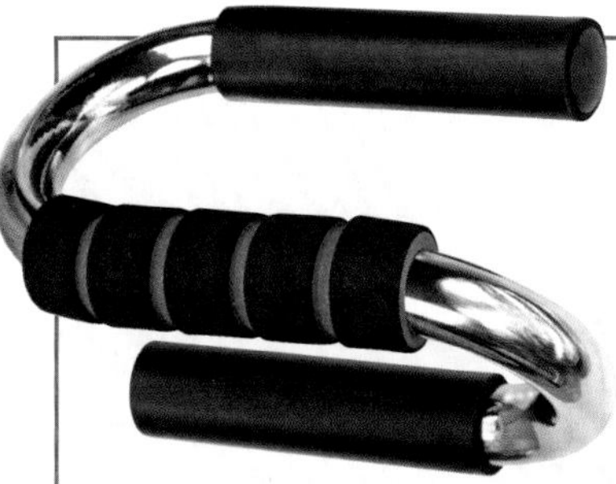

MAXIMIZE YOUR PUSH-UPS

You can perform push-ups on a variety of weighted props, from standard dumbbells to specially designed push-bars. These add-ons increase your range of motion, letting you go down slightly deeper, and they make the movement a little easier on your wrists. To perform, grasp the prop, and move up and down as you would during the Basic Push-Up (#226).

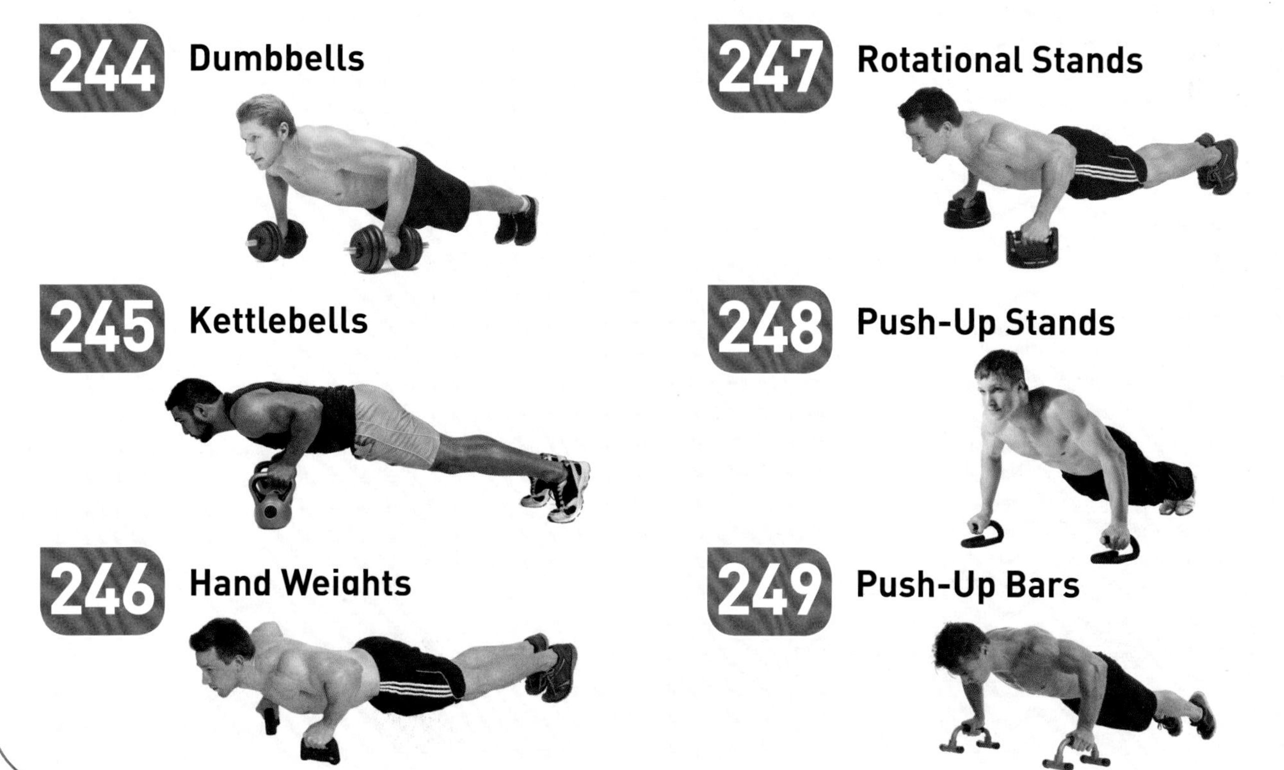

244 Dumbbells

245 Kettlebells

246 Hand Weights

247 Rotational Stands

248 Push-Up Stands

249 Push-Up Bars

Weighted Santana Push-Up

The Santana Push-Up, also called a Handstand or T-Stabilization Push-Up, is a great way to combine a strength exercise and a rotational movement. This push-up variation will rev up your metabolism and increase balance and coordination.

- Assume the drop position, with your hands grasping a set of dumbbells. Bend your arms, and lower your torso until your chest touches the floor.
- Straighten your arms, and at the top of the push-up, lift your right arm straight up, rotating your torso to stack your shoulders, and turn your heels to the left so that your body and arms form a T.
- Lower the right dumbbell to the floor, and push off your feet, rotating your whole body in the opposite direction as you jump up. Land on your feet facing the opposite direction. This counts as one rep. Repeat all steps, this time raising your left arm.

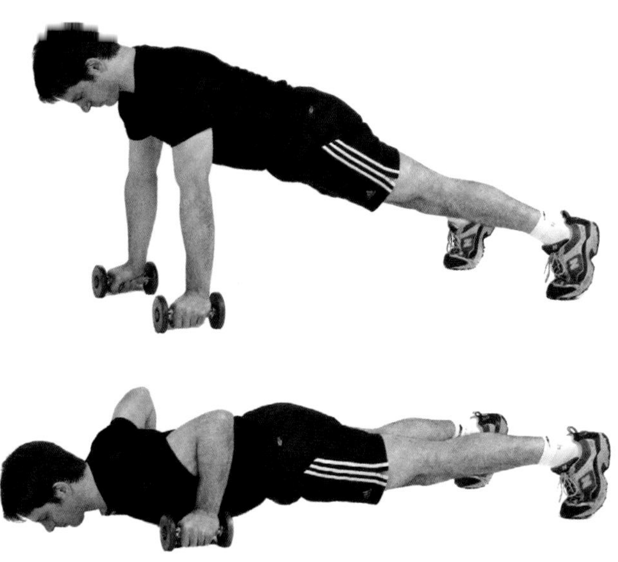

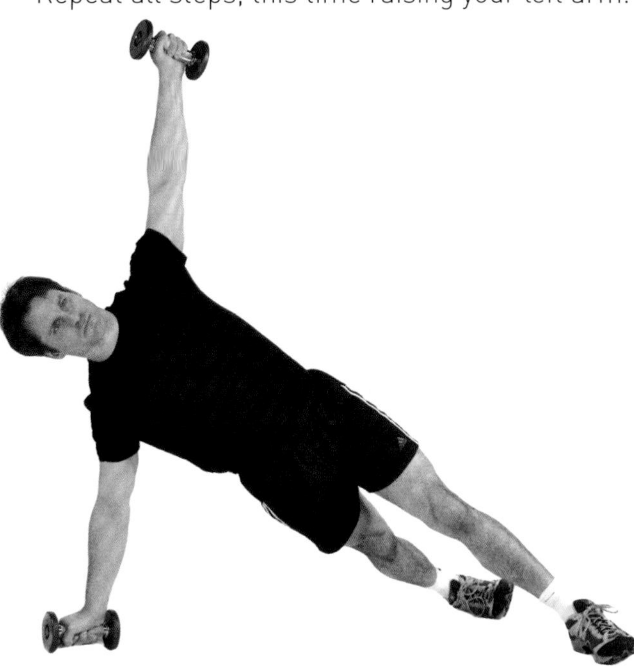

251 Santana Push-Up

Stand with your feet hip-width apart. Squat down, and put your hands on the ground in front of you. Jump your feet back into the drop position, and bend your arms, lowering your torso until your chest touches the floor. Straighten your arms, and at the top of the push-up, lift your right arm straight up, rotating your torso to stack your shoulders, and turn your heels to the left so that your body and arms for a T. Lower your raised hand to the floor, and return to the drop position. Push off your feet, and rotate your whole body in the opposite direction as you jump up. Land on your feet facing the opposite direction. This counts as one rep. Repeat all steps, this time raising your left arm.

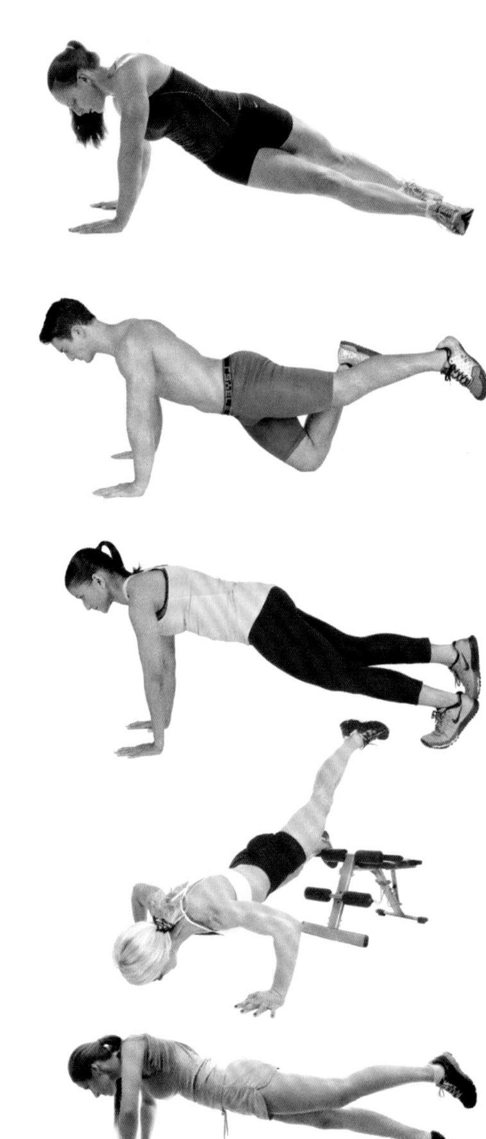

252 Push-Up with Lower-Body Rotation

Assume the drop position, and then rotate your lower body with either your feet split and your bottom foot forward, or with one foot on top of the other. Perform as your would a Basic Push-Up (#226).

253 Single-Leg Knee Push-Up

Begin on your hands and knees, and then walk your hands forward, dropping your hips so that your body forms a straight line from shoulders to knees. Raise one leg, and perform as you would a Basic Knee Push-Up (#227).

254 Single-Leg Push-Up

Assume the drop position, raise one leg, and perform as you would a Basic Push-Up (#226).

255 Single-Leg Decline Push-Up

Begin on your hands and knees, with your hands spread wide, and then prop your feet on an elevated surface. Raise one leg, and with your back flat, bend your elbows to touch your chest to the floor, and then extend your arms back to the upright position.

256 Single-Leg Roller Push-Up

Begin on your hands and knees, with your hands spread wide, and then prop your feet on an elevated surface. Raise one leg, and with your back flat, bend your elbows to touch your chest to the floor, and then extend your arms back to the upright position.

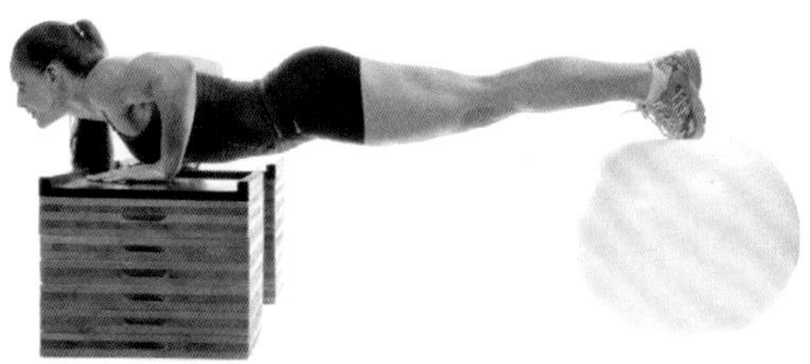

257 Push-Up on Swiss Ball and Blocks

With your hands shoulder-width and fingertips parallel to your collarbone, place your hands on blocks, and place your feet with ankles fixed at 90-degree angles, toes down on a Swiss ball so that your body is horizontal. Bend your elbows to lower your torso until your chest is level with your hands. Return by extending your elbows and pushing into the blocks, elevating your entire body simultaneously.

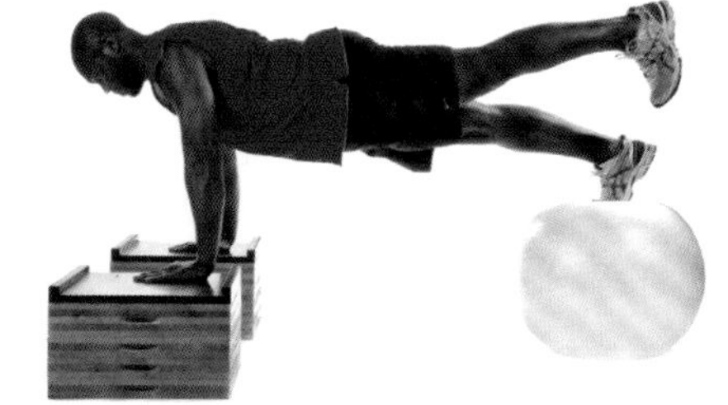

258 Single-Leg Push-Up on Swiss Ball and Blocks

Keeping the toes of one foot on a Swiss ball, elevate your other leg. Perform as your would a Push-Up on Swiss Ball and Blocks (#257).

259 Box Push-Up

Place one hand on the floor and the other on a box. Bend your arms, and lower your torso until your chest is level with the box. Press forcefully back to the starting position.

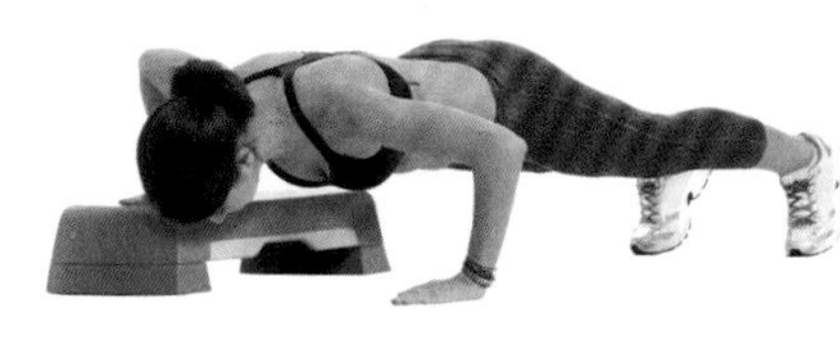

260 Crossover Box Push-Up

Place your left hand on the box and your right on the floor, perform as you would a box push-up, and then lift your right hand and place it beside your left hand on top of the box. Move your left hand down to the floor so your hands are shoulder-width apart again. Perform another push-up to complete the repetition.

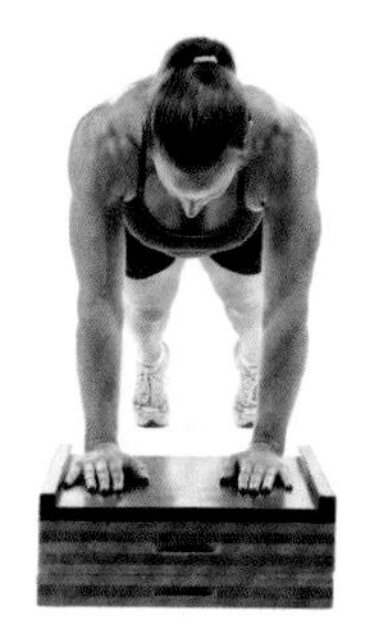

261 Single-Arm Push-Up

Assume a drop position with your legs spread wide. Rest one arm on the small of your back. Lower with control, turning your torso slightly away from the supporting arm so that your arm and both feet form a triangle. When your chin is about a fist's width above the floor, push your body upward to the starting position.

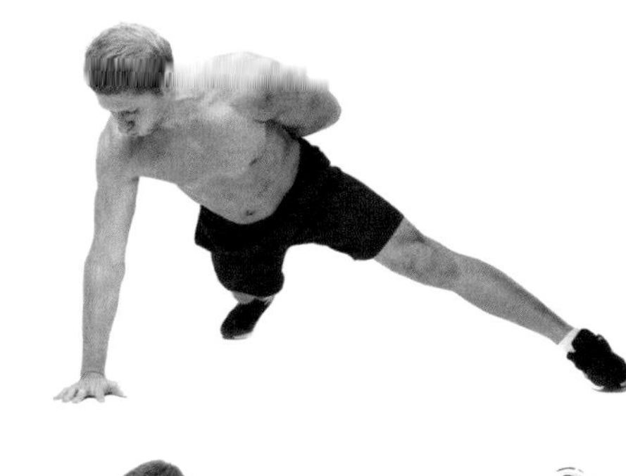

262 Single-Arm, Single-Leg Push-Up

Assume the drop position, and perform as you would the Basic Push-Up (#226), but at the top of the movement, raise your opposite leg and arm, pause, and then lower your arm and leg to the starting position.

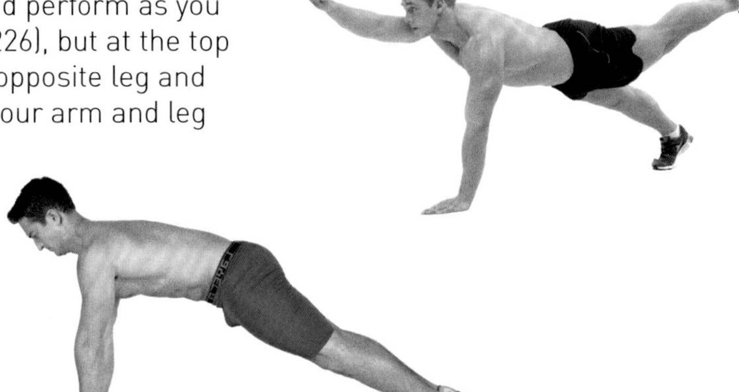

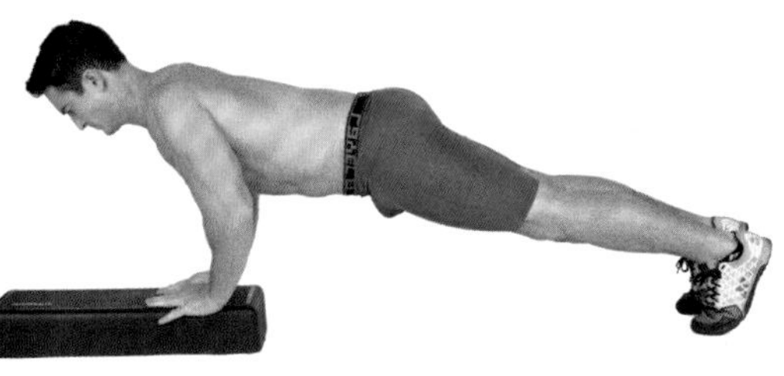

263 Dynamic Box Push-Up

Assume the drop position, with your hands on a box, placed closed together so that your thumbs and index fingers touch. Lower your body, and then press explosively off the box, your hands landing on the floor on either side of the box. Immediately lower your body, and then press up explosively so that your hands land back on the box in the starting position to complete the repetition.

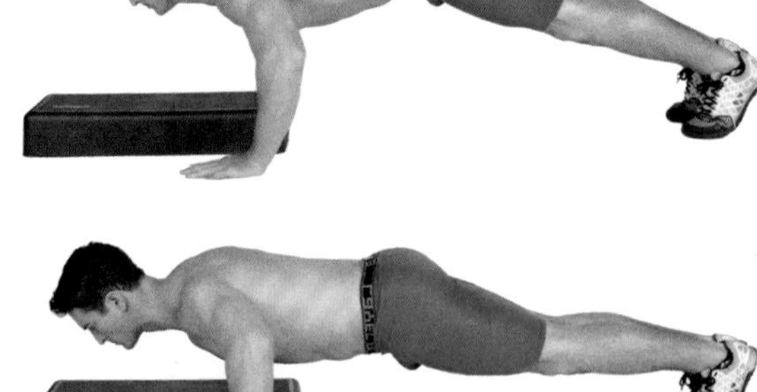

264 Alternating Shuffle Push-Up

Assume the drop position, and then move your right hand to the left until both hands are next to each other. Now slide your left hand farther left until your hands are shoulder-width apart again. Do a push-up, and then repeat the process, moving to the right and doing another push-up.

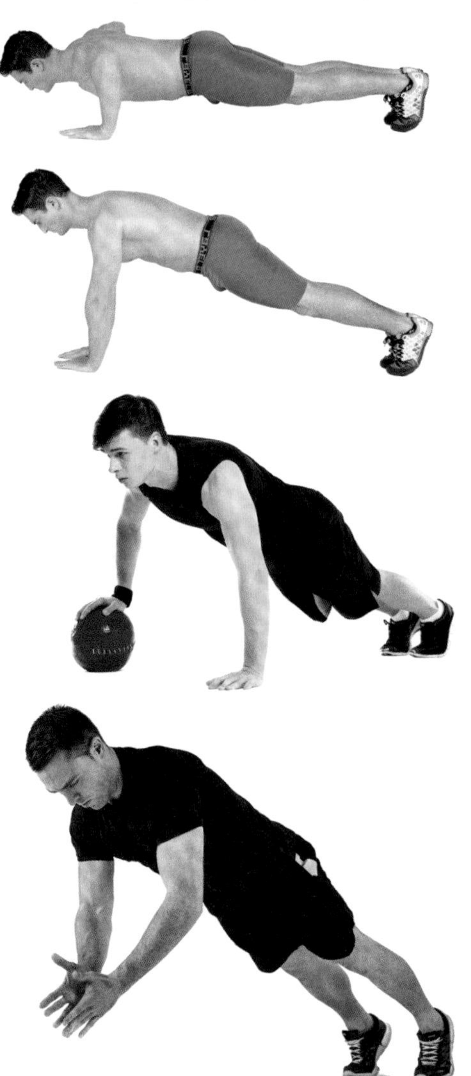

265 Alternating Medicine Ball Push-Up

Assume the drop position with one hand on the floor and the other hand on top of a medicine ball. Lower your torso toward the floor, pause, and then press back up to the starting position. Roll the medicine ball beneath the other hand before repeating the movement.

266 Push-Up with Clap

Lie flat on the floor, face down. Place your hands slightly outside of your shoulders and your fingertips parallel to your collarbone so that your elbows are at 45-degree angles to your torso. Place both feet on tiptoes. Keeping your body rigid, forcefully and quickly push your hands into the floor so that you generate enough momentum to come off the floor. Just as your body reaches its highest point, clap them directly underneath your chest, and immediately return them to the starting position, decelerating so that your body descends to a position just above the floor.

267 Plyo Kettlebell Push-Up

Assume the drop position with one hand planted on the floor and the other gripping a kettlebell. Lower yourself until your upper arms are parallel to the floor. Next, quickly push your arms to full extension. As you do so, switch hands on the kettlebell. Lower yourself again, switching sides each time you push yourself back up.

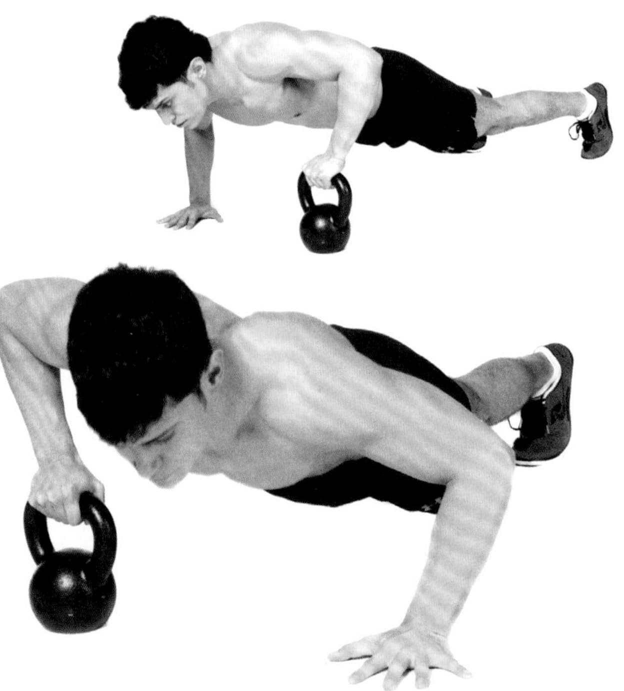

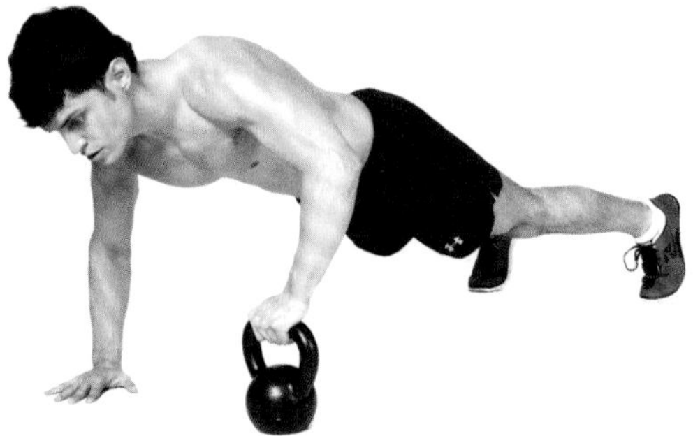

268 Diver Bomber

The Dive Bomber is a high-intensity plyometric push-up variation that places a lot of body weight on the shoulders and arms. The sliding position of the body mimics a bomber aircraft diving toward the ground and then swooping back upward.

- Assume the drop position, with your hands grasping the drop position.
- Spread your feet, and then walk your hands toward your feet until your butt is up in the air and your shoulders are placed above and slightly behind your hands.
- Lower your chest in between your hands to the floor while keep your butt in the air.
- Arch your lower back, and push your body weight out in front of your arms and elevate your chest and straighten your arms. Reverse this movement to the starting position.

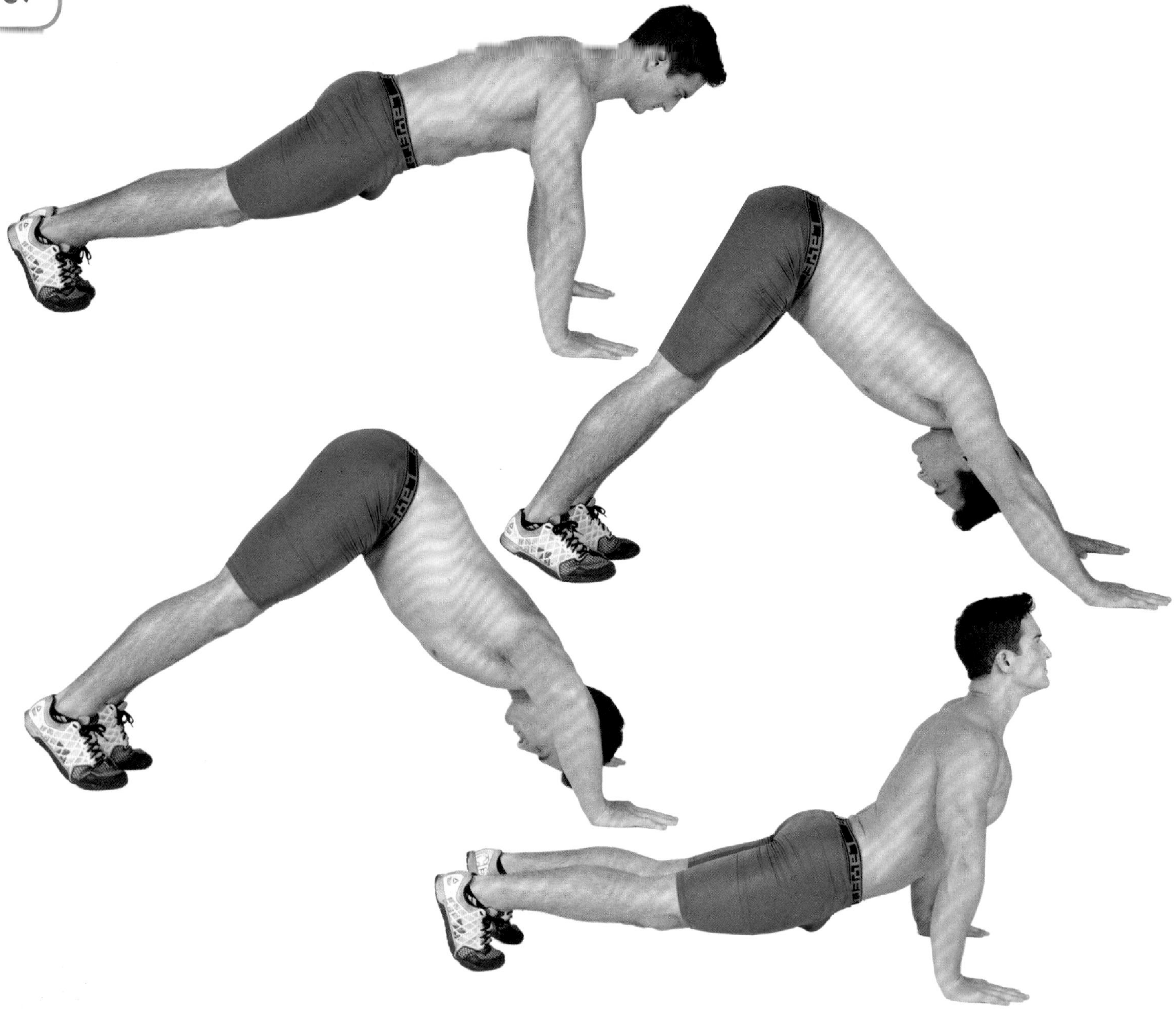

269 Knee Push-Up & Roll-Out

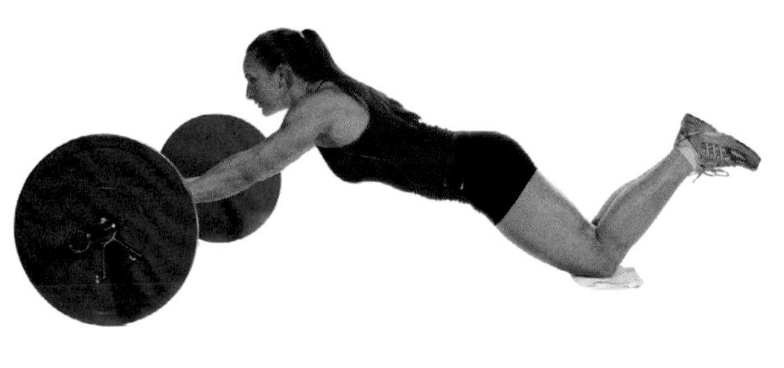

Place a barbell on the floor so that the bar is horizontal to your torso. Grasp the bar with your elbows extended, your arms straight, and the bar beneath your chest. With your body rigid, bend your knees to the floor. Keeping your elbows at 45-degree angles to your torso, use your knees as a fulcrum and let your body drop until your chest touches the bar. Extend your elbows, and push up and away until your arms are fully extended. Pause. then push on the bar, rolling it forward with your arms remaining extended. Pause briefly, and pull back on bar, returning it to starting position.

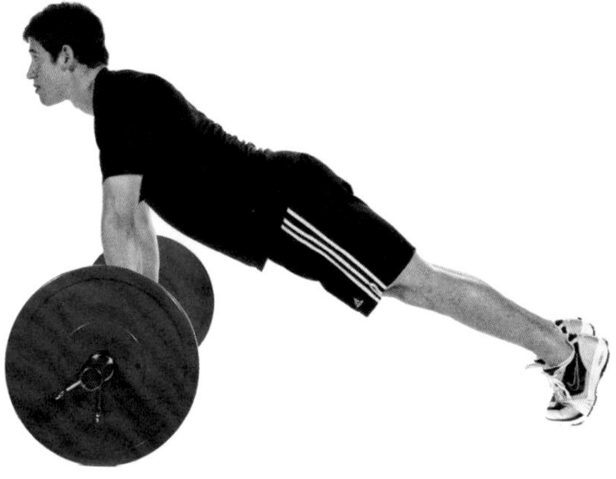

Push-Up and Roll-Out

Perform as you would a Knee Push-Up and Roll-Out (#269), but with your legs extended and your body rigid.

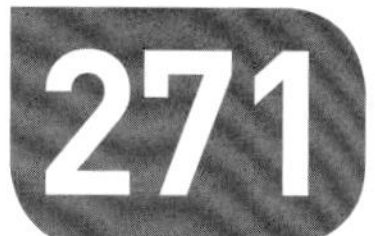

Suspended Push-Up

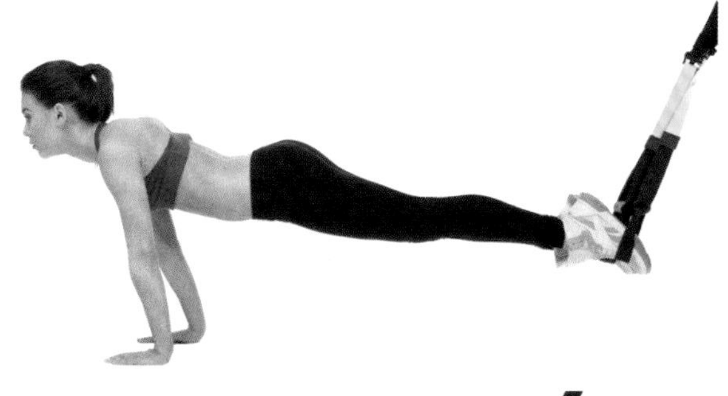

Place your feet securely into the foot cradles of a suspension trainer, positioning them directly under the anchor point, and assume the drop position with your feet together, your back flat, and your core tight. Bend your arms, and lower your torso until your chest touches the floor. Straighten your arms to rise back up to the starting position to complete the repetition.

Suspended Atomic Push-Up

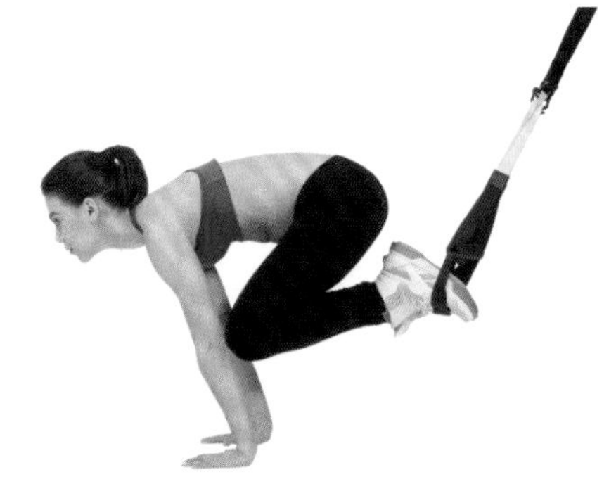

Kneel facing away from the anchor point with your feet in the foot cradles. Place your hands on the floor slightly wider than shoulders width, and lift up to the drop position. Bend your elbows to 90 degrees to lower your body toward the ground. Press back up, lift your hips slightly and crunch, bringing your knees to your chest.

Ring Push-Up

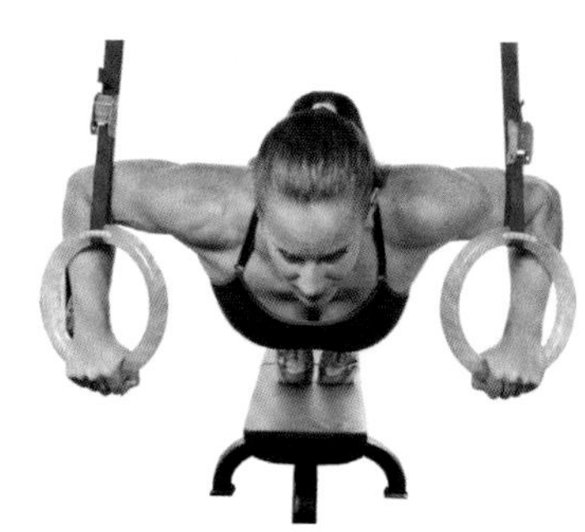

With your body rigid, grasp rings slightly wider than shoulder-width apart with a palms-down grip, so that the rings are parallel to your chest. Using your toes as a fulcrum, bend your elbows to lower your body chest-first. While descending, move your hands apart laterally, until your chest is directly between your= hands at ring level, and your elbows are bent to 90 degrees. Return by extending your arms and pushing toward the floor until your elbows are straight.

274 DFRB

This high-intensity multi-phase agility exercise comes straight from special forces boot camp training grounds. "DFRB" stands for Drop, Face, Recover, and Back. "Drop" means to get into a starting push-up position. "Face" means to lower your body until your chest touches the floor. "Recover" means to jump both feet to your chest, and quickly stand up. "Back" means to flip onto your back. To perform this exercise, you move through these four positions in rapid succession. Begin by performing them in DFRB order, but as you develop strength and endurance, you can repeat the moves in any order, keeping in mind that performing all four equals one repetition.

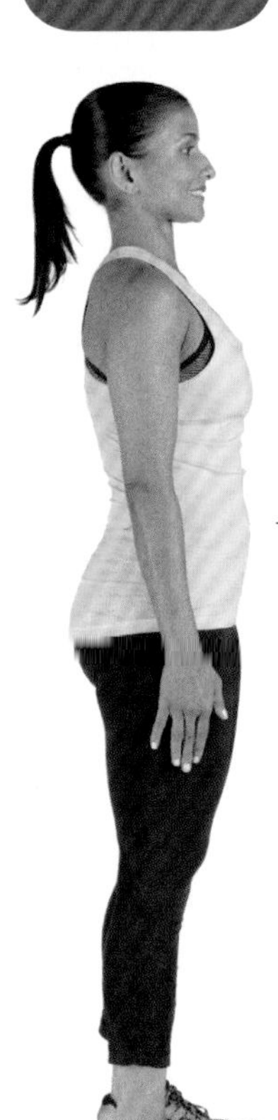

- Stand tall, with your arms at your sides.
- Drop forward into a push-up position.
- Lower your chest to the floor to assume the Face position.

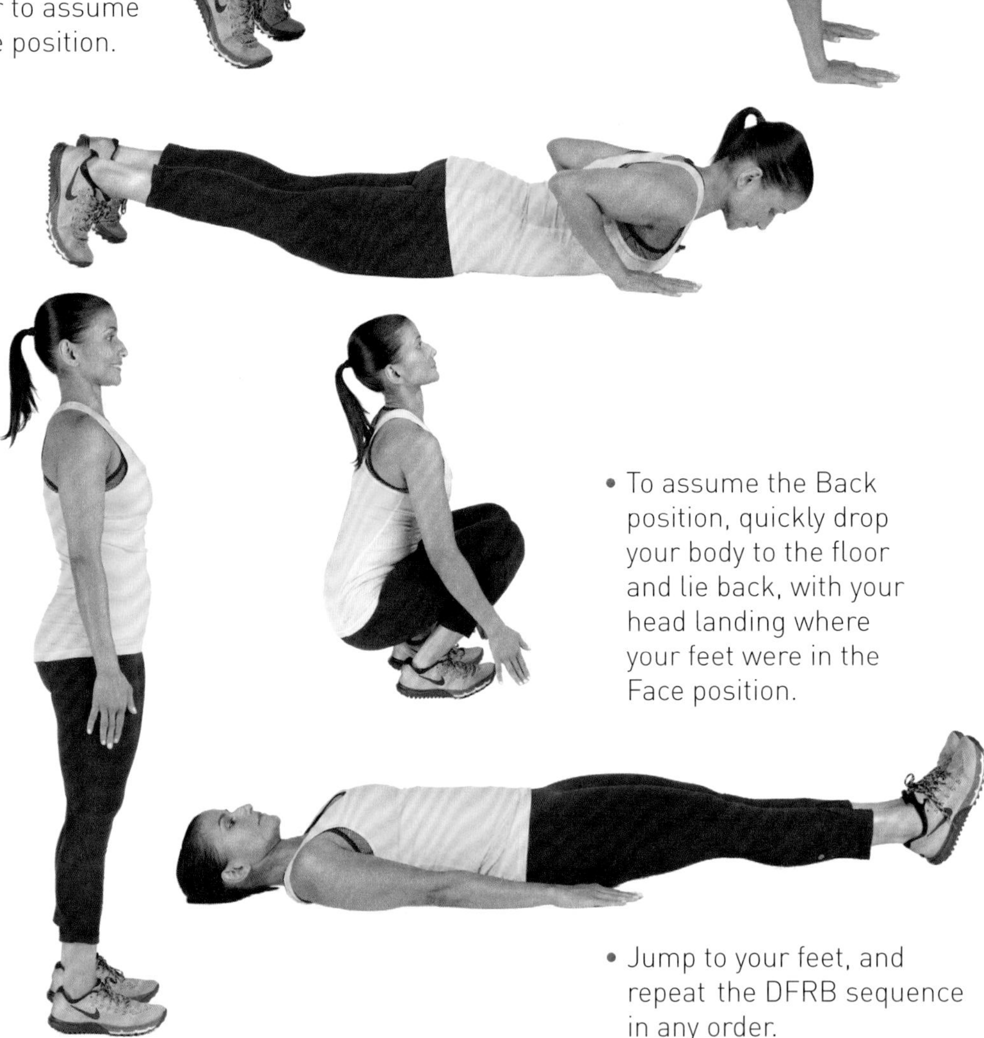

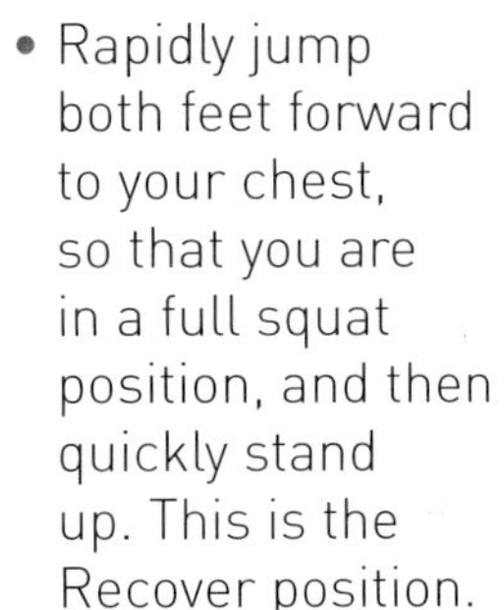

- Rapidly jump both feet forward to your chest, so that you are in a full squat position, and then quickly stand up. This is the Recover position.

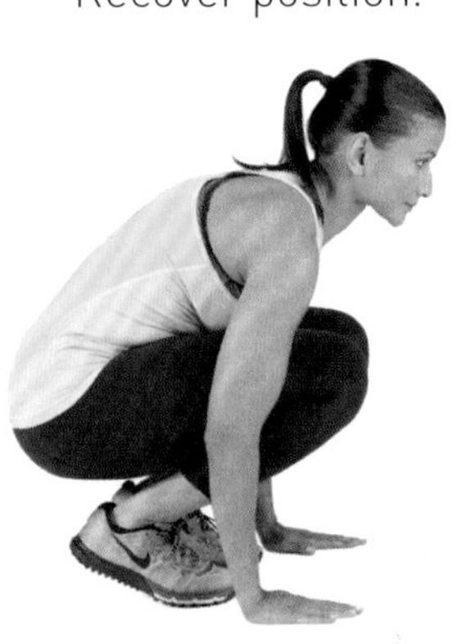

- To assume the Back position, quickly drop your body to the floor and lie back, with your head landing where your feet were in the Face position.
- Jump to your feet, and repeat the DFRB sequence in any order.

275 Towel Fly

The Towel Fly is an advanced modification of a push-up that calls for you to move your arms in and out rather than up and down. Utilizing your body weight, it gives your chest muscles an efficient workout while also recruiting muscles of your arms, back, hips, and abdomen to keep your body stabilized. Try to perform as many as 20 in row for a high-intensity challenge. You can use a single towel, two small towels, or even paper plates under your hands—anything that will slide smoothly on the floor.

- Place a towel on the floor in front of you. Assume the drop position, with your elbows fully extended, and the towel under your hands.
- Maintaining a rigid drop position, with your abdominals braced and your weight on your feet, move your hands together. The towel should bunch together below your sternum.

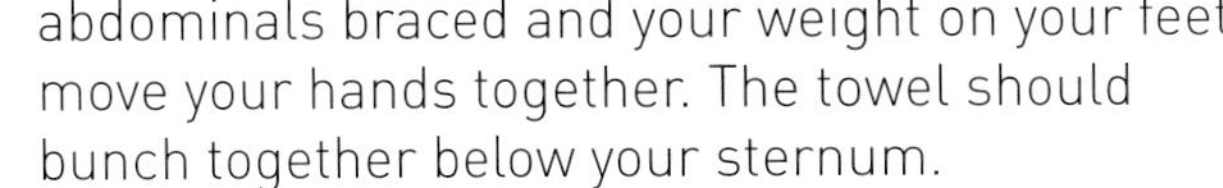

- Straighten out the towel by pressing outward with your arms, returning to the starting position.

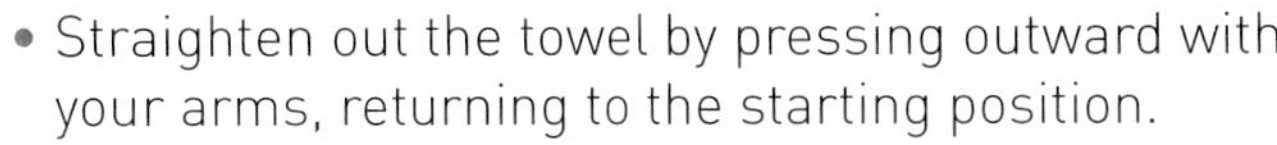

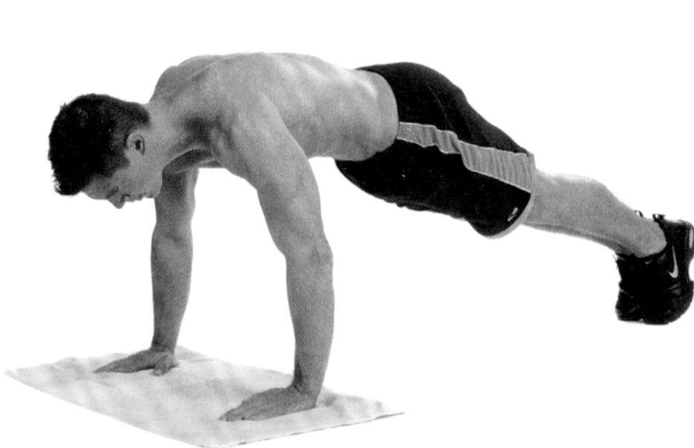

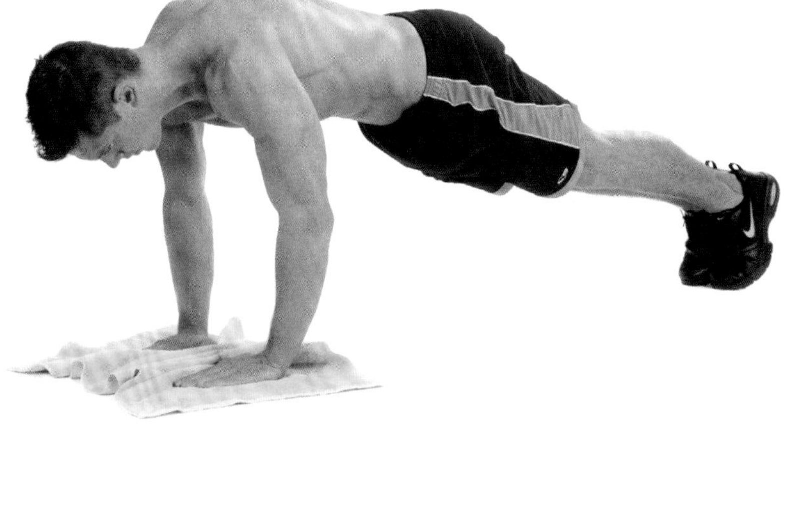

276 Single-Arm Forward Slide

On a smooth flat surface (preferably wood) assume the drop position with legs straight and each hand placed on a small individual towel. Bend one elbow and simultaneously slide the other hand upward, keeping that elbow straight to cause your torso to descend. Return by pushing into the floor with the bent arm and pulling downward with the overhead, straightened one, until torso returns to original position. Alternate arms.

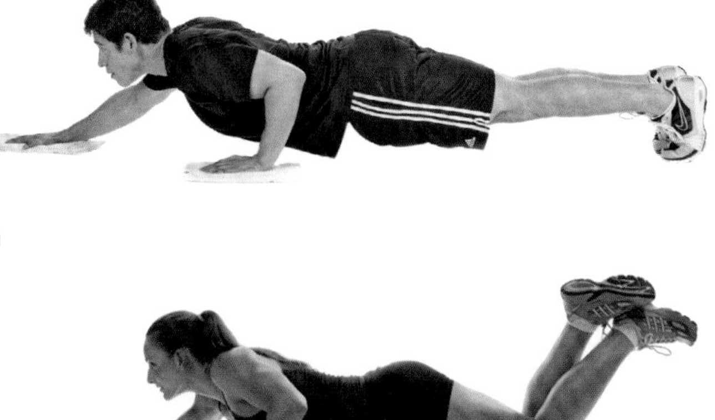

277 Single-Arm Forward Knee Slide

Assume a bent-knee drop position, and perform as you would the Single-Arm Forward Slide (#276).

278 Up-Down

The Up-Down exercise gets your blood pumping and the fat burning. This multiphase exercise is meant to tax your cardiovascular system by working almost all of your muscles, and it has the added benefit of increasing your coordination and agility. You can add another element of upper-body conditioning by performing the Up-Down with Push-Up variation. Sport teams and military personnel rely on these exercises to develop nimbleness and speed.

- Run in place, bringing your knees waist-high with each step.
- Drop down, and touch your chest to the floor.
- Immediately stand back up, and resume running with high knees as quickly as possible. Perform for the desired reps and sets.

➔ FIND YOUR FORM

Keep your knees at waist level while running in place. Avoid landing on your chest—allow your hands to contact the floor first, and then lower onto your chest. Don't flop—move with control.

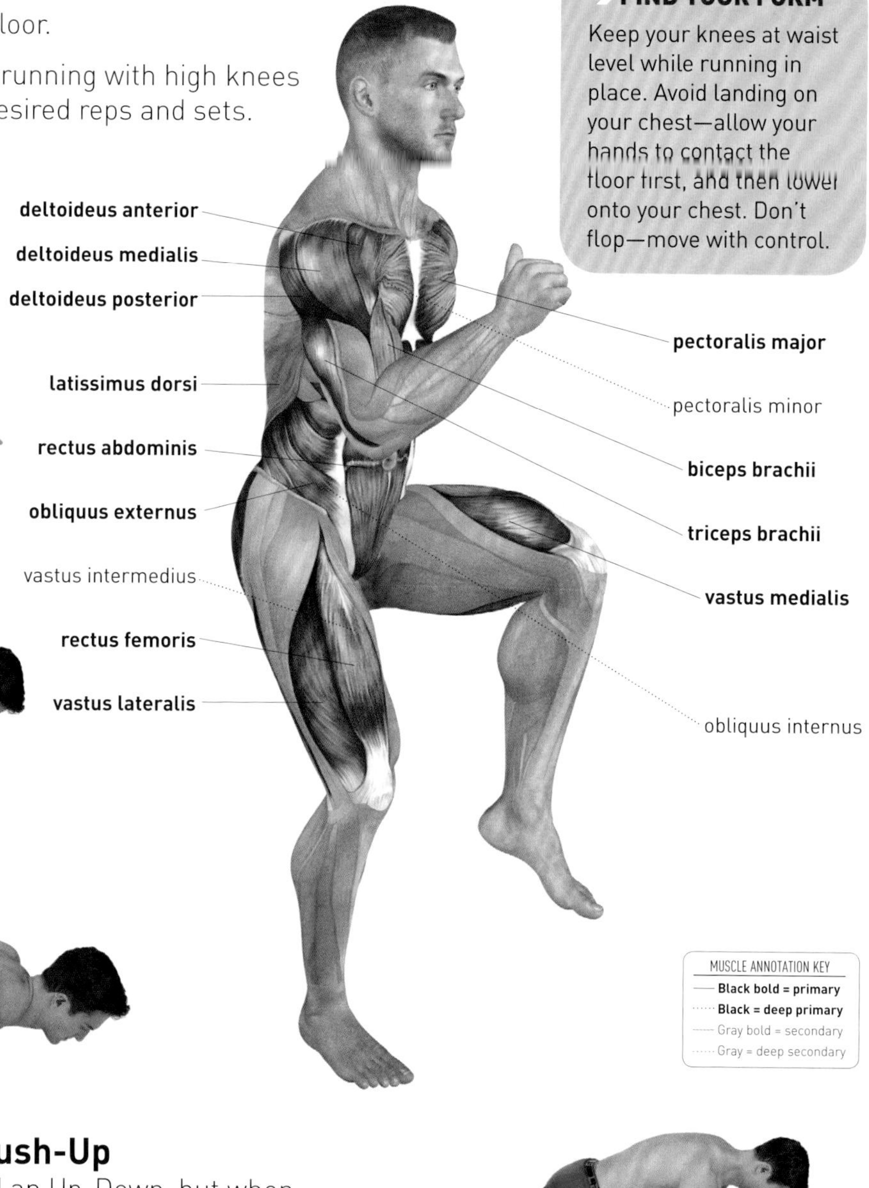

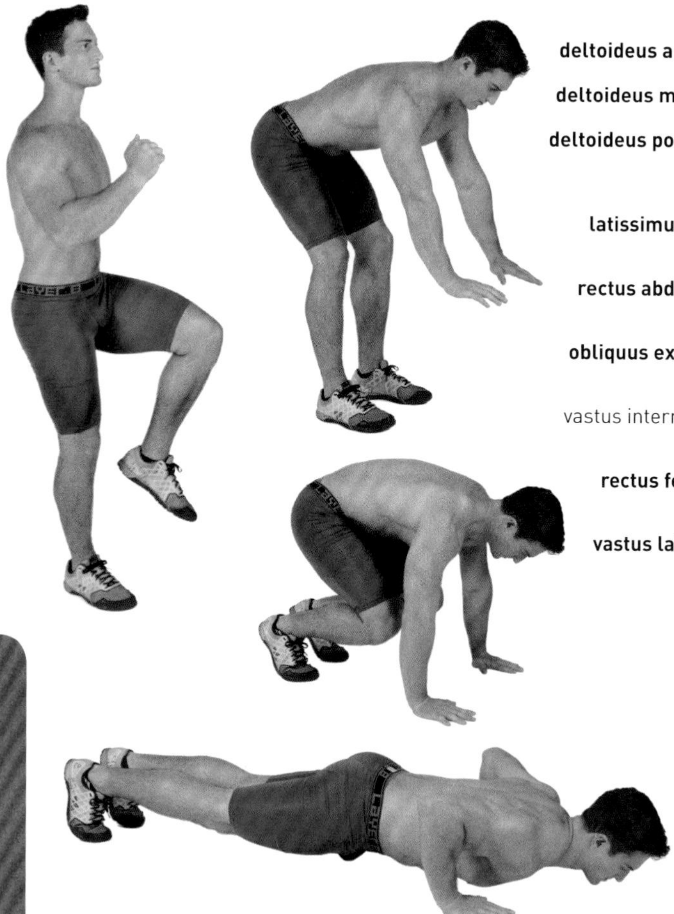

deltoideus anterior
deltoideus medialis
deltoideus posterior
latissimus dorsi
rectus abdominis
obliquus externus
vastus intermedius
rectus femoris
vastus lateralis
pectoralis major
pectoralis minor
biceps brachii
triceps brachii
vastus medialis
obliquus internus

MUSCLE ANNOTATION KEY
Black bold = primary
Black = deep primary
Gray bold = secondary
Gray = deep secondary

279 Up-Down with Push-Up

Perform as you would an Up-Down, but when you drop down to touch your chest to the floor, raise your torso to perform a push-up. Immediately jump back up to your feet, and. resume running with high knees.

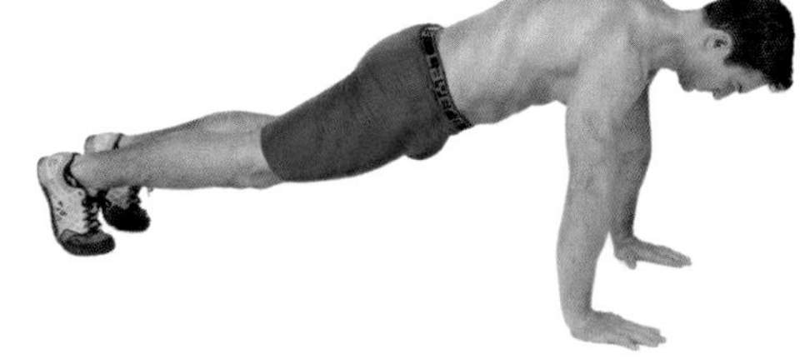

280 Alternating Renegade Row

The Renegade Row is a hardworking exercise that combines the benefits of an explosive upper-body move with a powerful core strengthener.

- With a kettlebell in each hand, assume the drop position.
- While staying on your toes and keeping your core stable and parallel to the floor, pull the kettlebell in your right hand up toward your chest while straightening your left arm and pushing that kettlebell into the floor.
- Lower your right arm, then repeat the movement with the left. Continue alternating sides for the desired repetitions.

➔ FIND YOUR FORM

Keep your hips level and square to the floor, and fully engage your core muscles so that your body is in the same position throughout, whether you are balancing on one arm or have both weights on the floor.

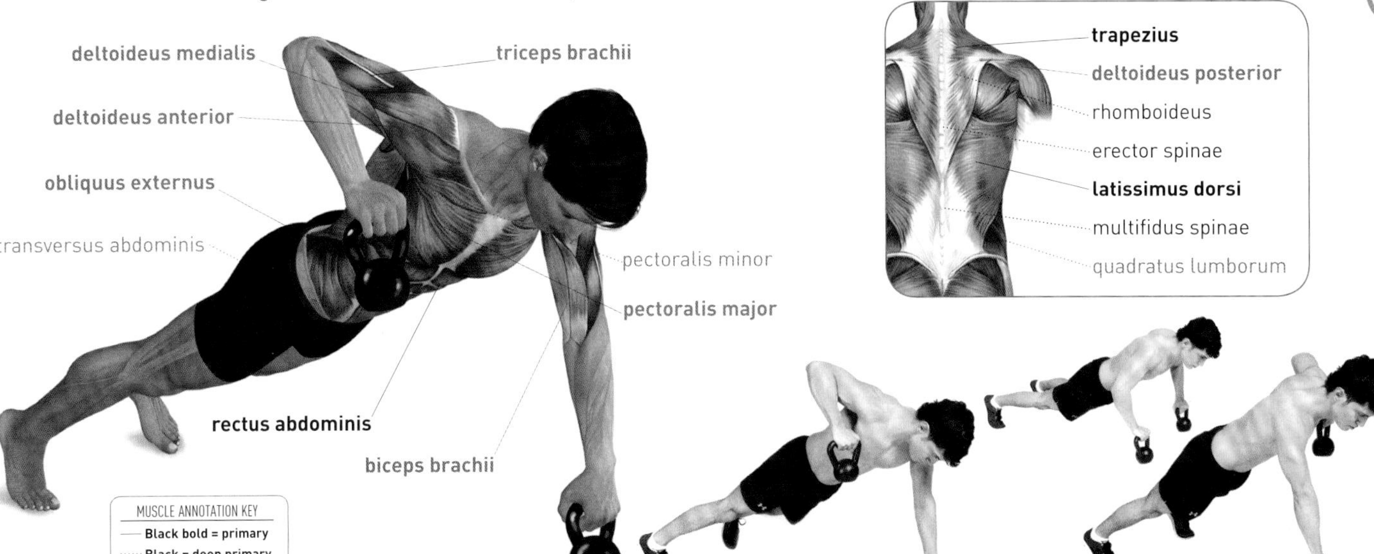

281 Single-Leg Renegade Row

Perform as you would the Alternating Renegade Row (#280), but raise one leg off the floor for a tougher challenge.

282 Tractor Tire Renegade Row

To challenge your balance and stability, perform a Renegade Row (#280) with your feet and hands propped on either side of a tractor tire.

283 Single-Arm T-Row

Start in the drop position, taking a wide stance with your legs and holding a dumbbell in each hand. Pull one of the dumbbells to chest level. Rotate your torso while raising your arm toward the ceiling. Slowly lower the weight back to the floor to return to the drop position. Repeat with the other arm to complete one repetition.

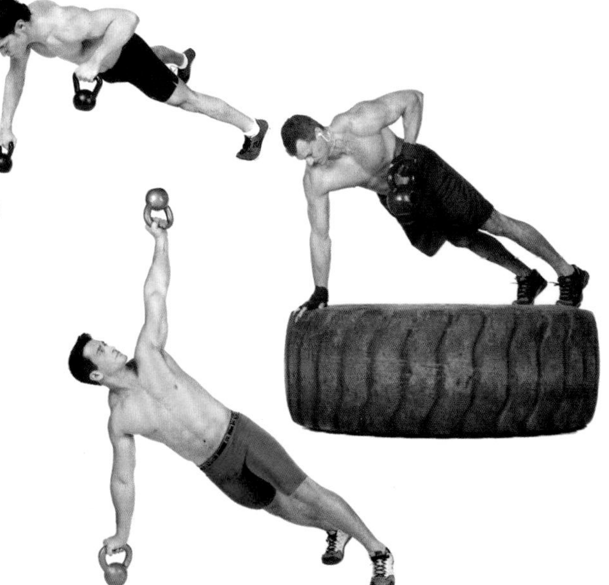

284 Crane Handstand

The Crane Handstand, also known as the Crane or Crow Pose, is a foundational arm-balancing yoga pose. It strengthens your upper arms, forearms, and wrists, while it also strengthens your abs and stretches your upper back and groins. Mastering this move improves balance and coordination—your goal is to pull your knees up near your armpits and lift your butt as high as possible while remaining balanced enough to keep your full weight off your wrists. For any handstand moves, until you have the strength and skill, working with a spotter is essential.

- Squat deeply until your buttocks are just above your heels. and then lean your torso forward, and extend your arms to place your hands on the floor in front of you. Turn your hands inward slightly, and widen your fingers.
- Bend your elbows, resting your knees against your upper arms. Lifting up on the balls of your feet and leaning forward with your torso, bring your thighs toward your chest and your shins to your upper arms. Round your back as you feel your weight transfer to your wrists.
- Exhale, and slowly lift your feet off the floor one at a time. Keep your head position neutral, and find your balance point.

FIND YOUR FORM

To help quell your fear of falling on your face, keep your breath even and keep your mind calm.

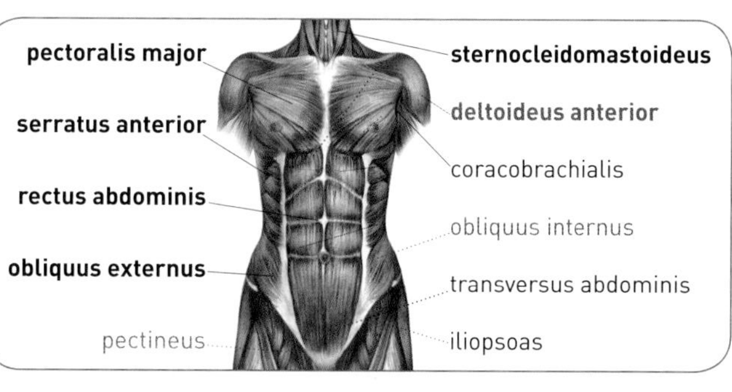

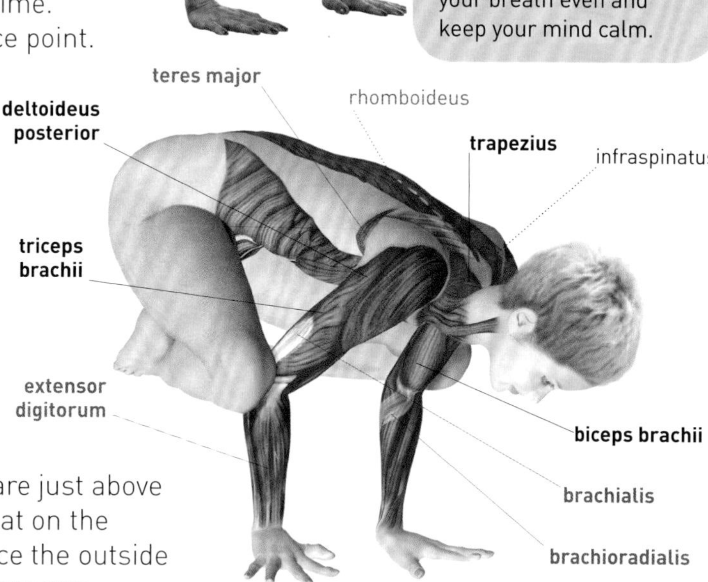

MUSCLE ANNOTATION KEY
- **Black bold = primary**
- Black = deep primary
- Gray bold = secondary
- Gray = deep secondary

285 Side Crane Handstand

Squat deeply until your buttocks are just above your heels. Place your left hand flat on the floor outside your right thigh. Place the outside of your right thigh on your left upper arm. Lean to the right until you can place your right hand flat on the floor so that your hands are shoulder-width apart. Slowly lift your pelvis as you shift your weight toward your hands, using your left arm as a support for your right thigh. Continue shifting to the right, drawing your abs toward your spine. Keep your feet together as you raise them off the floor toward your butt. Hold for the desired time, breathing through the balance. Exhale as you bring your feet to the floor. Repeat on the other side.

286 Crane Handstand Push-Up

To add a further balance challenge, perform a Crane Handstand (#284) on push-ups bars.

287 Handstand

Stand up straight, and raise your arms straight over your head. Kick straight forward with your dominant leg, and as you fall into a lunge position, tip your body forward. Hold your arms straight and move your head toward the ground. Straighten your legs and torso toward the sky, balancing your weight on your hands. To release the handstand, split your legs and drop your dominant leg to the ground. Start to stand up and as you do put your other leg on the ground. You can perform this free-standing or against a wall.

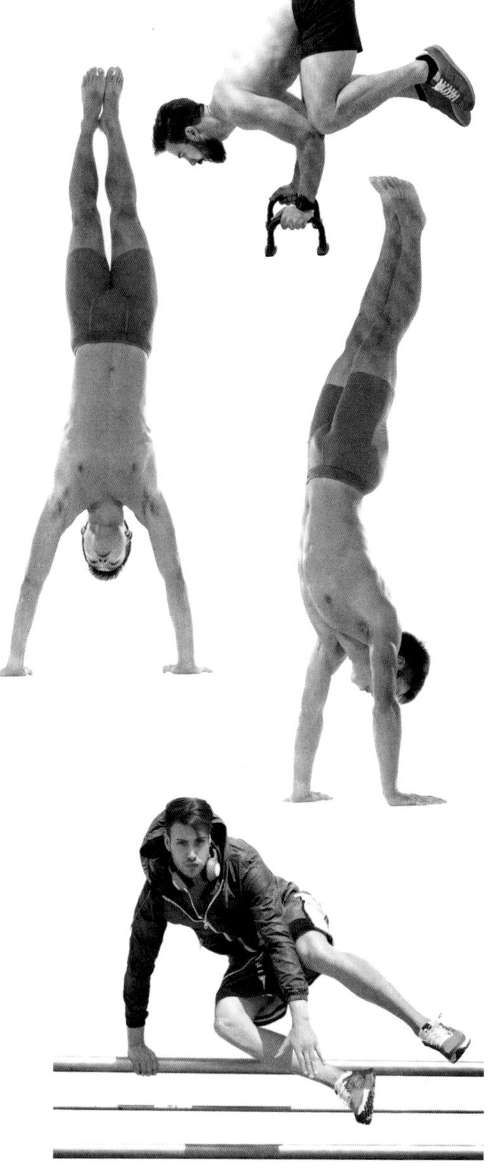

288 Handstand Walk

Perform a Handstand (#287), and then walk your hands forward while maintaining balance.

289 Parkour Vault

Approach an obstacle, such as a railing, in a direct line. Reach one arm forward, place your hand flat on the top of the obstacle, and shift your weight off your feet onto your shoulder. Launch your body off the ground, and kick your outer leg sideways as you vault over the obstacle. Reach your inner (bottom) foot to the floor, release your hand, and continue stepping forward. Repeat in the opposite direction,leading with your other arm.

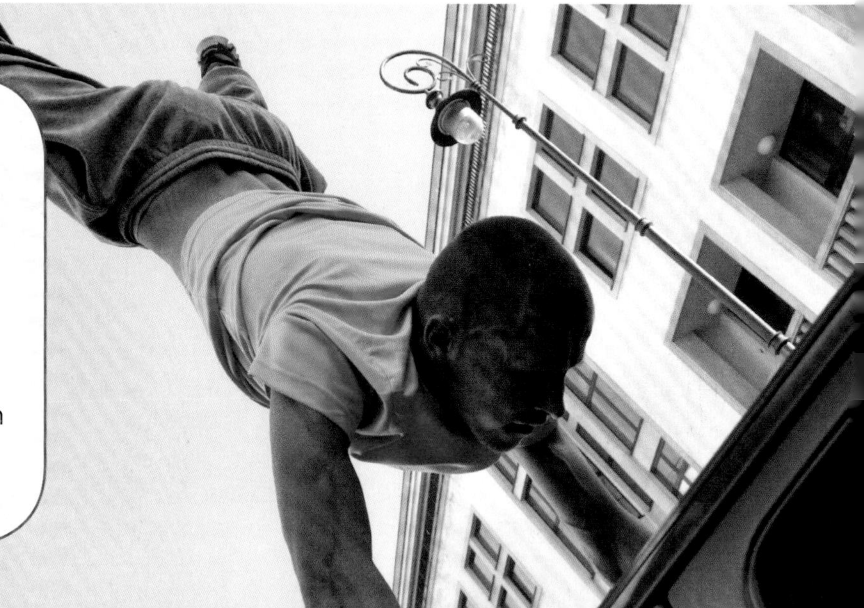

PARKOUR TRAINING

One of the most intense forms of fitness training has to be Parkour, a high-energy discipline inspired by military obstacle course training. The goal—practitioners must move through a complex obstacle-filled course as efficiently and quickly as possible using no equipment. Commonly performed as an urban acrobatic workout, Parkour moves include vaults, rolls, jumps, handstands, and swings.

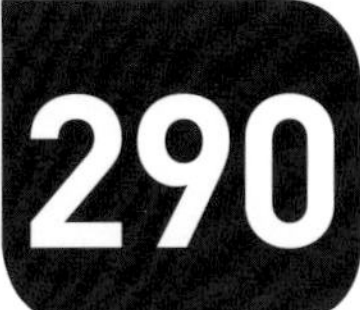

Bench Dip

The classic Bench Dip is a medium-intensity strength move that target the triceps. Like many strength moves, it can easily be incorporated into a high-intensity workout, you can do it just about anywhere and on any elevated surface, from a flat bench at the gym, the park bench in the square, or the storage bench in your living room. A slightly more difficult version of this exercise, the Triceps Dip, calls for you to lift your entire body weight, increasing the demand on your triceps.

- Sit up tall near the front of a sturdy chair. Place your hands beside your hips, wrapping your fingers over the front edge of the chair.
- Extend your legs in front of you slightly, and place your feet flat on the floor. Scoot off the edge of the chair until your knees align directly above your feet and your torso will be able to clear the chair as you dip down.
- Bending your elbows directly behind you, without splaying them out to the sides, lower your torso until your elbows make a 90-degree angle.
- Press into the chair, raising your body back to the starting position.

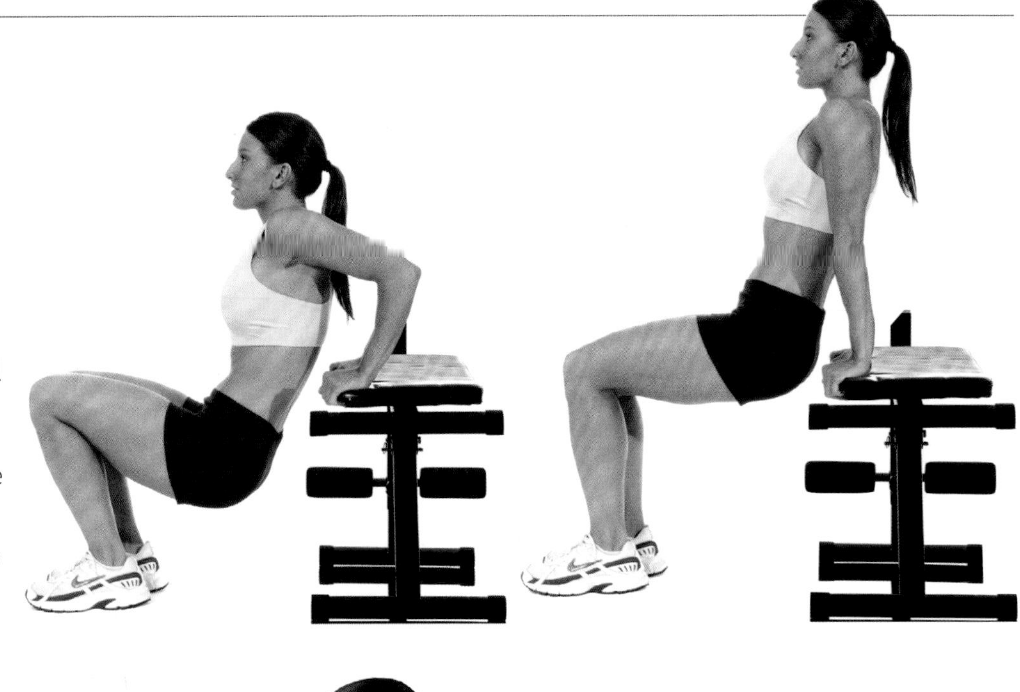

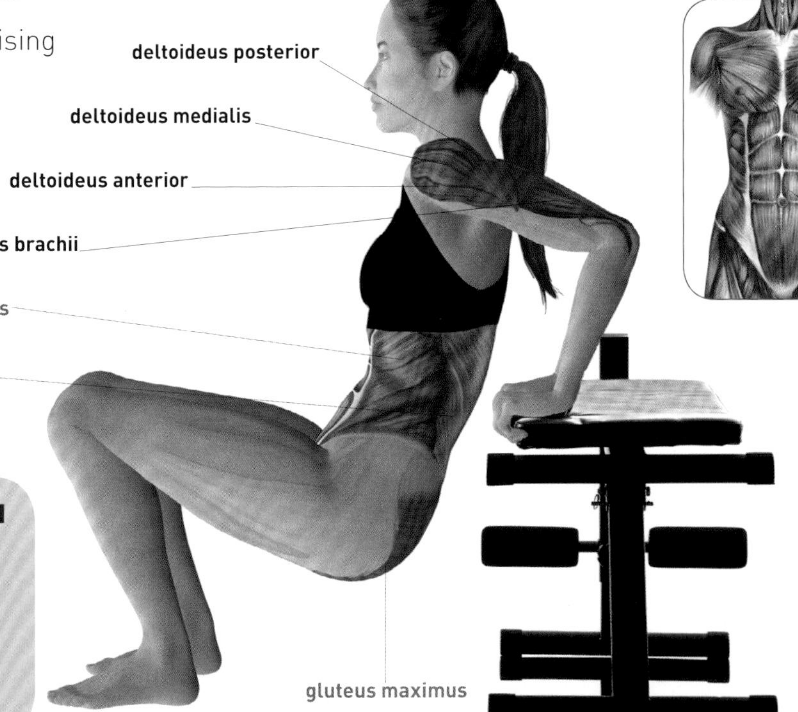

pectoralis minor
coracobrachialis
pectoralis major
serratus anterior
rectus abdominis

➔ FIND YOUR FORM

This is an easy move to master, but it can be hard on the shoulders, so be sure to keep our movements smooth and controlled.

MUSCLE ANNOTATION KEY
Black bold = primary
Black = deep primary
Gray bold = secondary
Gray = deep secondary

291 Triceps Dip

Begin standing in front of a dip station or parallel bars. Place one hand on each bar, and grip as you push and extend your arms to full lockout. Lower yourself until your upper arms are parallel to the ground, then push back up to the starting position.

292 Assisted Bench Dip

Perform as you would a Bench Dip (#290), placing your feet directly in front of your torso and planting them firmly on the assist bench.

293 Roller Triceps Dip

Sit on the floor with your legs outstretched, the foam roller behind you. Place both hands on the foam roller, with your fingers facing toward your buttocks, elbows bent. Press through your legs and straighten your arms to lift your hips and shoulders. Keeping your shoulders pressed down away from your ears, bend your elbows and dip your trunk up and down. The foam roller should not move.

294 Single-Leg Bench Dip

Perform as you would a Bench Dip (#290) with one leg lifted straight out, parallel to the floor, and your knees squeezed together. Perform the desired repetitions, and then switch sides.

295 Floor Dip

Sit with your feet flexed in front of you and your heels touching the floor. Place your hands on the floor next to you so that your fingertips point towards your hips and your elbows point behind you. Lift your hips off the floor until your shoulders are directly over your wrists and your arms are nearly straight. Bend your elbows, and dip your torso up and down without letting your buttocks touch the floor.

296 Single-Leg Floor Dip

Perform as you would a Floor Dip (#295) while keeping one leg elevated and extended straight out in front of you.

297 Dip to Kick

Perform as you would a Floor Dip (#295), but at the top of the movement, kick one leg upward while reaching for your toes with the opposite hand. Switch sides, and repeat.

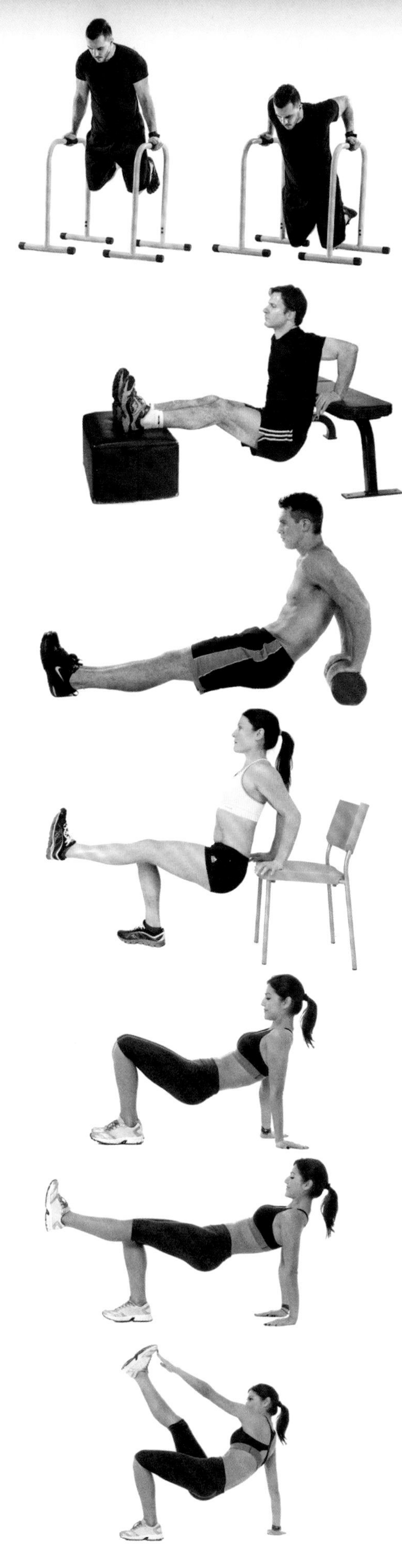

Upward Plank

The Upward Plank is known by many names— Reverse Plank, Incline Plank, Inclined Plane, and Upward Plane. A basic back-bending yoga pose, it strengthens your core, shoulders, arm, wrist, and leg muscles. It also stretches your shoulders, chest, and ankles while helping you to hone your balance and flexibility.

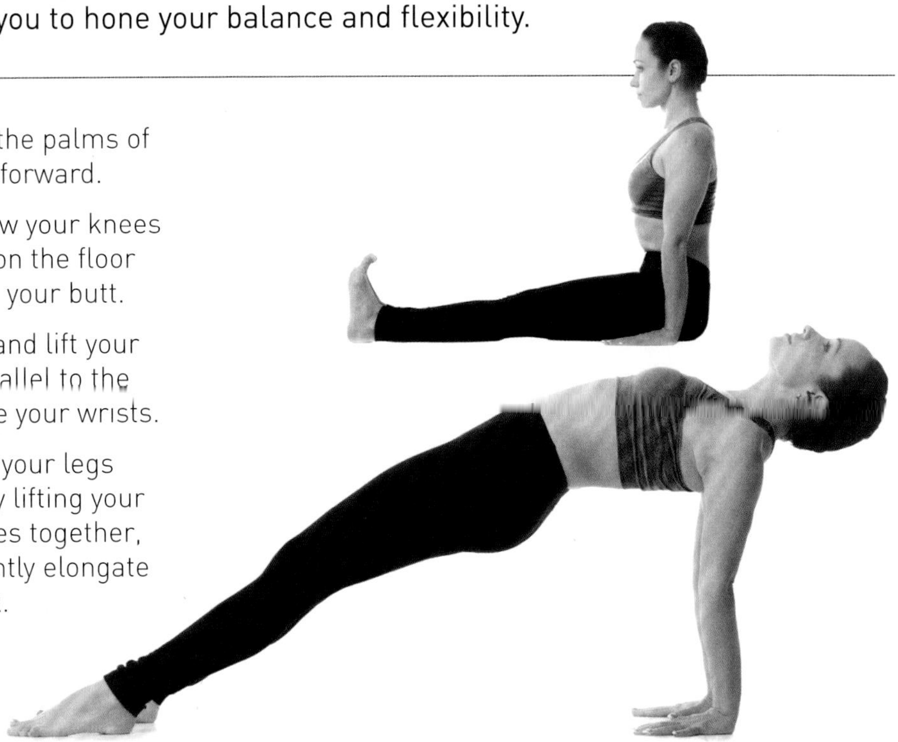

- Sit with your legs extended, and place the palms of your hands on the floor, fingers facing forward.
- Move your hands behind your hips, draw your knees toward your chest,and place your feet on the floor with your heels about a foot away from your butt.
- Press down with your hands and feet, and lift your hips until your back and thighs are parallel to the floor with your shoulders directly above your wrists.
- Without lowering your hips, straighten your legs one at a time. Push your hips higher by lifting your chest and bringing your shoulder blades together, creating a slight arch in your back. Gently elongate your neck, and let your head drop back.
- Hold for the desired time, and then return to the starting position.

➔ FIND YOUR FORM

Keep your shoulders above your wrists, and lengthen your spine, neck and arms.

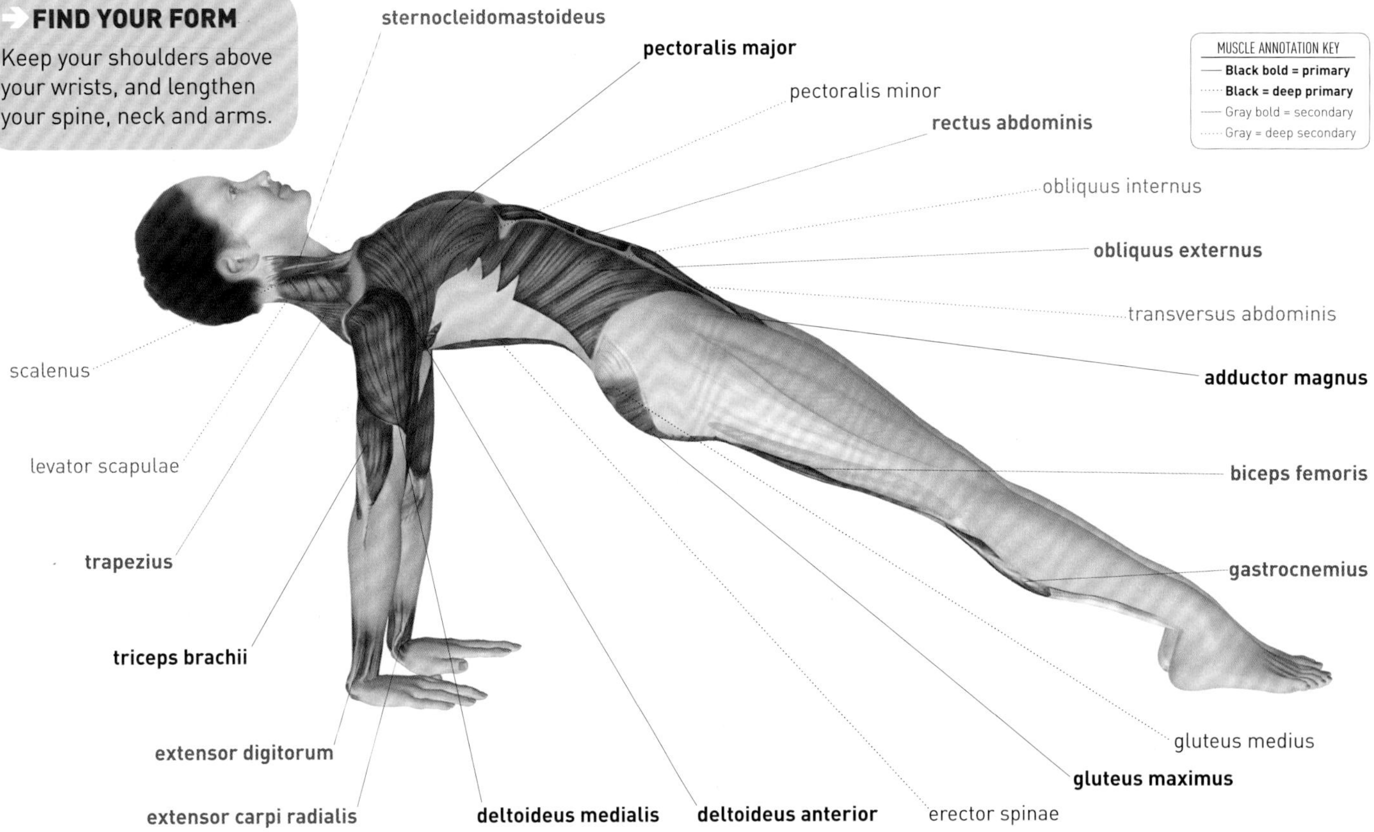

MUSCLE ANNOTATION KEY
Black bold = primary
Black = deep primary
Gray bold = secondary
Gray = deep secondary

sternocleidomastoideus
pectoralis major
pectoralis minor
rectus abdominis
obliquus internus
obliquus externus
transversus abdominis
adductor magnus
biceps femoris
gastrocnemius
gluteus medius
gluteus maximus
erector spinae
deltoideus anterior
deltoideus medialis
extensor carpi radialis
extensor digitorum
triceps brachii
trapezius
levator scapulae
scalenus

Upward Plank Kick

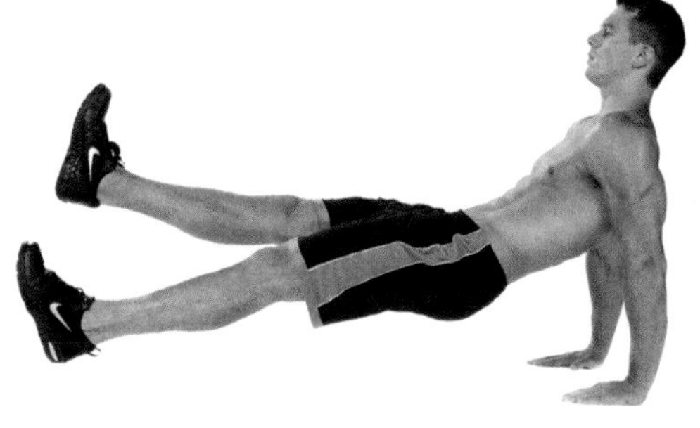

Sit with your legs parallel and stretched out in front of you. Place your hands behind you with your fingers pointed toward your hips. Press up through your arms, and lift your chest up, squeezing your buttocks and lifting your hips while pressing your heels into the floor. Continue lifting your pelvis until your body forms a long line from your shoulders to your feet. Without allowing your pelvis to drop, raise your right leg straight up. Slowly lower your leg to the floor, and switch to the left leg. Continue alternating legs for the desired repetitions.

Upward Plank Hip Lift

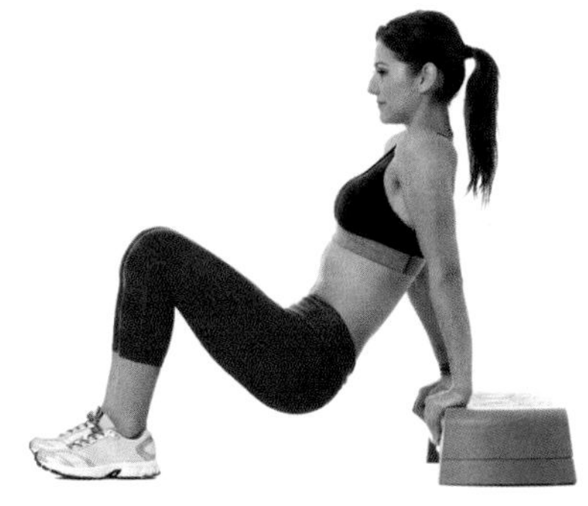

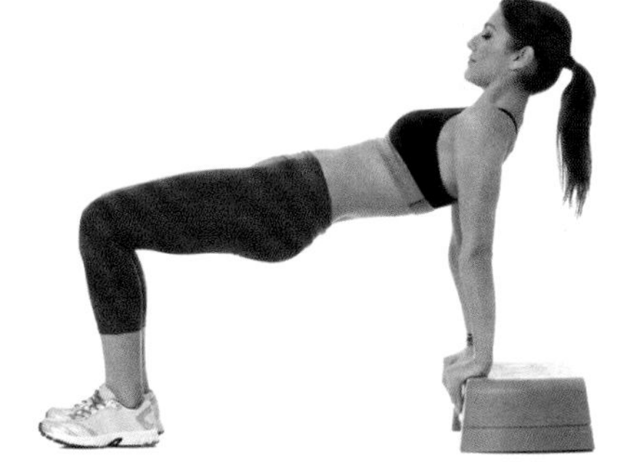

Place an aerobic step behind, and then sit with your legs parallel and stretched out in front of you. Place your hands on the step behind you with your fingers pointed toward your hips. Lift your hips slightly so that your butt is a few inches above the floor. This is your starting position. Press up through your arms, and lift your chest up, squeezing your buttocks and lifting your hips while pressing your heels into the floor. Continue lifting your pelvis until your body forms a long line from your shoulders to your feet. Pause, and then lower yourself back to the starting position, and then repeat for the desired repetitions.

301

Upward Plank March

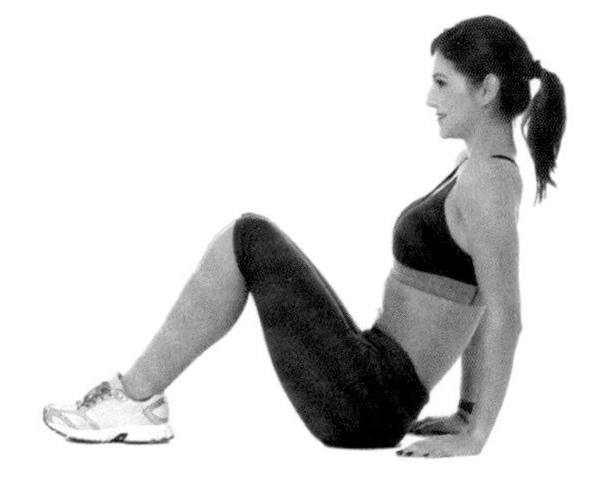

Perform you would the Upward Plank Kick (#299), but instead of keeping your leg straight, bend it to a 90-degree angle. Alternate lifting and lowering your knees as if you were marching, using a 4-count rhythm to keep a steady pace. Continue marching for the desired time or repetitions.

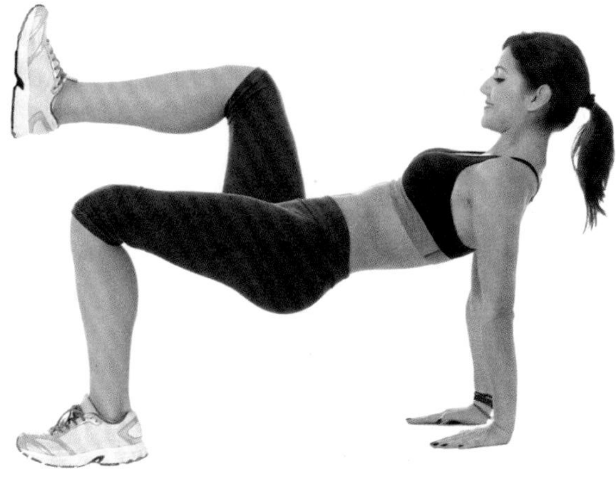

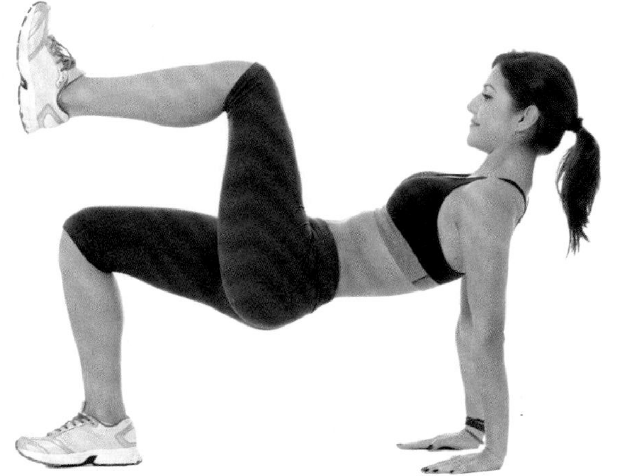

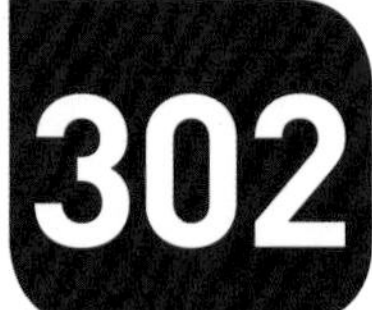

302 Forearm Plank

The Forearm Plank is an isometric, or contracted, exercise, designed to work your entire core. There are many versions of the plank, and they are performed everywhere from yoga and Pilates studios to hard-core gyms for a good reason: it is a reliable way to build endurance in your abs and back, as well as in the core stabilizer muscles.

- Lie on your stomach, with your legs extended behind you. Bend your arms so that your forearms rest flat on the floor. Keep your palms flat or make fists.
- Bend your knees, supporting your weight between your knees and your forearms, and then push through with your forearms to bring your shoulders up toward the ceiling as you straighten your legs.
- With control, lower your shoulders until you feel them coming together at your back. Hold for the desired time.

trapezius
infraspinatus
supraspinatus
teres minor
subscapularis
rhomboideus
erector spinae

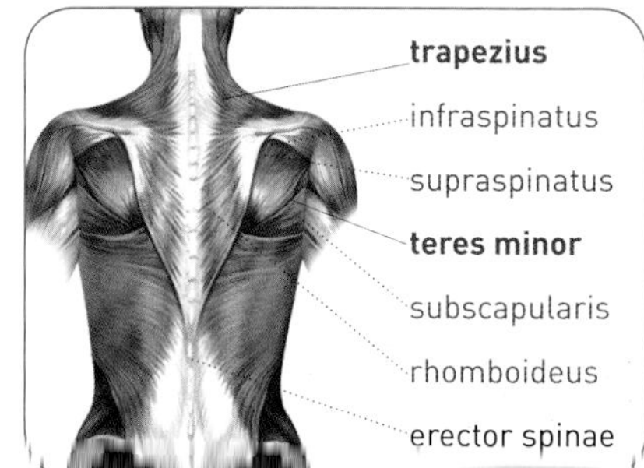

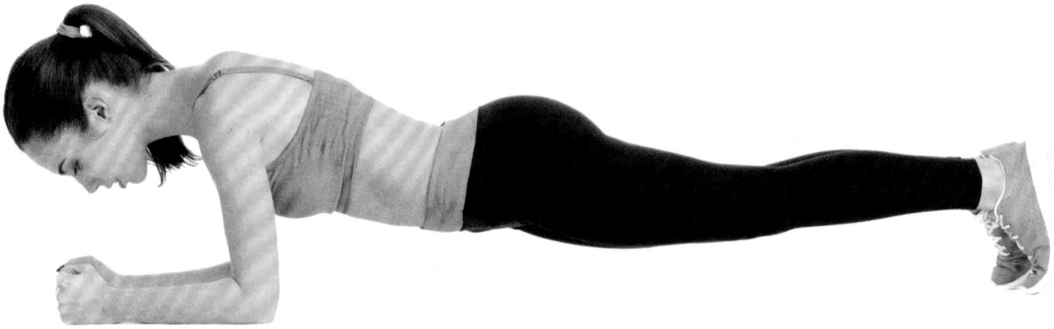

➔ FIND YOUR FORM
Fully engage your abs so that your butt doesn't rise or sink.

MUSCLE ANNOTATION KEY
— **Black bold = primary**
⋯ Black = deep primary
— Gray bold = secondary
⋯ Gray = deep secondary

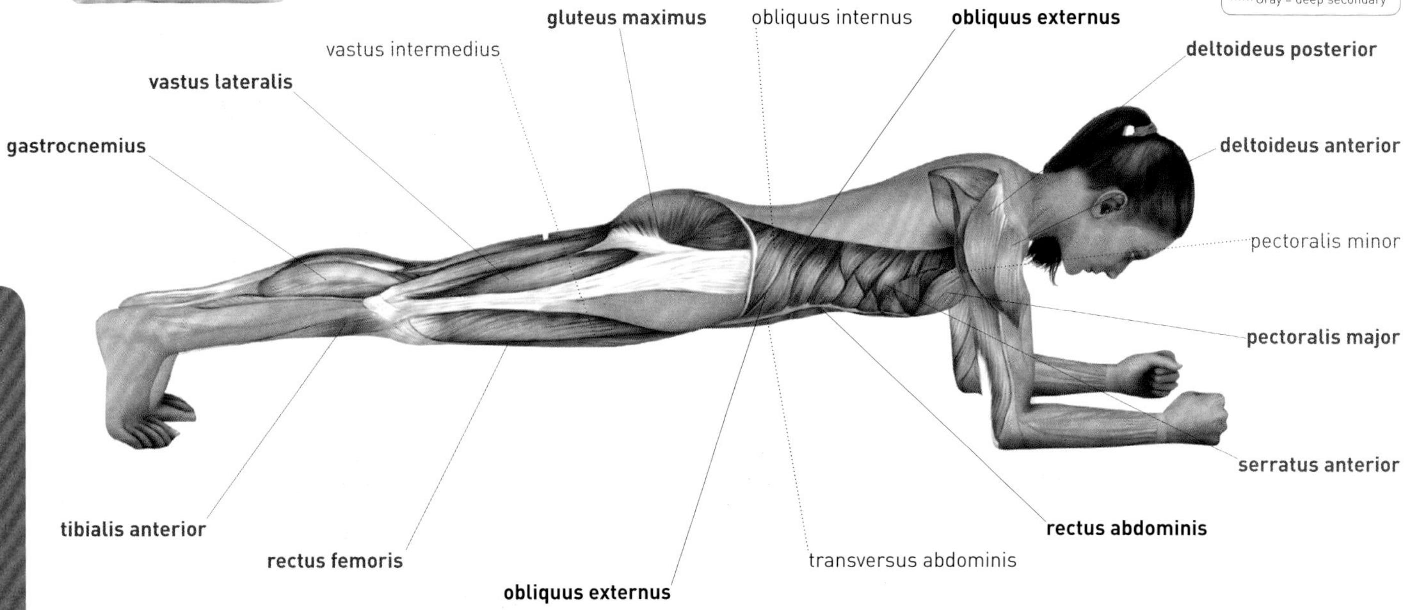

gluteus maximus
obliquus internus
obliquus externus
vastus intermedius
vastus lateralis
deltoideus posterior
gastrocnemius
deltoideus anterior
pectoralis minor
pectoralis major
serratus anterior
tibialis anterior
rectus abdominis
rectus femoris
transversus abdominis
obliquus externus

303 Forearm Plank Leg Extension

Assume the Forearm Plank position (#302), and then lift and lower your legs one at a time. Keep the rest of your body still, and your abs engaged throughout.

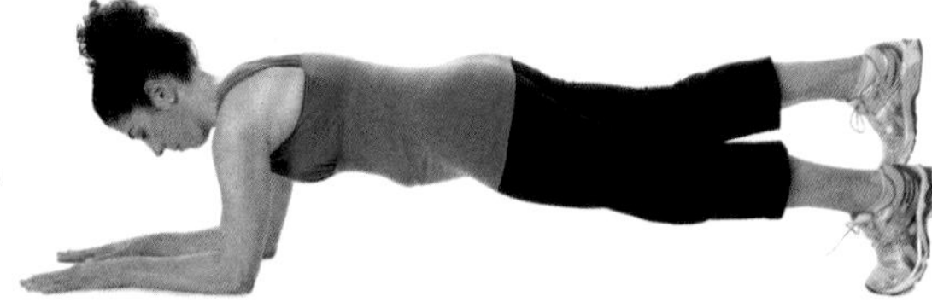

304 Forearm Plank Knee Drops

Assume the Forearm Plank position (#302), and keeping your hips level and parallel to the floor, flex your right knee toward the floor as you inhale, and extend it again as you exhale. Alternate sides for the desired repetitions.

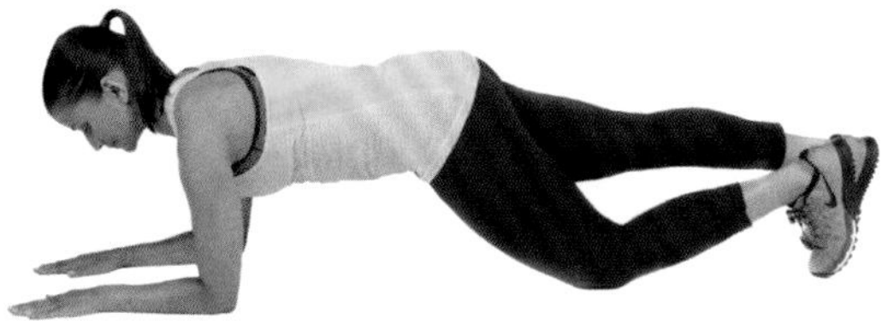

305 Chaturanga

From the High Plank position (#314) open your chest, and broaden your shoulder blades while tucking in your tailbone. With your legs turned slightly inward, lower yourself to the floor until your upper arms are parallel to your spine. Tuck your tailbone under, and draw your abdominals in toward your spine to maintain the straight line from your shoulders to your heels.

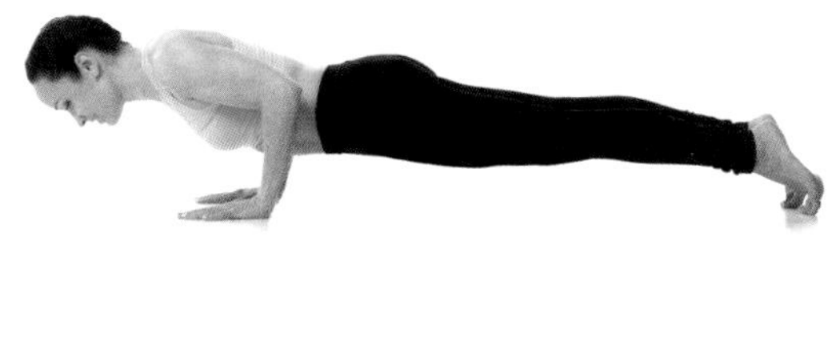

306 Suspended Forearm Plank

Face away from the anchor point, place your toes in the foot cradles, and assume a tabletop position with your hands under your shoulders, your forearms flat on the floor. Keeping a tight core, press your feet into the foot cradles and lift up into a plank position. Continue as long as you can maintain a perfect plank.

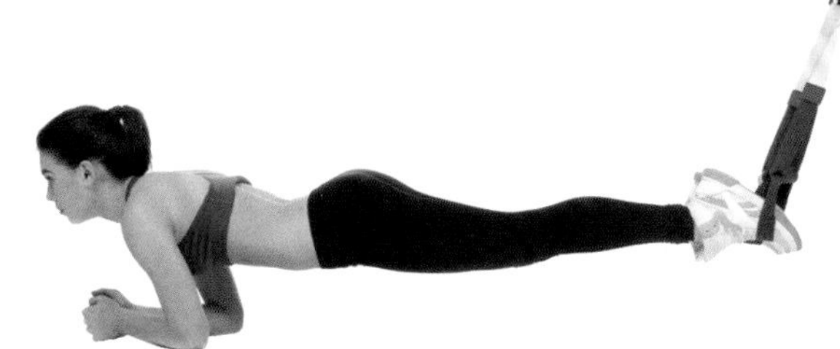

307 Spiderman Plank

Assume the Forearm Plank position (#302). Keeping your body in a straight line, bring your right knee to your right elbow. Hold, return to the starting position, and then repeat with the left leg. Continue alternating legs for as long as you can while maintain proper form.

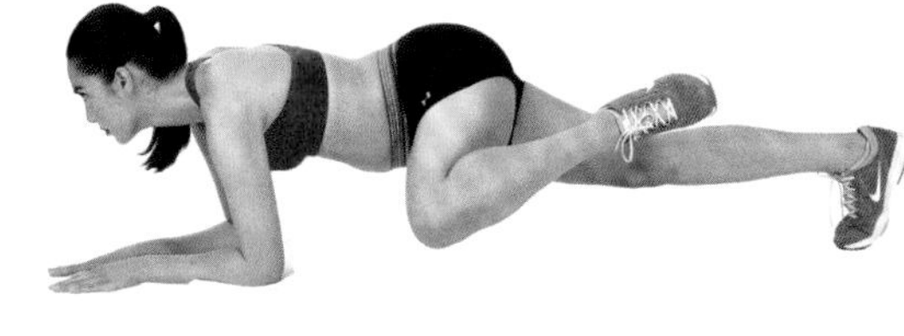

308 Arm-Reach Plank

Assume the Forearm Plank position (#302). Engage your abdominals, and lift your right arm off the floor. Hold for the desired time, and then release to return to the starting position. Switch arms and repeat.

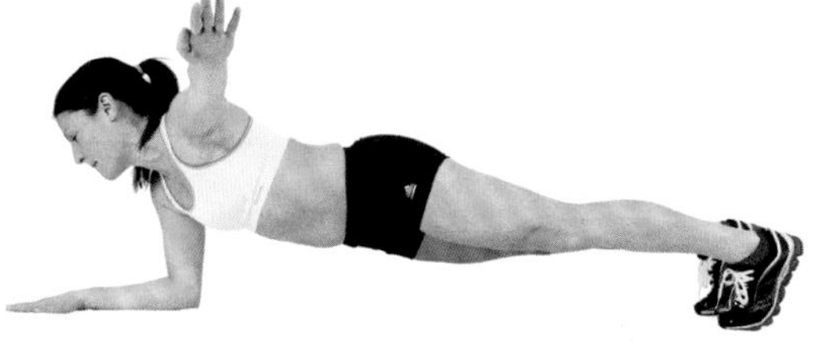

309 Plank-Up

Assume the Forearm Plank position (#302), and then lift up with your right arm until it is fully extended, and then straighten your left arm until you are balanced on both arms in a High Plank (#314). Reverse one arm at a time, lowering from the planted hand to forearm until back in the initial Forearm Plank. Repeat for the desired repetitions, trying to maintain a steady rhythm as you move from one arm to the other.

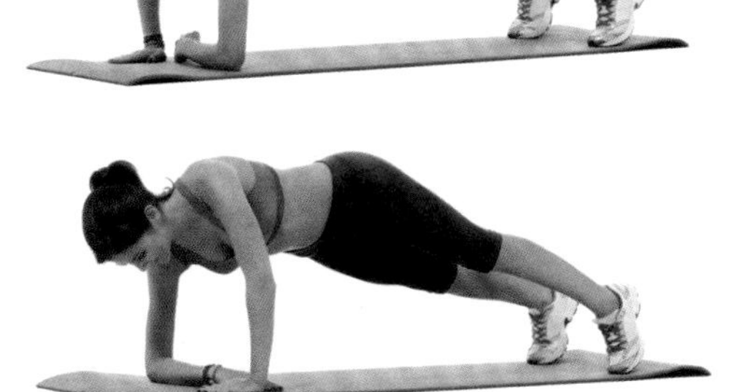

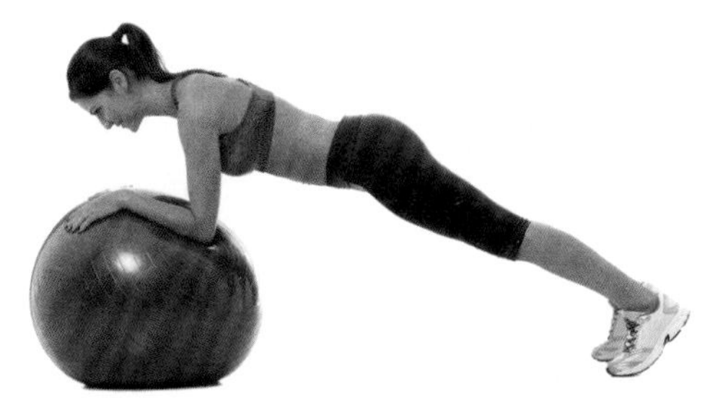

310 Swiss Ball Forearm Plank

Position yourself on your toes with your arms bent and forearms resting on top of a Swiss ball. Form a long, straight line from your ankles to your shoulders. Hold this position for as long as you can.

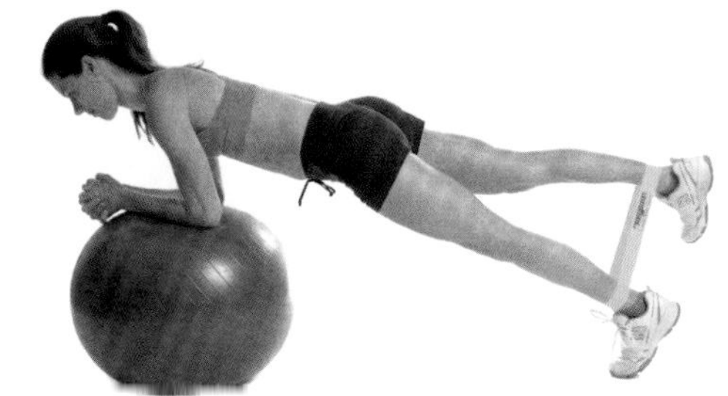

311 Swiss Ball Loop Extension

With a resistance loop or a resistance band tied around your ankles, assume the Forearm Plank position (#302) with your arms propped on a Swiss ball. Keeping your abs tight, exhale, and squeeze your glutes to raise your right leg, lengthening your body as your weight transfers from your arms to your left foot. Return your right foot to the floor. Repeat for the desired reps, switch legs, and repeat on the other side.

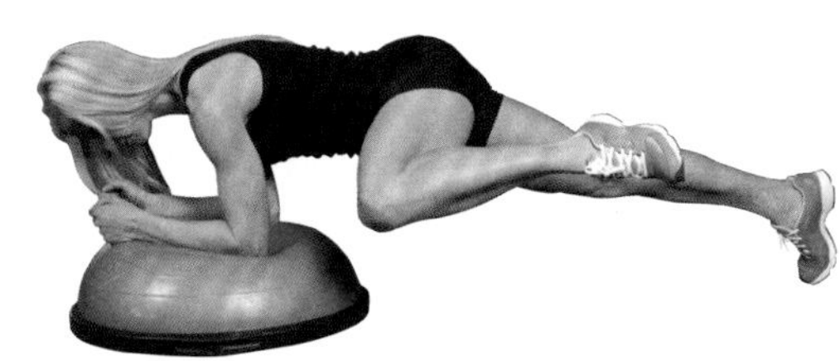

312 BOSU Spiderman Plank

Assume the Forearm Plank position (#302) with your arms propped on the dome side of a BOSU. While keeping your body in a straight line, bring your right knee to your right elbow. Hold for one second, return to the starting position, and repeat with the left leg. Continue alternating legs for as long as you can while maintaining proper form.

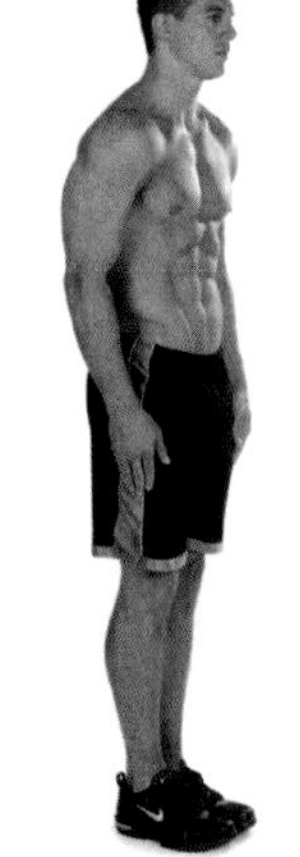

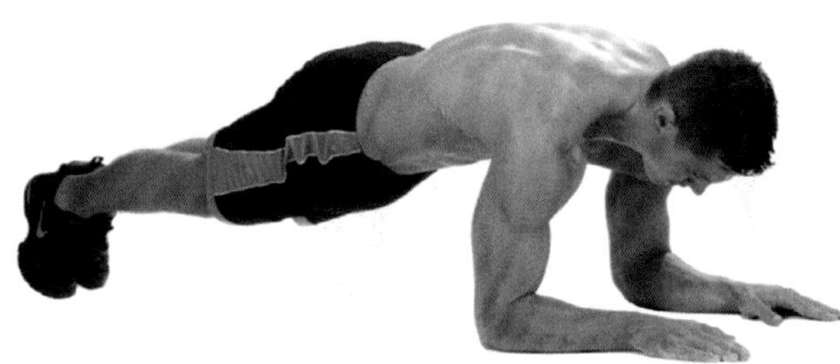

313 Forearm Plank Roll-Down

Stand tall with your weight equally distributed between your feet. Bend from your waist to place your hands flat on the floor in front of your feet. Walk your hands away from your feet until your body reaches the Forearm Plank position (#302), forming a straight line from your shoulders to your heels. Keeping your arms straight, dip your shoulders three times. Walk your hands back to your feet, and return to an upright position. Perform the desired reps at a rapid pace.

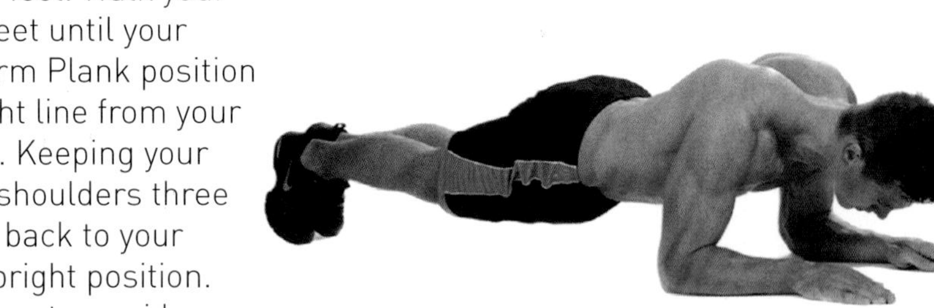

314 High Plank

The High Plank is the same as a push-up's "drop" starting position—you prop your elongated body on your extended legs and straight arms. Like the drop position, it is the launching point for numerous power exercises, and in yoga, the High Plank is a base position from which you move into many other poses.

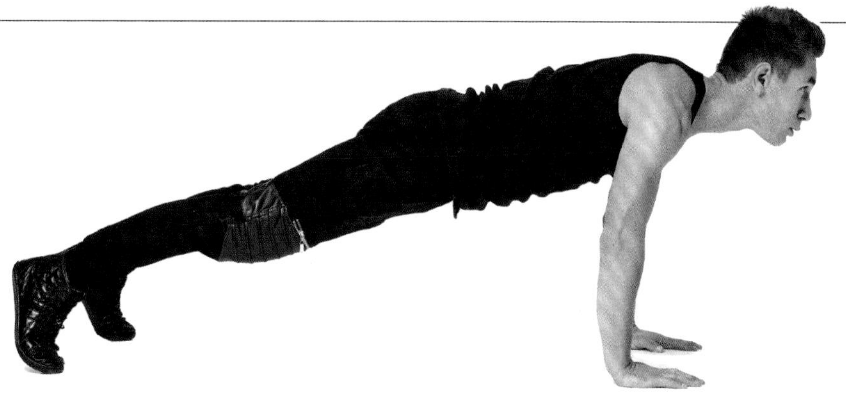

- With your hands shoulder-width apart, place your palms on the floor, keeping your feet together and back straight.
- Push your body up until your arms are straight. Hold for the desired time.

315 High Plank with Leg Extension

Assume the High Plank position (#314), with your shoulders directly over your hands, your torso straight. Lift your left leg straight toward the ceiling. Return to the High Plank, and repeat with the other leg.

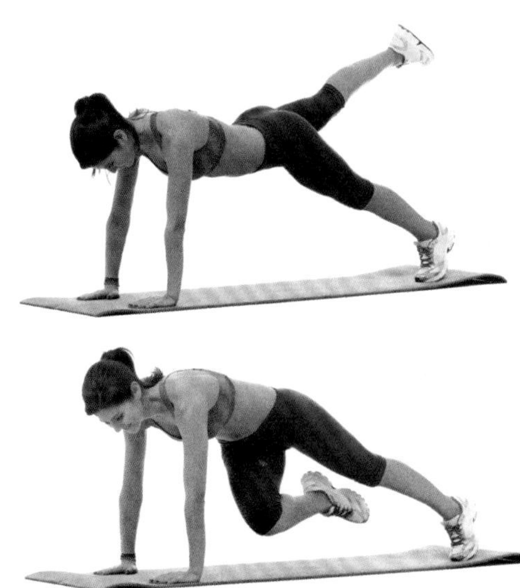

316 High Plank Knee Pull-In

Assume the High Plank position (#314), with your shoulders directly over your hands, your torso straight. Draw your left leg upward toward your chest. Return to the High Plank, and repeat with the other leg.

317 Plank Roll-Down

Perform as your would a Forearm Plank Roll-Down (#313), walking your hands out to the High Plank position (#314), rather than the Forearm Plank.

318 High Plank Knee Pull-In with Extension

Assume the High Plank position (#314), with your shoulders directly over your hands, your torso straight. Draw your left knee into your chest, flexing the foot while rocking your body forward over your hands. You should come up on the toes of your right foot. Extend your left knee backward, rocking the body back, and shifting your weight onto your heel. With your head in between your hands, straighten your right leg and lift it toward the ceiling.

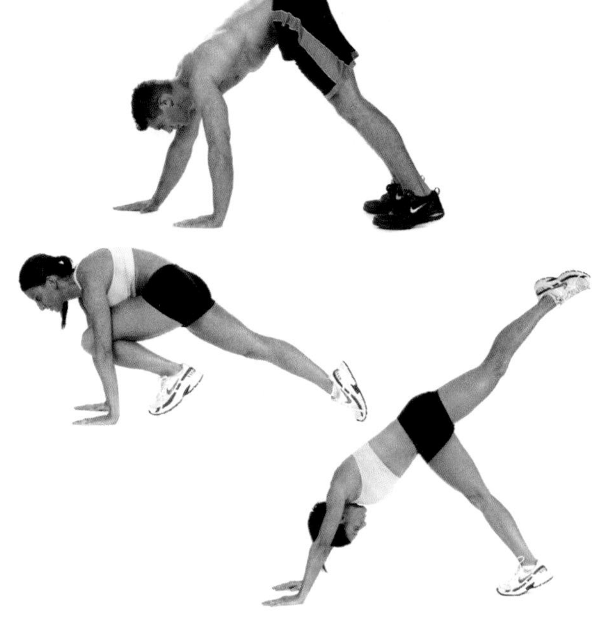

319 Swiss Ball Shin Plank

This version of a plank on a Swiss ball is slightly easier than a forearm version. The Swiss Ball Shin Plank is still an effective exercise, helping to stabilize and strengthen your core, back, shoulders, and chest muscles. It also forms the foundation of many other plank moves, preparing you for higher intensity exercises.

- Kneel on your hands and knee with a Swiss ball behind you. Raise your legs to rest your shins and ankles on the ball.
- Push the ball back to lift and straighten your knees until your body forms a straight line from shoulders to feet.
- Hold this position for as long as possible, while still maintaining good form.

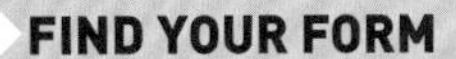

FIND YOUR FORM

To challenge yourself, prop as little of your legs on the ball as possible—the more of your legs which are supported on the ball, this exercise will be.

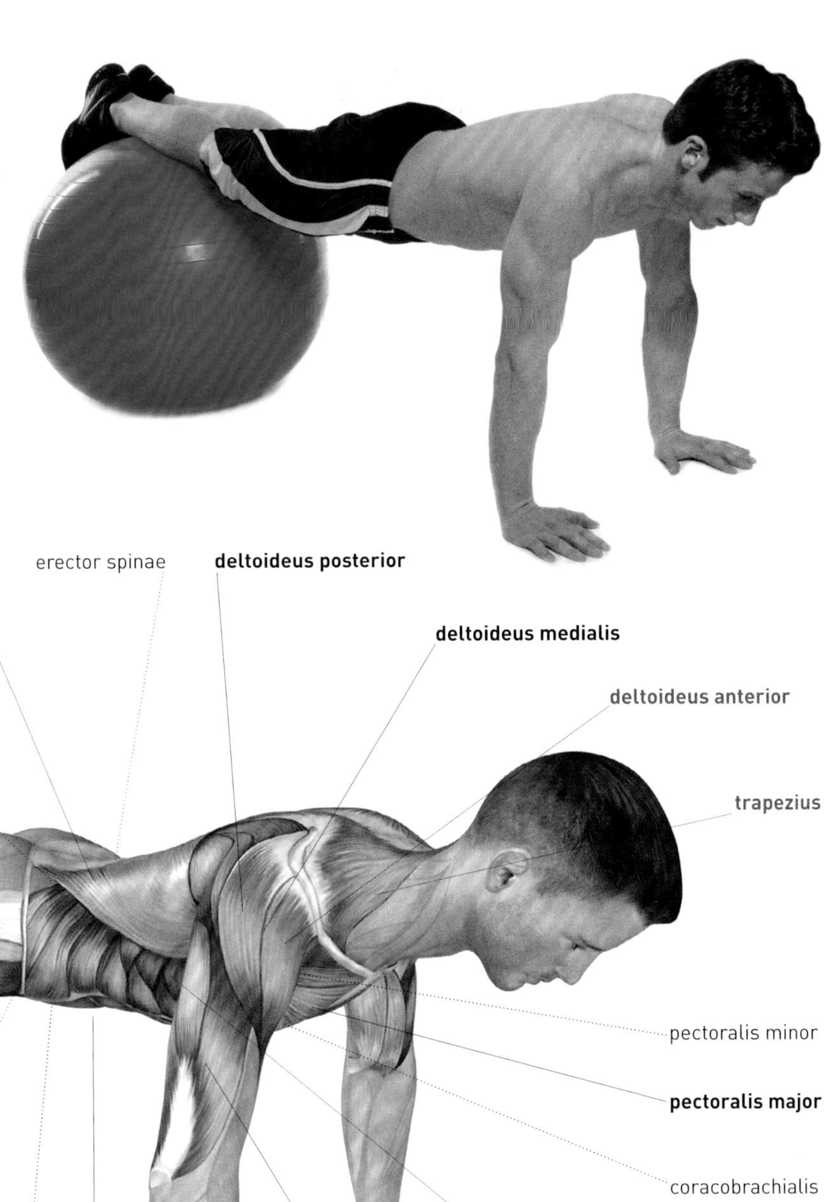

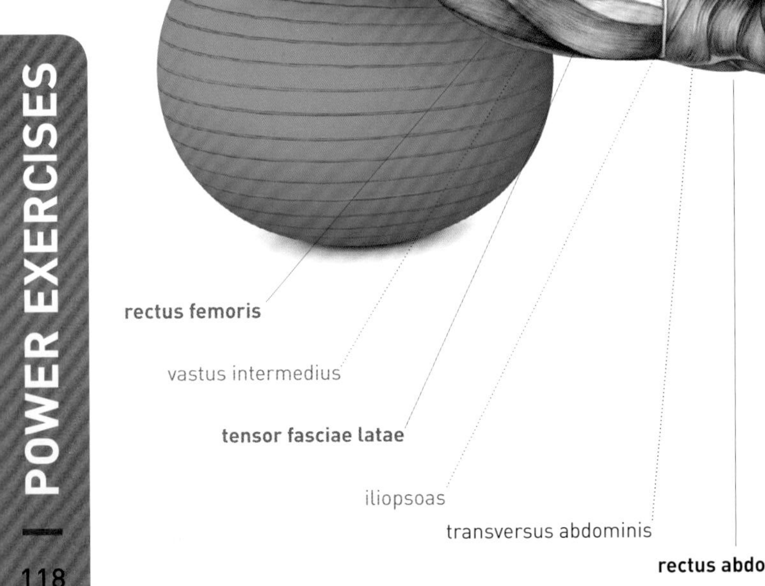

320 Swiss Ball Hand Walk-Around

Assume the Swiss Ball Shin Plank Position (#319), and then lift, reach, and place your left hand to the side, followed by the right hand, as you "walk" in a circle. Rotate 90 degrees to your left, or a quarter turn, and then hand walk back to the starting position. Repeat the entire sequence, moving to the right.

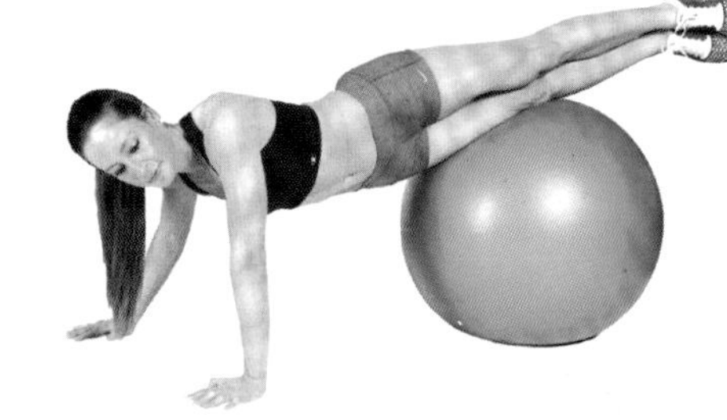

321 Swiss Ball Skier

Lie prone on a Swiss ball, and move forward until your thighs are resting on the top of the ball. While maintaining your core position, rotate your trunk quickly to the left so that your legs are stacked on top of each other. Return to the starting position, and perform the same movement to the right.

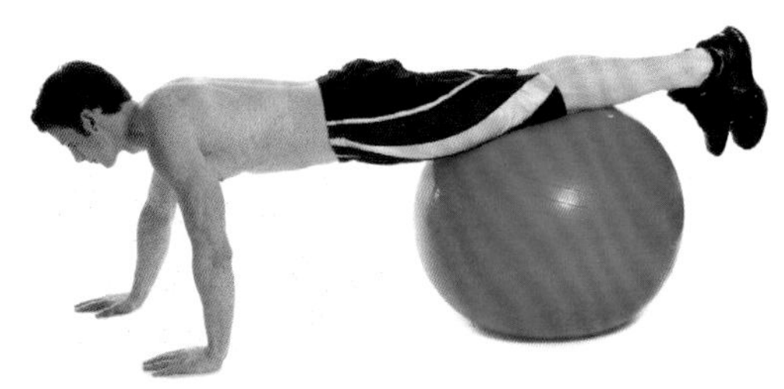

322 Swiss Ball Hand Walkout

Lie prone on a Swiss ball, with your hips over the center of the ball as you support your weight on your arms. Your hands should be directly below your shoulders. Lift, reach, and place your left hand forward and then your right, rolling the ball underneath you until it reaches your feet.

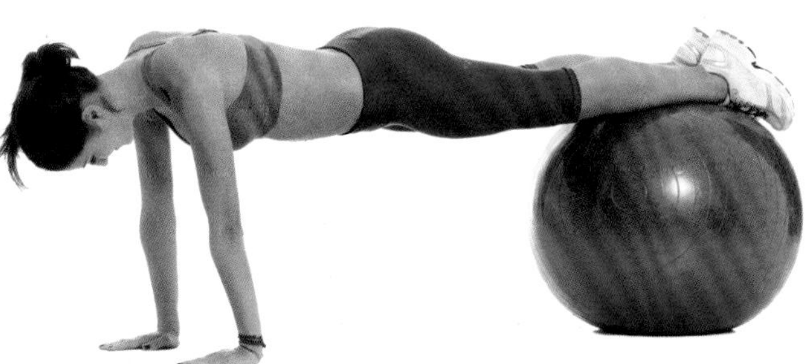

323 Swiss Ball Plank with In-Out

Assume the Swiss Ball Shin Plank Position (#319), and then extend your right leg to the side and downward off the ball. Return your leg to the ball, and then repeat on the other side.

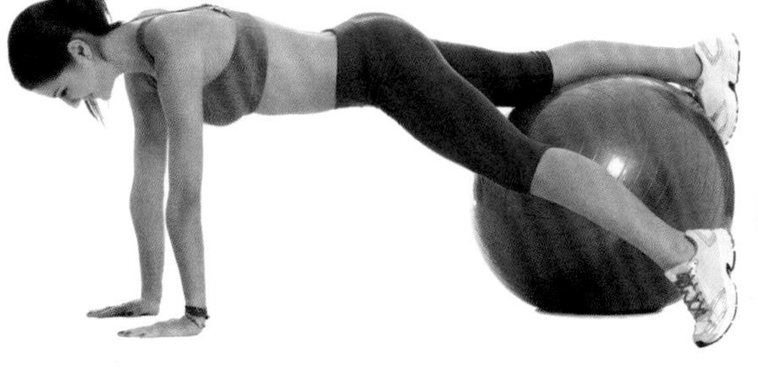

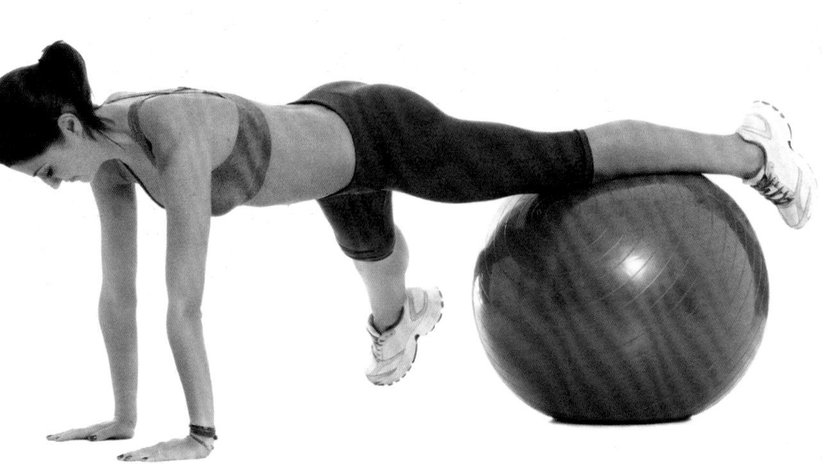

324 Side Plank

The Side Plank is a superb move to tone your midsection while shoring up the strength of your lower back. To get the most of this exercise, aim to hold it with flawless form for at least a minute—and then repeat for three sets on both sides. Once you have mastered this strategy, add in one of its many variations to your core-training drills.

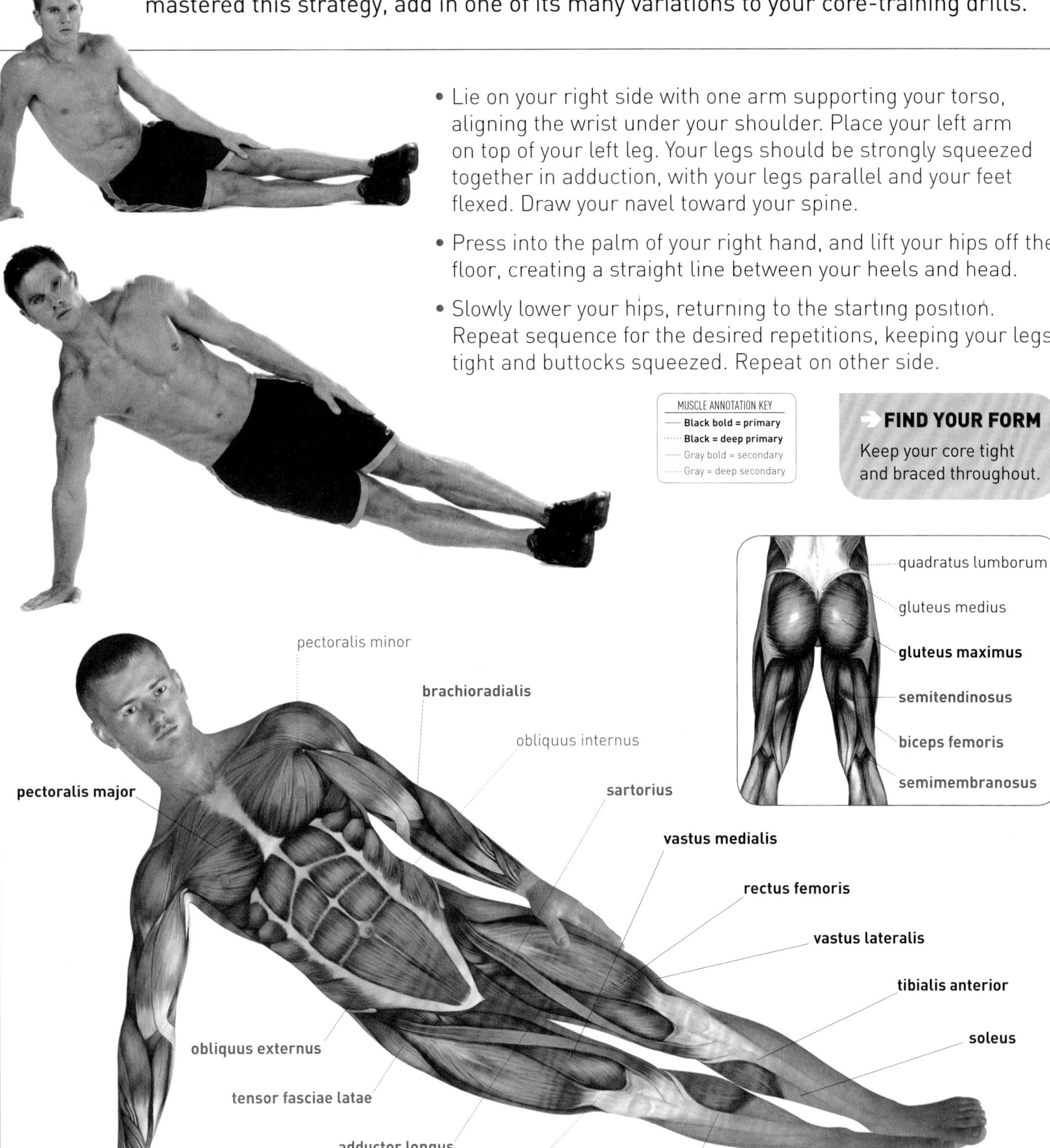

- Lie on your right side with one arm supporting your torso, aligning the wrist under your shoulder. Place your left arm on top of your left leg. Your legs should be strongly squeezed together in adduction, with your legs parallel and your feet flexed. Draw your navel toward your spine.
- Press into the palm of your right hand, and lift your hips off the floor, creating a straight line between your heels and head.
- Slowly lower your hips, returning to the starting position. Repeat sequence for the desired repetitions, keeping your legs tight and buttocks squeezed. Repeat on other side.

MUSCLE ANNOTATION KEY

- **Black bold = primary**
- Black = deep primary
- Gray bold = secondary
- Gray = deep secondary

FIND YOUR FORM

Keep your core tight and braced throughout.

325

Forearm Side Plank

Lie on your right side with your arm bent so that your are resting on your forearm, supporting your torso. Pressing your left forearm into the floor, raise your hips off the floor until your body forms a long, straight line. Slowly lower your hips, returning to the starting position. Repeat sequence for the desired repetitions, keeping your legs tight and buttocks squeezed. Repeat on other side.

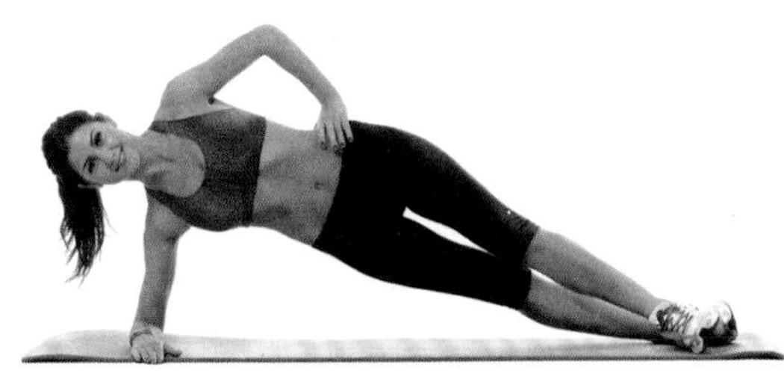

326

Forearm Side Plank with Hip Raise on Aerobic Step

With your feet propped on a step, perform a Forearm Side Plank (#325). Repeat on other side.

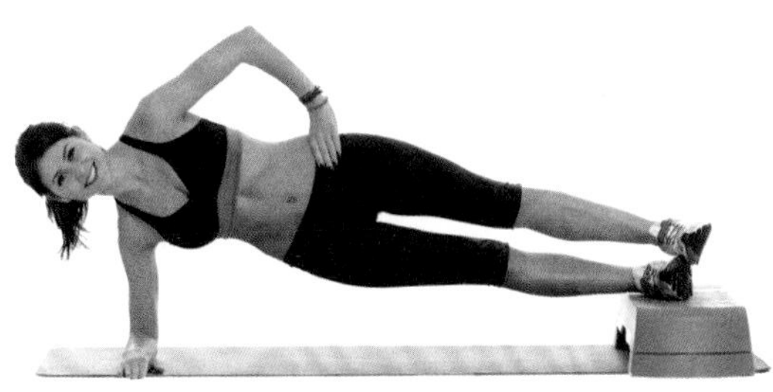

327

Forearm Side Plank with Knee Tuck

Perform as you would a Forearm Side Plank (#325), and bend your top knee to a 90-desgree angle, and lift it toward your chest. Repeat on other side.

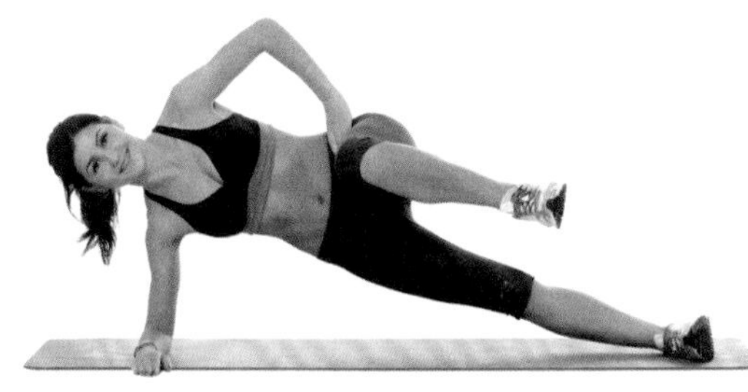

328

Forearm Side Plank with Toe Touch

Perform as you would a Forearm Side Plank (#325), and then extend your bottom leg upward as you extend your top arm to touch your fingers to your toes. Repeat on other side.

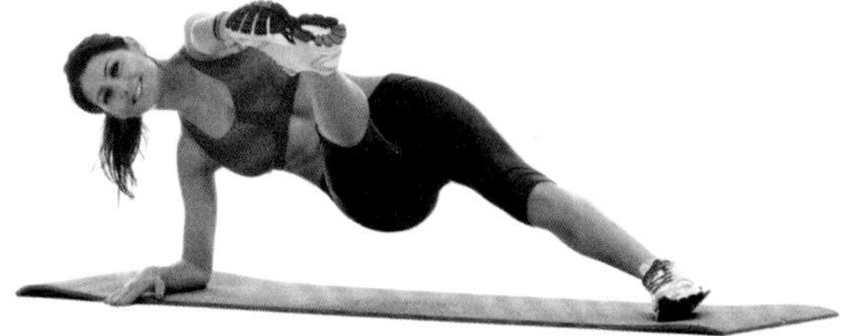

329

Side-Bend Lift

Lie on your right side with your right hand behind your hand and extend your left arm along the side of your body. Keeping your feet together, lift both legs upward. Repeat on the other side.

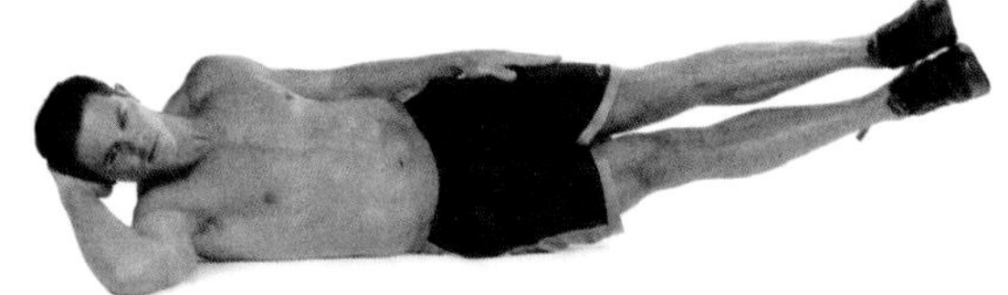

330

Lying Abduction

Lie on your right side with your arm bent so that your are resting on your forearm, supporting your torso. Extend your left arm along the side of your body, a dumbbell in your hand. Maintaining the position of the rest of your body, smoothly raise your top leg. Lower to the starting position. Repeat for the desired repetitions, and then repeat on the other side.

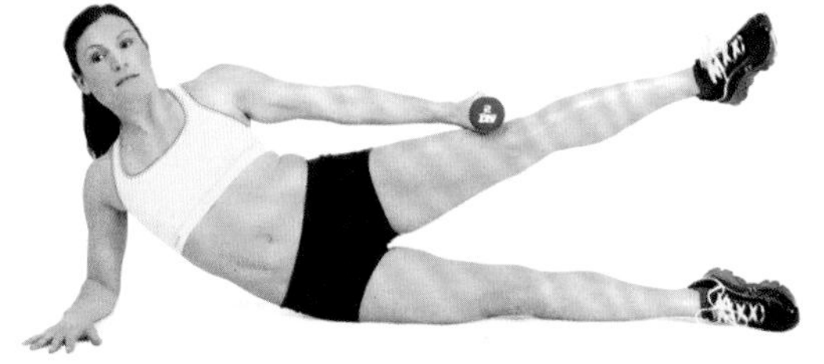

331

Lying Abduction into Side Plank

Perform as you Lying Abduction (#330), but when you return to the starting position, lift your hips to move into the Forearm Side Plank (#325). Lower to the starting position. Repeat on the other side.

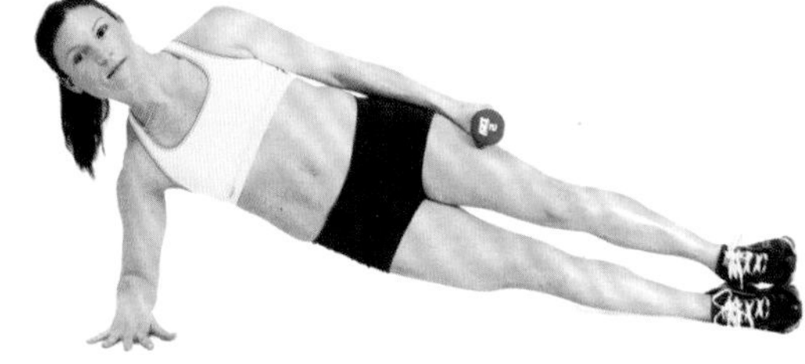

T-Stabilization

T-Stabilization is advanced variation of a High Plank exercise that effectively targets your abdominal, hip, lower-back, and oblique muscles. It also helps you work on improving your balance and coordination.

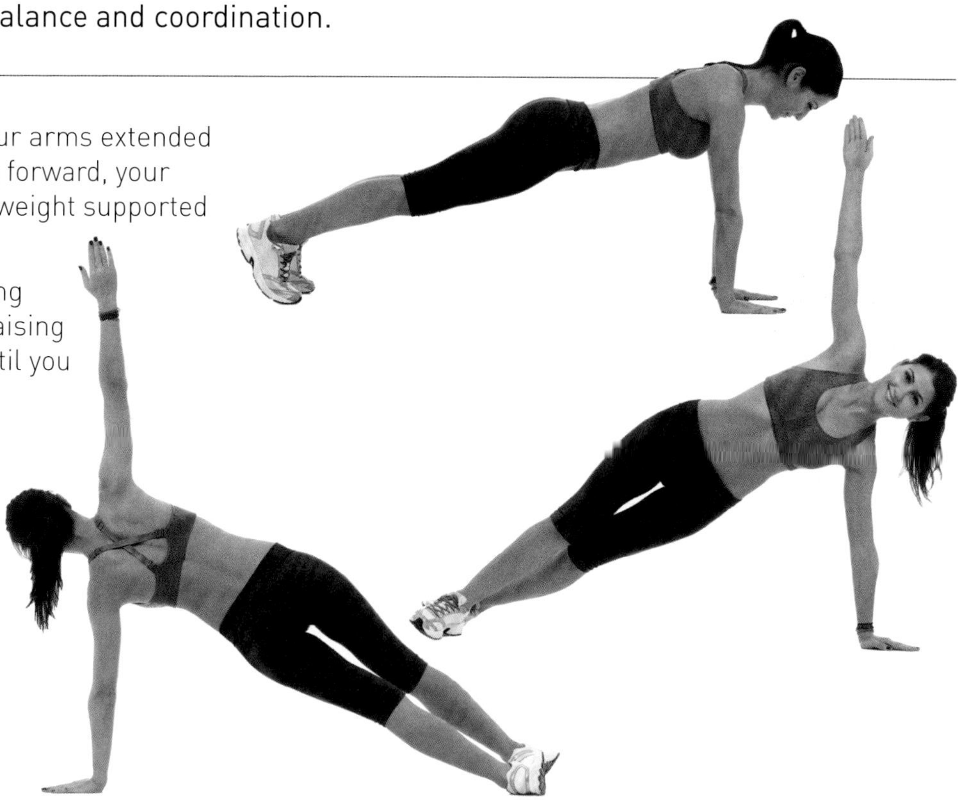

- Assume the drop position with your arms extended to full lockout, your fingers facing forward, your legs outstretched, and your body weight supported on your toes.
- Turn your hips to one side, stacking one foot on top of the other and raising your top arm across your body until you are pointing toward the ceiling.
- Hold for the desired time, lower, and then repeat on the other side to complete one rep.

FIND YOUR FORM

Engage your core, keeping your body in one straight line and avoiding arching or bridging your back.

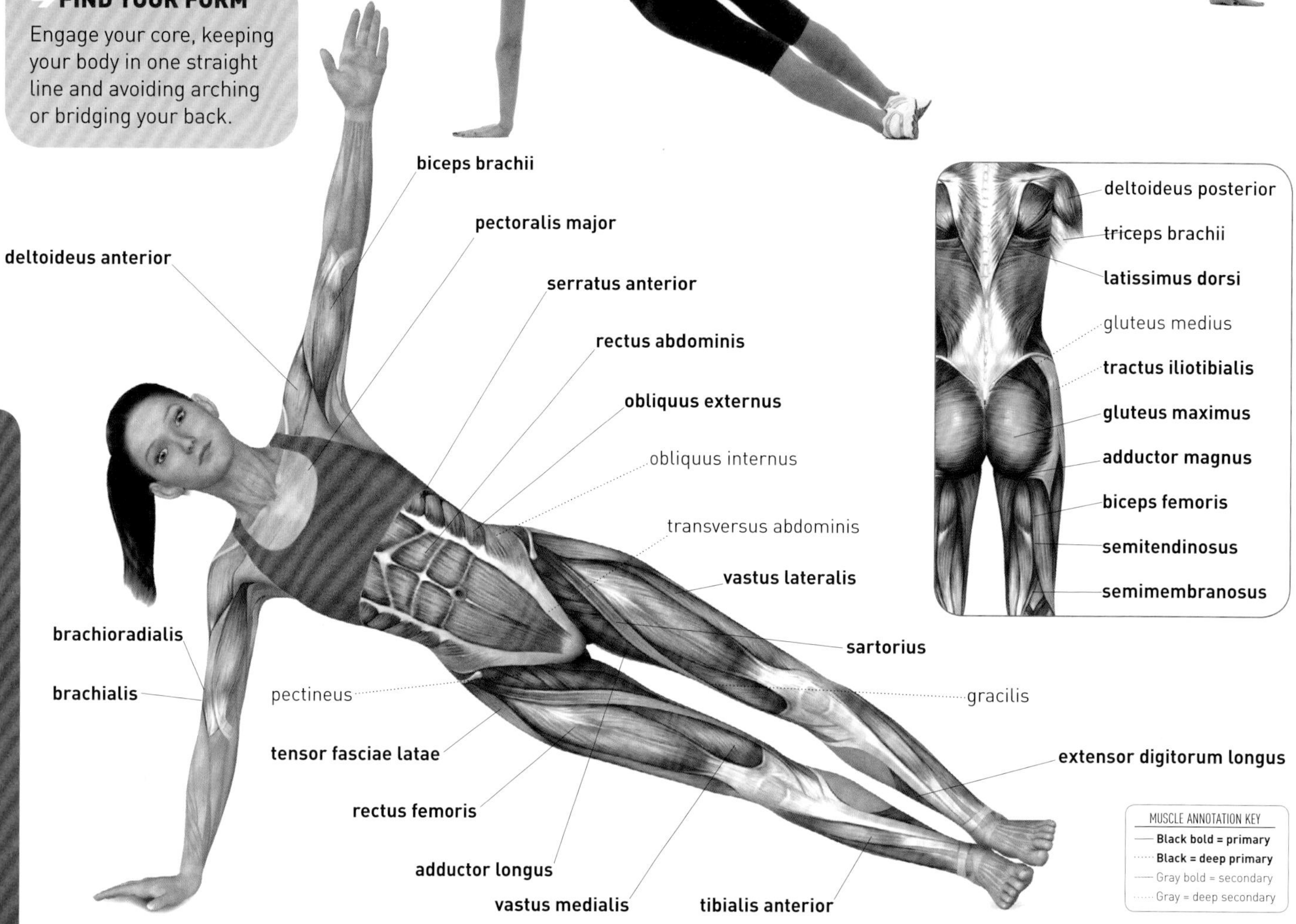

biceps brachii
pectoralis major
deltoideus anterior
serratus anterior
rectus abdominis
obliquus externus
obliquus internus
transversus abdominis
vastus lateralis
brachioradialis
sartorius
brachialis
pectineus
gracilis
tensor fasciae latae
extensor digitorum longus
rectus femoris
adductor longus
vastus medialis
tibialis anterior

deltoideus posterior
triceps brachii
latissimus dorsi
gluteus medius
tractus iliotibialis
gluteus maximus
adductor magnus
biceps femoris
semitendinosus
semimembranosus

MUSCLE ANNOTATION KEY
Black bold = primary
Black = deep primary
Gray bold = secondary
Gray = deep secondary

333 Suspended T-Stabilization

Face away from the anchor point, and place your toes in the foot cradles, and assume the drop position. Perform as you would the T-Stabilization (#332). Repeat on the other side.

334 Kneeling Forearm T-Stabilization

Assume the Forearm Side Plank position (#325). Pressing your forearm into the floor, raise your hips off the floor until your body forms a long, straight line. Repeat on the other side.

335 T-Stabilization with Leg Raise

Assume the Forearm Side Plank position (#325). Raise your top leg toward the ceiling while extending your top arm to reach for your toes. Repeat on the other side.

336 Plank with Rotation

Assume the drop position with your hands slightly wider than shoulder-width with both feet on one towel. Draw both knees upward while simultaneously rotating your hips and lower body until your ankles are rotated 90 degrees and both feet are stacked and pointing to one side. Extend your knees and hips, and rotate back. Repeat on the other side.

337 T-Stabilization Twist

Lie on your right side with your legs extended and pressed firmly together. Press your right hip into the floor. Position your right hand directly beneath your shoulder, and press your body upward until you form a straight line from shoulder to feet. Extend your left arm toward the ceiling, and then bring your left arm down and across your torso, rotating your upper body to the right. Return to the starting position, and then repeat the on the other side.

338 T-Stabilization with Reach-Under

Assume the Forearm Side Plank position (#325), propped on your left arm. Pressing your left forearm into the floor, raise your hips off the floor until your body forms a long, straight line. Twist your upper torso toward the floor as you reach your right arm under your chest as far as you can stretch. Twist your upper torso back to front as you extend your right arm toward the ceiling. Complete the desired repetitions, and then switch sides.

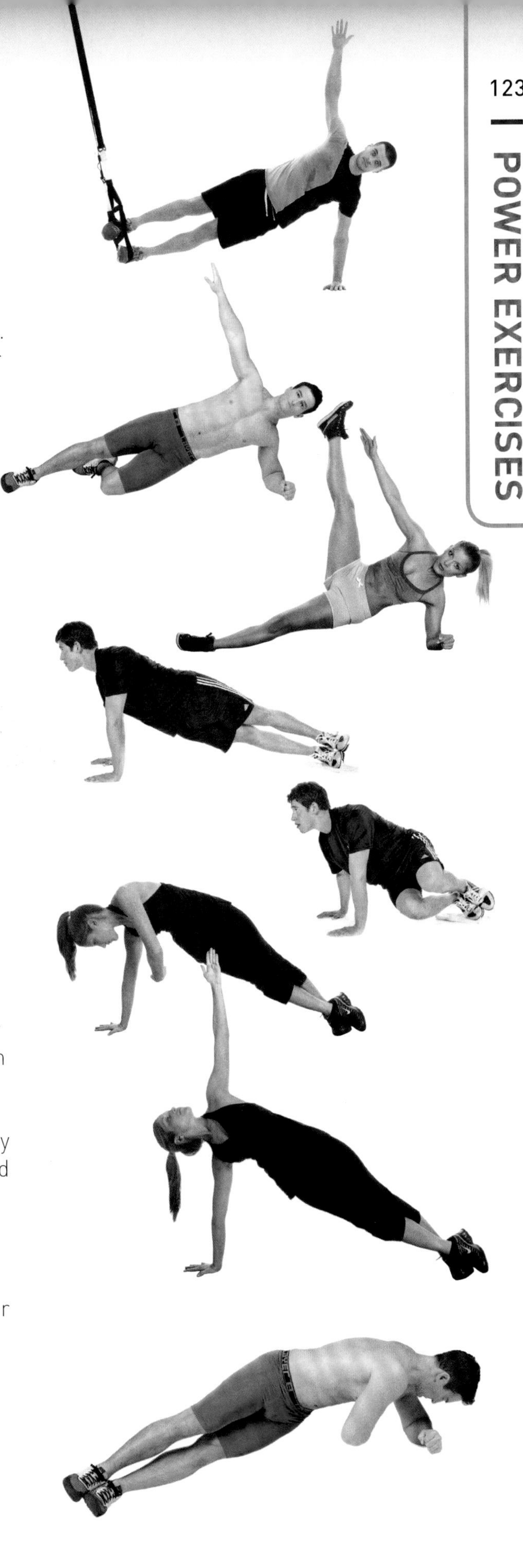

Kneeling Side Kick

To strengthen your glutes, the Kneeling Side Kick is a can't-miss exercise. It particularly targets the hard-to-work gluteus medius (the smallest of the gluteal muscles). Strong glutes are essential for balanced movement during high-intensity workouts.

- Kneel with your right hand on the floor directly below your shoulder, with the fingers pointing outward. Place your left hand behind your head.
- Lift your left leg to hip level and straighten it, reaching out of your heel. Keep your whole body aligned in one plane so that there is no rotation.
- Kick your left leg straight out in front of you, flexing your foot and trying not to move at your waist.
- Pull your left leg behind you, pointing your toes and keeping your leg at hip l. Repeat sequence for the desired reps, and then repeat with the other leg.

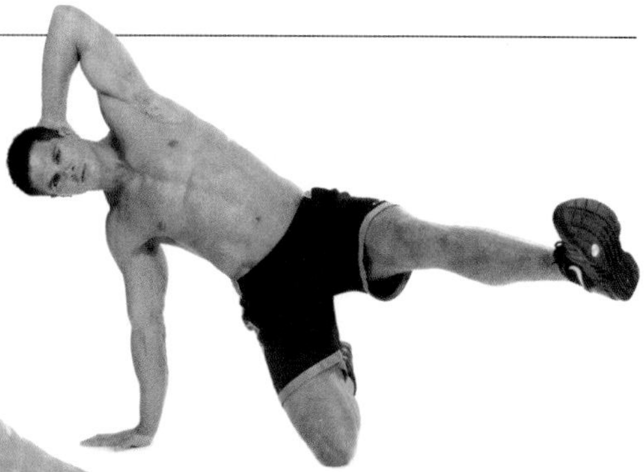

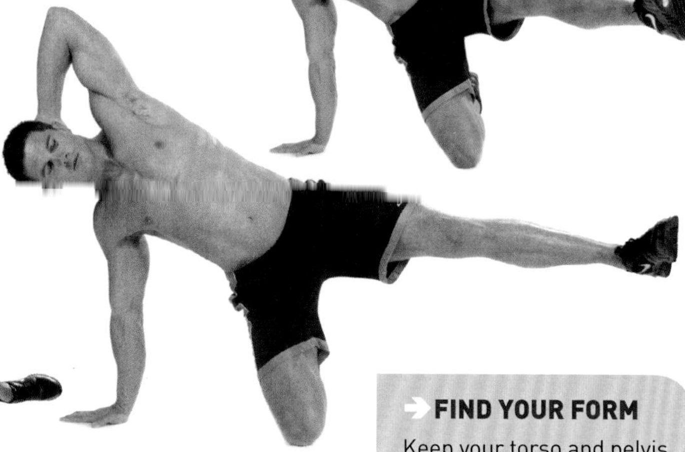

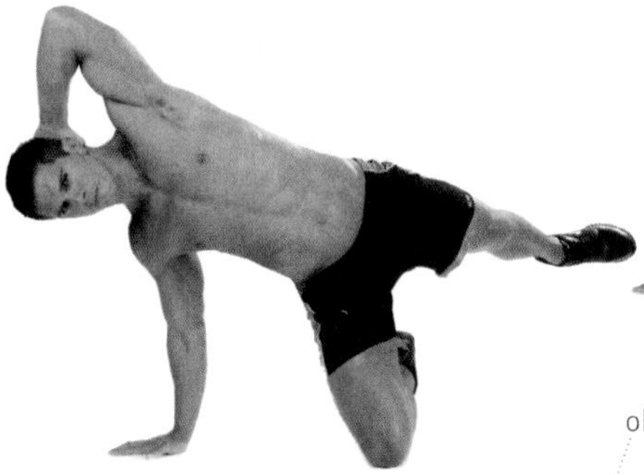

FIND YOUR FORM

Keep your torso and pelvis stable as your move your leg back and forth.

MUSCLE ANNOTATION KEY
- **Black bold = primary**
- Black = deep primary
- Gray bold = secondary
- Gray = deep secondary

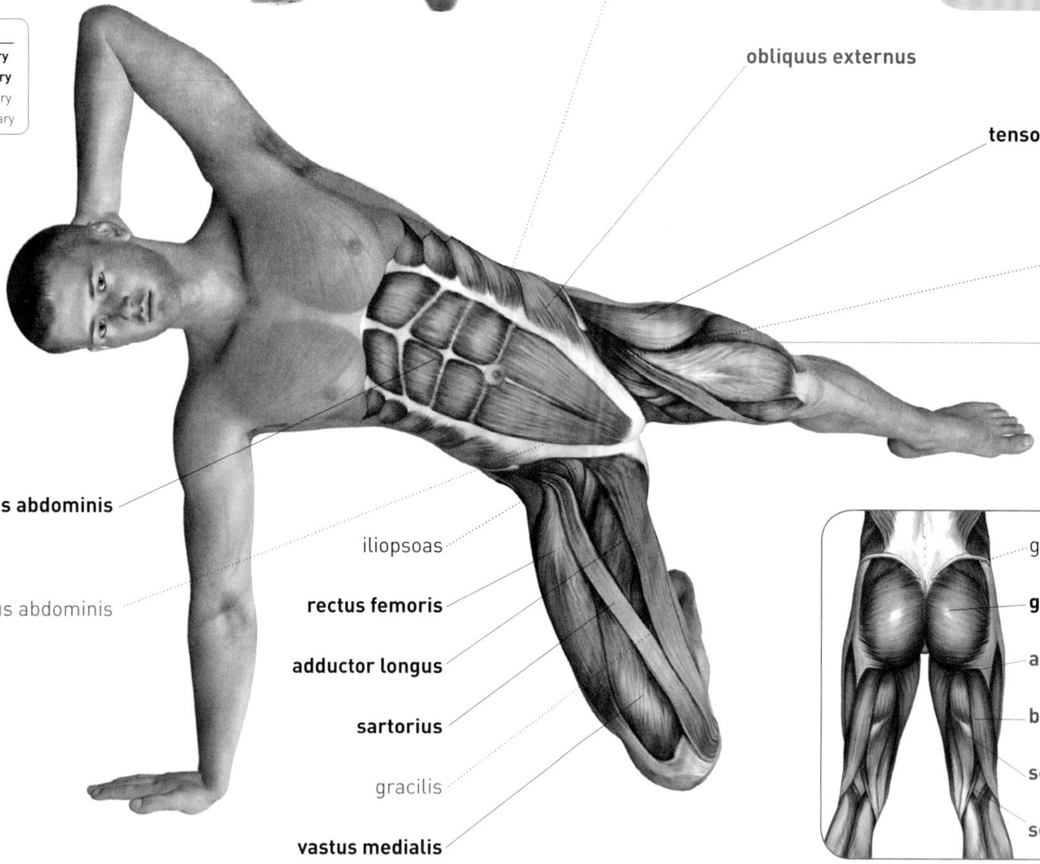

340 Swiss Ball Kneeling Side Lift

Prop your right arm on top of a Swiss ball, and place your left hand on your hip. Begin leaning your torso to the right, and then lift your left leg as high as you can while keeping it in line with your hips. Kick your left leg straight out in front of you, flexing your foot and trying not to move at your waist. Pull your left leg behind you, pointing your toes and keeping your leg at hip height. Repeat sequence for the desired reps, and then repeat with the other leg.

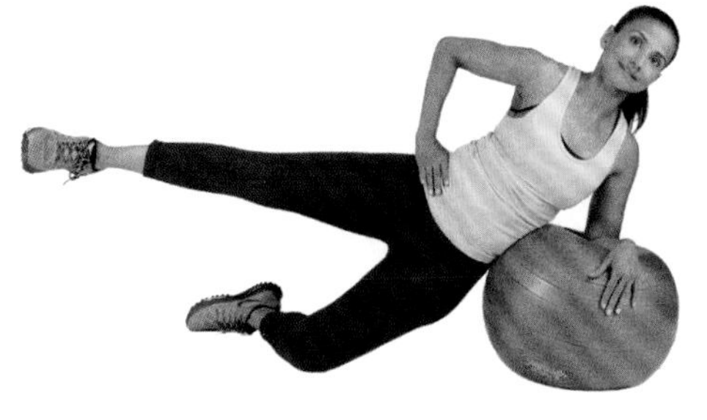

341 Kneeling Side Raise

Kneel on the floor and balance on your left knee with your left hand on the floor directly under your left shoulder. Extend your right leg out to the side, with your toes touching floor and your right fingertips behind head. Keeping your right leg straight, kick it forward at hip height, flex your right foot, hold it for a second. Repeat sequence for the desired reps, and then repeat with the other leg.

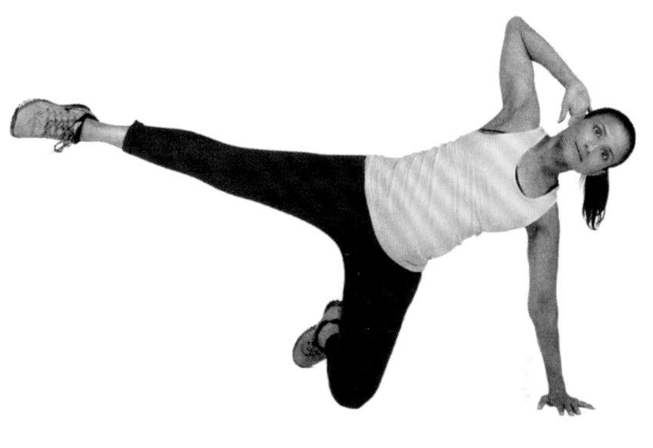

342 Kneeling Side Circles

Kneel on the floor with your right leg outstretched to the side and your left leg lined up under your hips. Place your left palm or fingertips on the floor, and arch your arm over your head. Lift your right leg, and begin making small circles, gradually increasing to larger, sweeping circles. Perform the desired reps, switch sides, and repeat on the other leg.

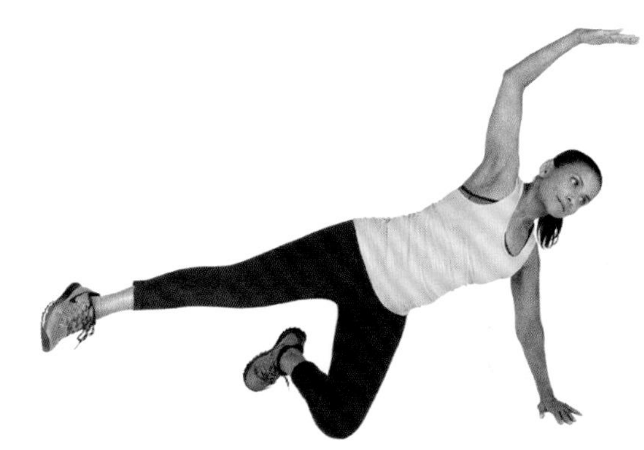

343 Kneeling Side Lift

Kneel on the floor with your right leg outstretched to the side and your left leg lined up under your hips. Place both hands behind your head, with your elbows extended out to the sides. Begin leaning your torso to the left, and then lift your right leg as high as you can while keeping it in line with your hips. Perform the desired reps,switch sides, and repeat on the other leg.

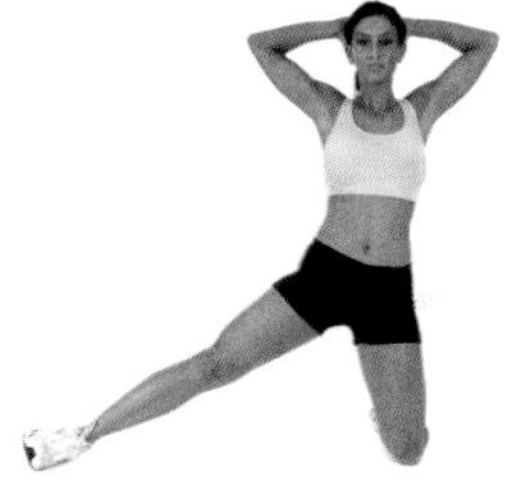

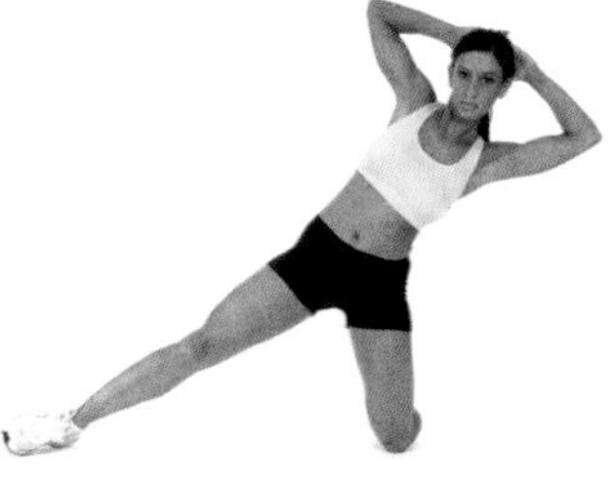

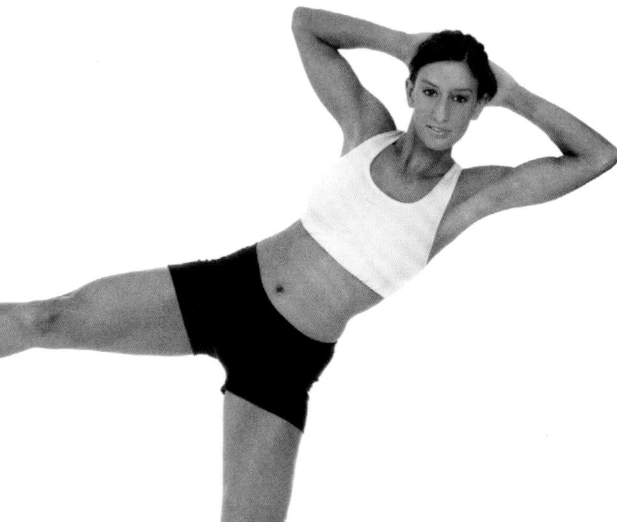

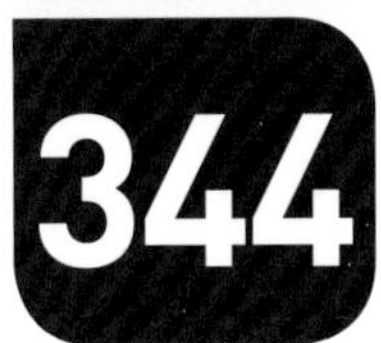

Swiss Ball Pike

Swiss Ball Pike is a demanding exercise—it requires balance, stability, and precision to complete with accuracy and proper form. It is a particularly effective core-strengthener that works the rectus abdominis, and it also targets your hip flexors, external obliques, and spinal erectors. In the starting position, your sense of balance comes into play, and as you raise your hips, the strength of your core muscles are greatly challenged. For best results, concentrate on keeping your movement smooth.

- Assume a drop position with your arms shoulder-width apart and your shins resting on a fitness ball.
- While keeping your legs straight, roll the ball toward your body while raising your hips as high as you are able. Lower, and repeat for the desired repetitions.

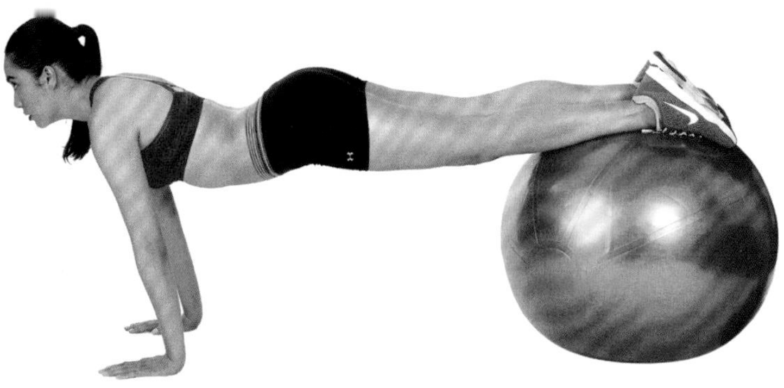

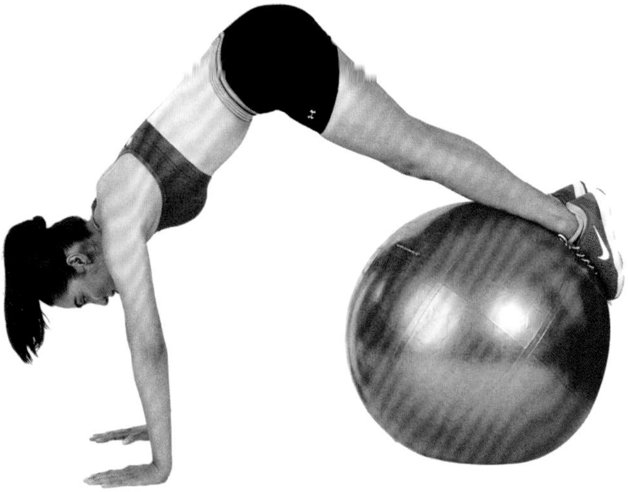

➔ FIND YOUR FORM

Position your hands so that they are directly below your shoulders.

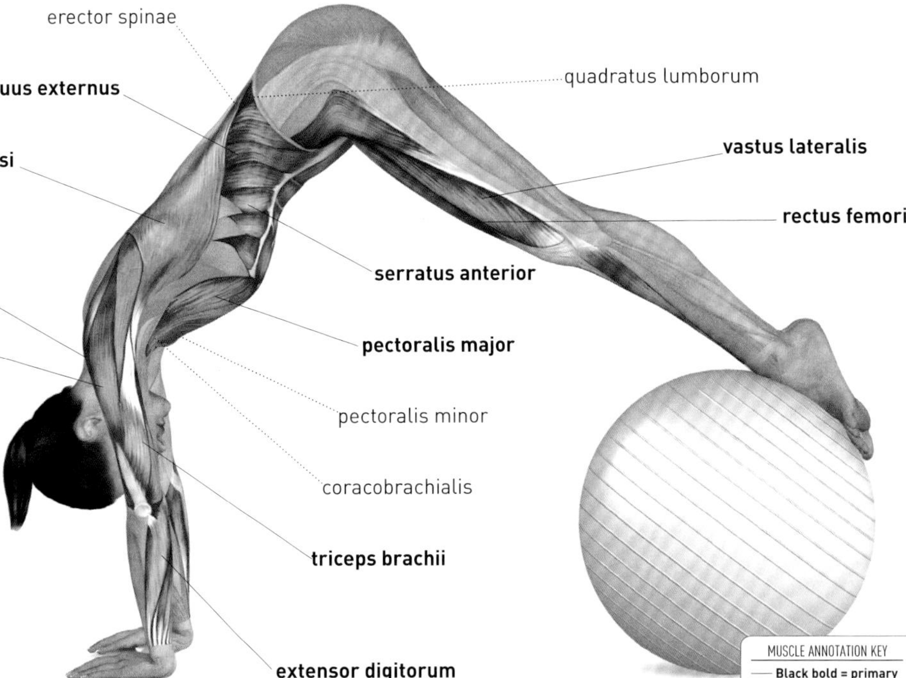

erector spinae
obliquus externus
quadratus lumborum
latissimus dorsi
vastus lateralis
rectus femoris
trapezius
serratus anterior
deltoideus anterior
pectoralis major
pectoralis minor
coracobrachialis
triceps brachii
extensor digitorum

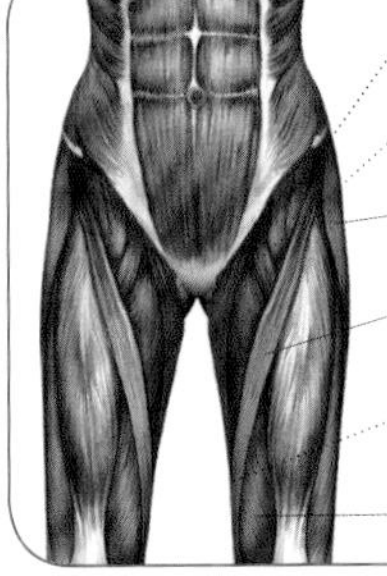

iliopsoas
pectineus
tensor fasciae latae
sartorius
gracilis
vastus medialis

MUSCLE ANNOTATION KEY
Black bold = primary
Black = deep primary
Gray bold = secondary
Gray = deep secondary

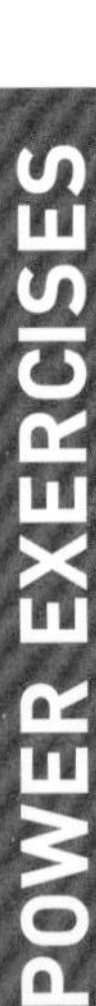

345

Pike

Start in a high plank position with the front of your body facing the floor in one long line with your weight on the balls of your feet. Keep your hands and feet solidly planted into the floor as you lift your hips toward the ceiling. Inhale in this inverted V position, extending your heels downward as you stretch your torso, arms and legs downward into your mat. Exhale as you return to the high plank position. Repeat for the desired repetitions and sets.

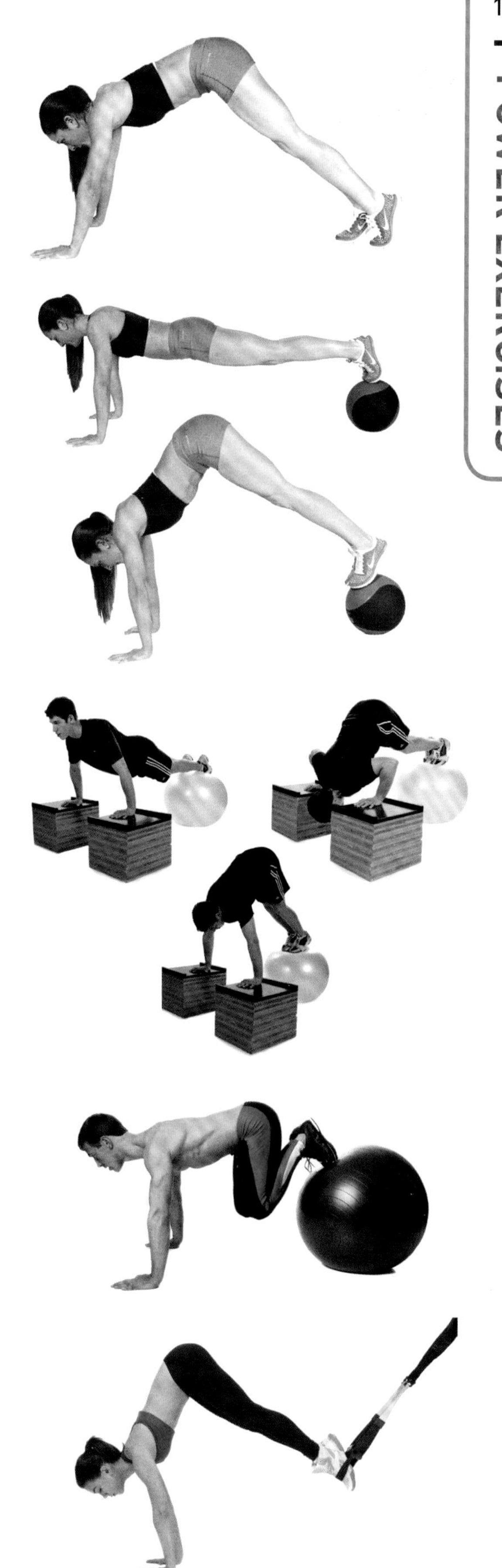

346

Medicine Ball Pike

Assume a drop position with your hands shoulder-width apart and your toes planted on a medicine ball. Raise your hips to the ceiling, rolling the medicine ball towards your hands as you do so. Reverse the movement, lowering yourself back down to the starting position. Repeat for the desired repetitions and sets.

347

Swiss Ball Pike and Press

Assume a drop position with your hands wider than shoulder-width apart on blocks (or a bench) and plant your toes on a Swiss ball. Raise your hips to the ceiling, rolling the ball toward your hands as you do so. Keeping your torso in that position, bend your elbows and drop your spine (head-first) between your hands. Return by pushing your hands into blocks until your elbows are fully extended. Then, drop hips and extend toes until body returns to horizontal. Repeat for the desired repetitions and sets.

348

Swiss Ball Jackknife

Assume a push-up position with your arms shoulder-width apart and your shins resting on a Swiss ball. Bend your knees, rolling the ball in toward your chest, keeping your arms straight the whole time. Extend your legs, and repeat for the desired repetitions and sets.

349

Suspended Pike

Kneel facing away from the anchor point with both feet in the foot cradles and place your hands under your shoulders. Lift your knees off the ground into plank position and raise your hips up, keeping legs straight. Lower your body back to plank position. Repeat for the desired repetitions and sets.

Plough

Known as Halasna in yoga, the Plough gets its name from the farming tool. It is an inverted forward-bending pose that challenges your flexibility and coordination. It also offers a thorough stretch from your shoulders and spine.

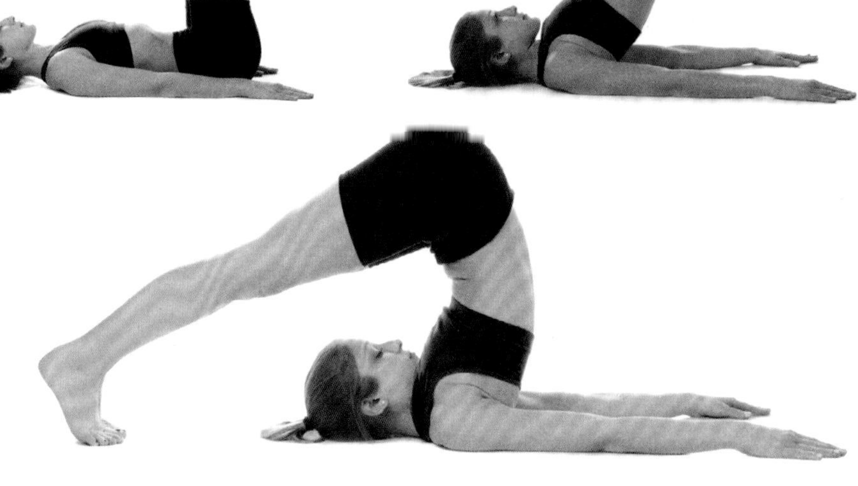

- Lie supine on the floor with your knees bent with your arms by your sides, your hands placed flat on the floor.
- Tighten your abdominals, and lift your knees off the floor. Exhale, press your arms into the floor, and lift your knees higher so that your buttocks and hips come off the floor.
- Continue lifting your knees toward your face, and roll your back off the mat from your hips to your shoulders. With your upper arms firmly planted on the floor, bend your elbows, and place your hands on your lower back. Draw your elbows in closer to your sides.
- Inhale, tuck your tailbone toward your pubis, and straighten your legs back toward your head until your torso is perpendicular to the floor.
- Exhale, and continue to extend you legs beyond your head. Squeeze your legs and bend at your waist until your toes touch the floor. Place your hands face down on the floor, pushing through your arms to maintain the lift in your hips. Hold for the desired time, and repeat.

FIND YOUR FORM

Avoid swinging your legs down quickly into the pose—move with precision and control. If the position feels hard on your neck, use a rolled-up blanket, foam pad, or other cushion to protect your vertebrae.

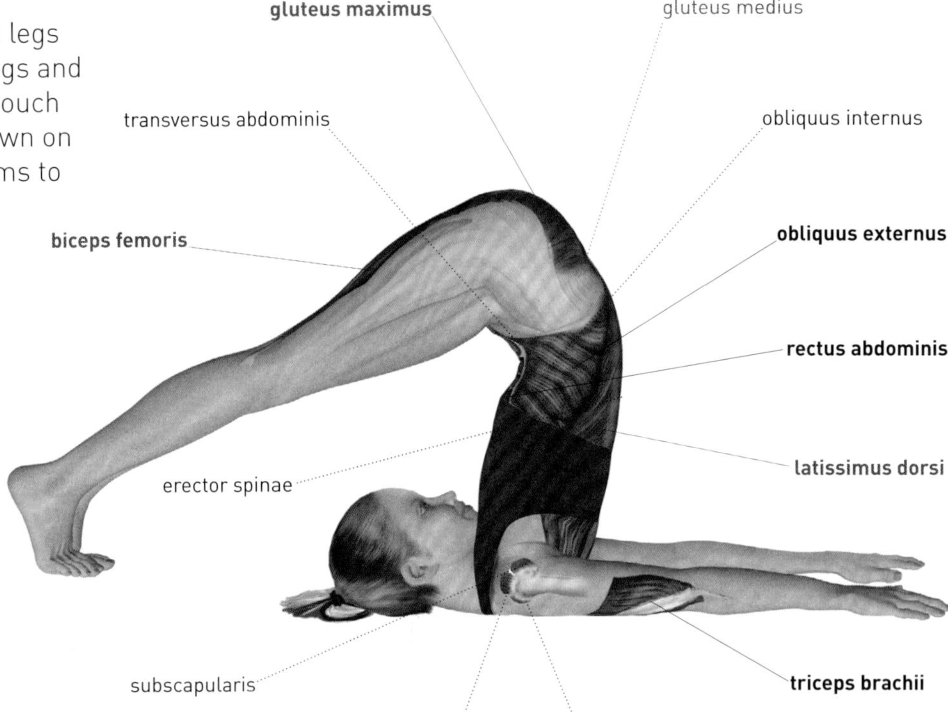

MUSCLE ANNOTATION KEY
Black bold = primary
Black = deep primary
Gray bold = secondary
Gray = deep secondary

Plough with Swiss Ball Adduction

Lie supine on the floor with your knees bent with your arms by your sides, your hands placed flat on the floor., grasping a Swiss ball between your feet. Perform as you would the Plough exercise (#350).

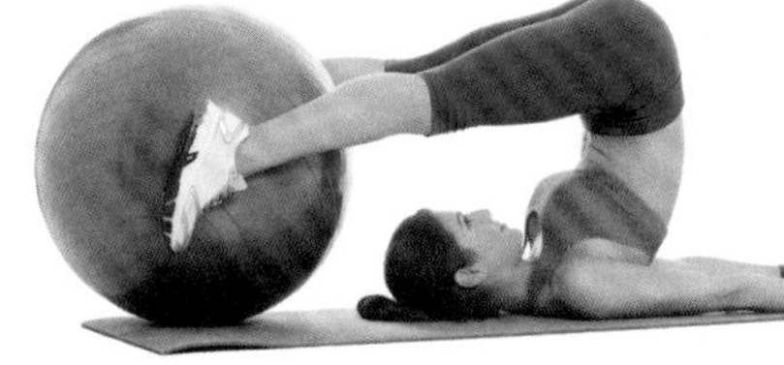

352 Swiss Ball Plough

Lie supine on the floor with your knees bent over a Swiss Ball, and then perform as you would the Plough exercise (#350).

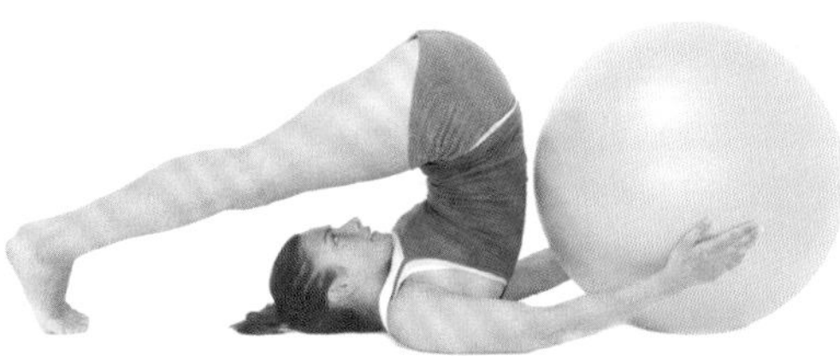

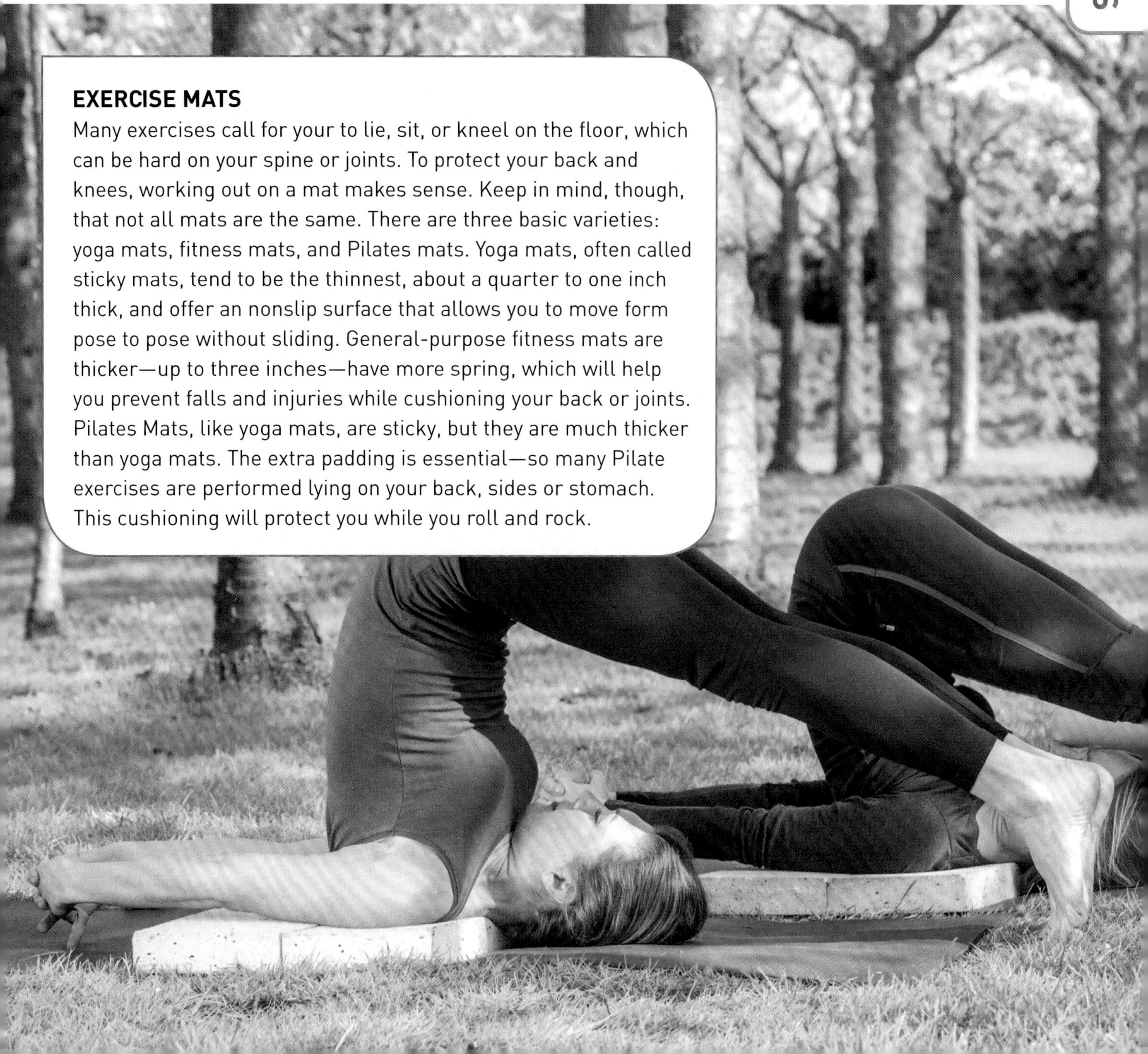

EXERCISE MATS

Many exercises call for your to lie, sit, or kneel on the floor, which can be hard on your spine or joints. To protect your back and knees, working out on a mat makes sense. Keep in mind, though, that not all mats are the same. There are three basic varieties: yoga mats, fitness mats, and Pilates mats. Yoga mats, often called sticky mats, tend to be the thinnest, about a quarter to one inch thick, and offer an nonslip surface that allows you to move form pose to pose without sliding. General-purpose fitness mats are thicker—up to three inches—have more spring, which will help you prevent falls and injuries while cushioning your back or joints. Pilates Mats, like yoga mats, are sticky, but they are much thicker than yoga mats. The extra padding is essential—so many Pilate exercises are performed lying on your back, sides or stomach. This cushioning will protect you while you roll and rock.

Bridge

The Bridge exercise functions as a core strengthener, a back bend, and enhances core stability. It is a great way to efficiently target your glutes and hamstrings. To perform the Bridge exercise correctly, you need to keep your body in proper alignment—your want to form a straight line from your shoulders to your knees. If you feel yourself sagging, lower to the starting position, and then try again.

- Lie on your back with your legs bent, your feet flat on the floor, and your arms extended on the floor, parallel to your body.
- Push through your heels while raising your pelvis until your torso is aligned with your thighs. Hold for the desired time, and then lower yourself back down.

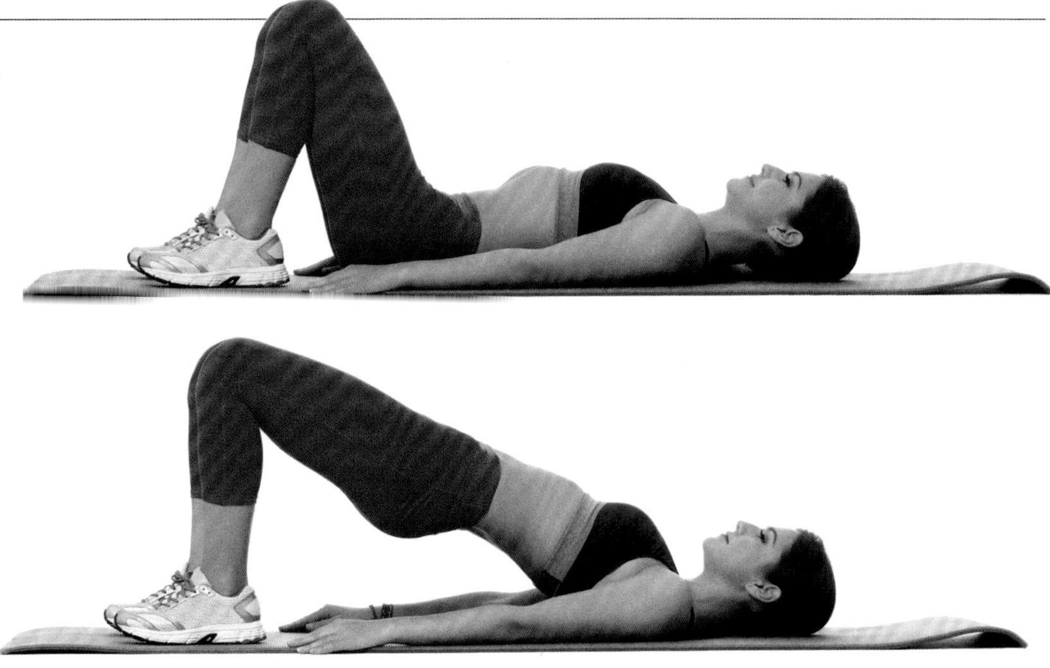

➔ FIND YOUR FORM

To fully engage your core, try to pull your navel back toward your spine.

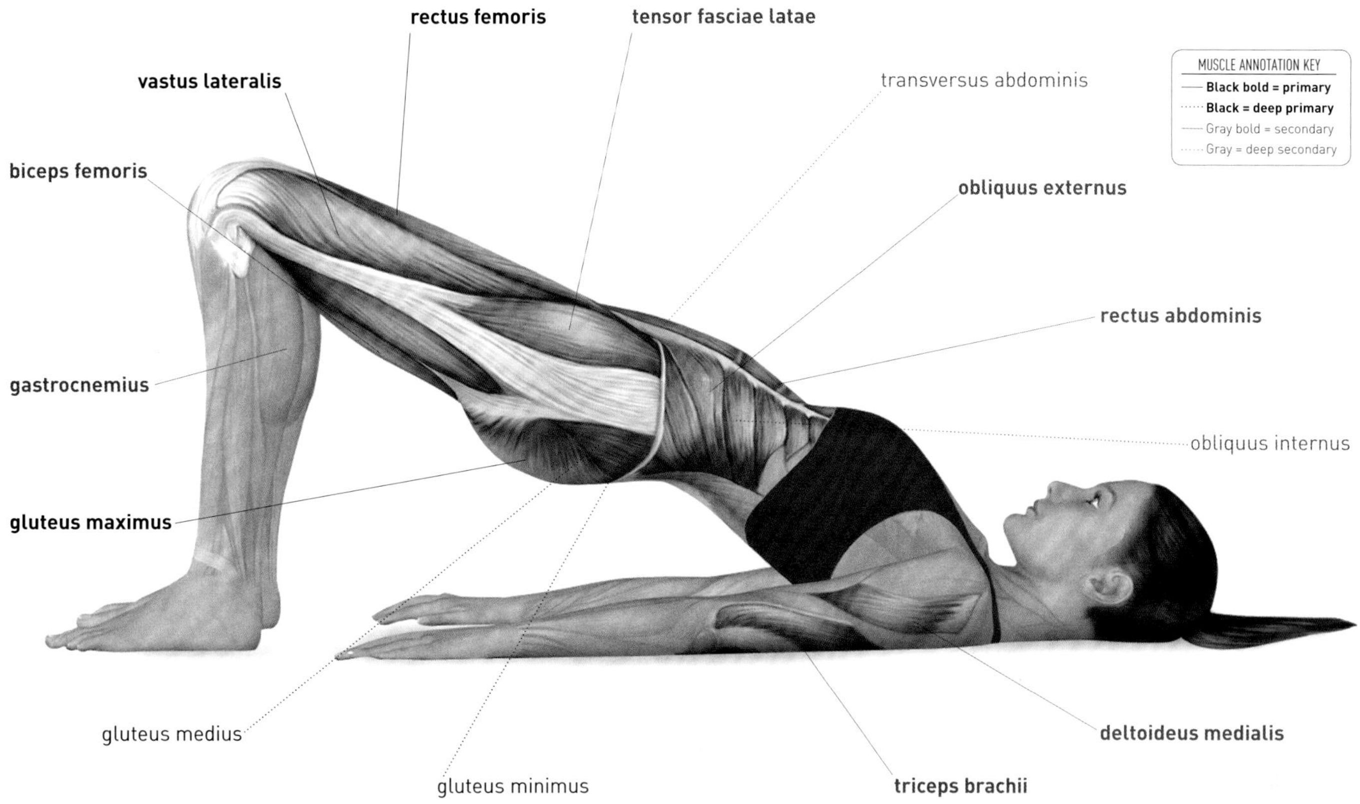

rectus femoris

tensor fasciae latae

vastus lateralis

transversus abdominis

biceps femoris

obliquus externus

rectus abdominis

gastrocnemius

obliquus internus

gluteus maximus

gluteus medius

gluteus minimus

triceps brachii

deltoideus medialis

MUSCLE ANNOTATION KEY

- **Black bold = primary**
- **Black = deep primary**
- Gray bold = secondary
- Gray = deep secondary

354 Piriformis Bridge

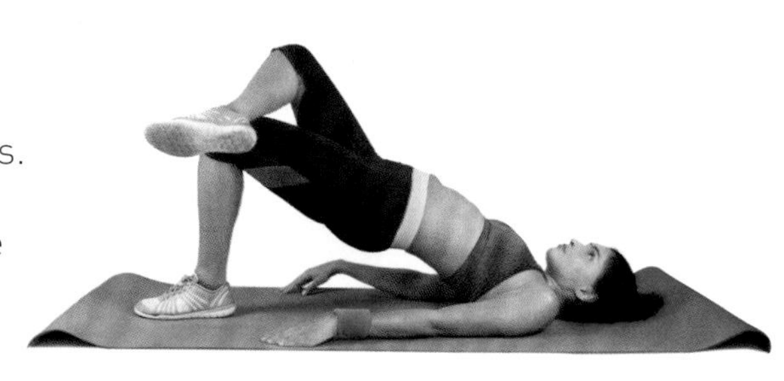

Lie on your back, arms extended at your sides. Your knees should be bent, with feet on the floor. Keeping the rest of your body still, raise your left leg to rest the ankle on your right knee. Press your palms into the floor and engage your abdominal muscles as you lift. Your body from shoulders to knees should form a diagonal line. Slowly and with control, return to starting position. Switch legs and repeat for the desired repetitions.

355 Bridge with High Knees

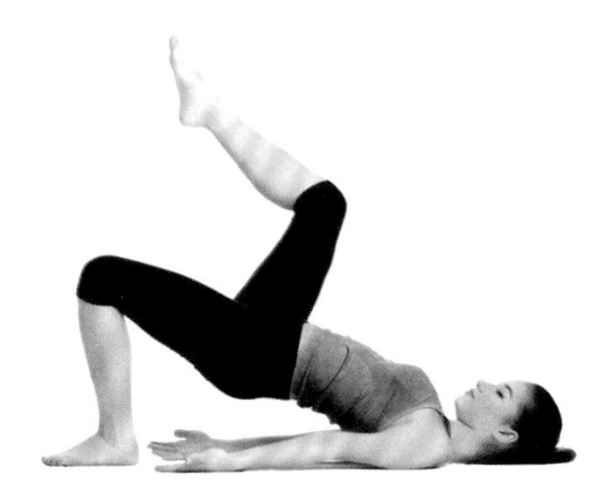

Perform the Bridge (#350), and then keeping your legs bent, draw your left knee back, bringing it as close to your chest as possible. Lower your left leg until your toe touches the mat. Be sure to keep your pelvis level. Bring your left knee toward your chest again. Repeat the sequence for the desired repetitions, and then lower your left leg to the floor, and repeat the exercise with your right leg. Repeat for the desired repetitions.

356 Bridge with Leg Lift

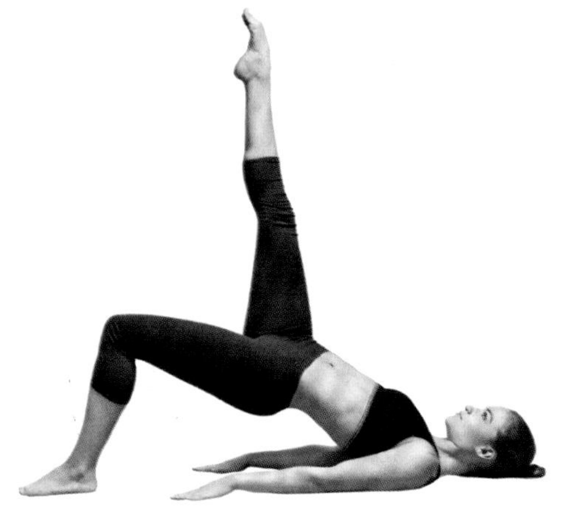

Perform the Bridge (#350), and then keeping one knee bent, extend the other straight to the ceiling. Hold, and then lower. Repeat sequence for the desired repetitions, and then lower your leg to the floor, and repeat the exercise with your other leg. Repeat for the desired repetitions.

357 Aerobic Step Bridge with Leg Lift and Chest Press

Holding a dumbbell or hand weight in each hand at chest level, lie on our back with your heals propped on an aerobic step and your knees bent. Extend one leg toward the ceiling. Push through the heel on the step while raising your pelvis until your torso is aligned with your thighs, while at the same time pressing the weights straight up. Lower to the starting position, and then repeat with the other leg. Repeat for the desired repetitions.

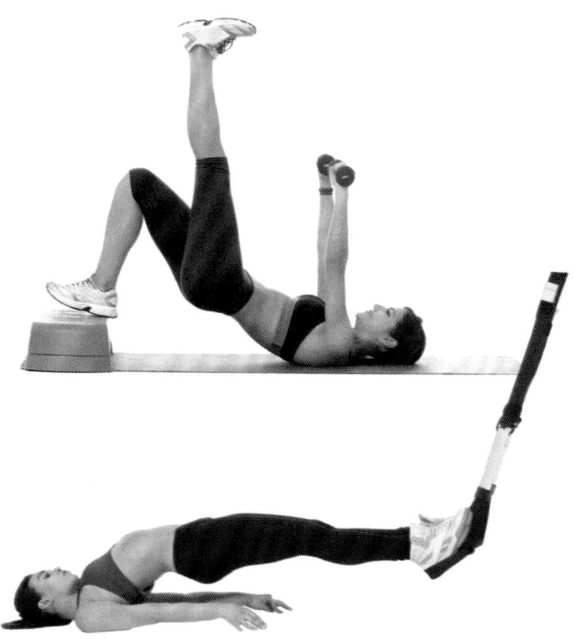

358 Suspended Bridge

Place both feet in the foot cradles of a suspension system, and then lie supine. Perform as you would the Bridge (#350). Repeat for the desired repetitions.

359 Roller Bridge with Leg Lift

Lie on your back, with the roller under your feet. Without moving the roller or arching your back, bridge up, and lift your hips into the air. Keeping your muscles firm, raise your right leg up to the height of your knees, and straighten your raised leg. Try to keep the roller from moving, and raise and lower your hips while keeping your outstretched leg raised. Repeat for the desired reps, and then switch legs.

360 Roller Bridge with Hamstring Pull-In

Lie supine on the floor, your knees bent and a foam roller under your feet. Perform as you would the Bridge (#353) lifting your hips so that they align with the shoulders in a neutral position. Squeeze your glutes, and pull your calves in and out as you roll the roller under your feet. Repeat for the desired repetitions.

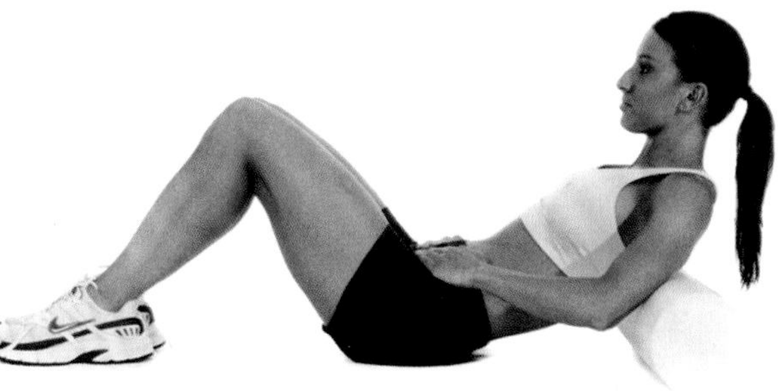

361 Roller Bridge with Leg Extension

Lie on your back, with the roller under your shoulders. Your butt should be on the floor, with your knees bent, and feet flat on the floor. Press into the floor with your feet, and bridge up, lifting your hips toward the ceiling until they are parallel to the floor. Extend your right leg, and then raise it up to the height of your knees. Keeping your leg straight and the roller still, raise and lower your hips. Return to Bridge position, and then repeat with the left leg.

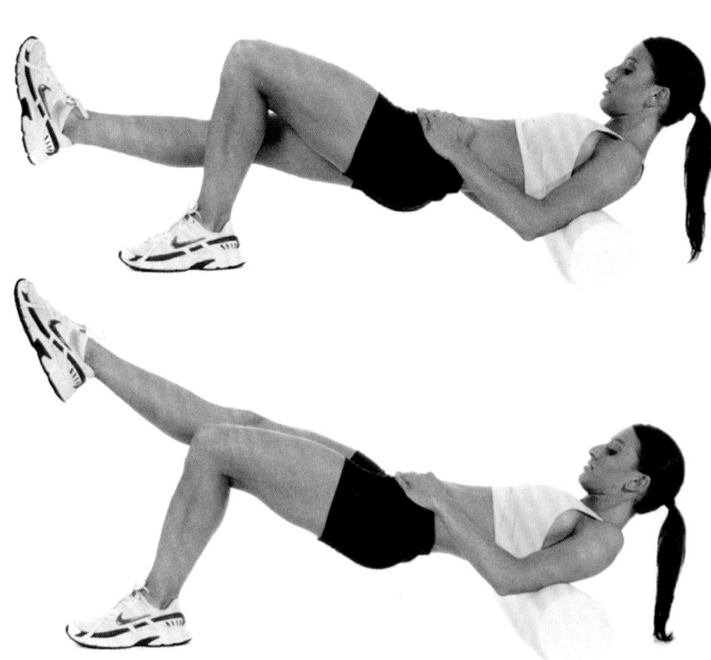

Swiss Ball Bridge

For many abdominal exercises, it is not the extent of your movements but the quality of them that makes the difference between an exercise that is effective and one that misses the target. The Swiss Ball Bridge is a perfect example—it is a powerful core exercise that also activates your glutes, lower back, and obliques.

- Sit on the floor with your back against a Swiss ball. Bend your knees to 90 degrees and spread your arms wide at shoulder height
- Push through your heels, and, using your glutes and hamstrings, raise your hips upward as you roll your back up the ball until your torso is aligned with your thighs.
- Hold for the desired time, and then lower yourself back down.

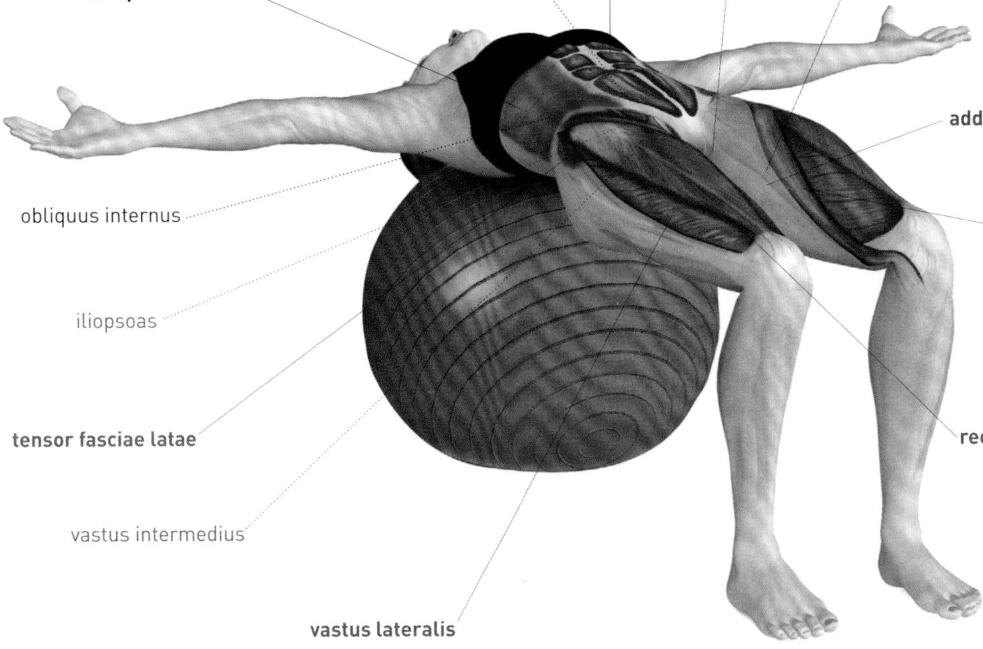

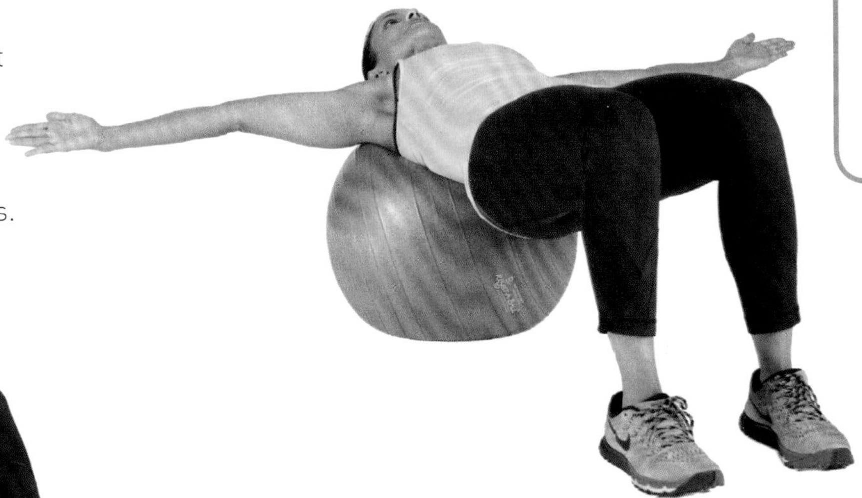

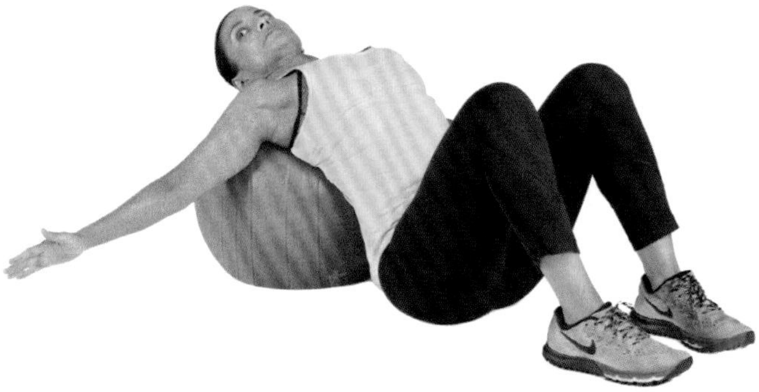

FIND YOUR FORM

Contract your glutes and hold your stomach tight to keep your hips and shoulders parallel to the floor. To maintain your upper-body form, you can hold a pole or broomstick with your arms outspread.

MUSCLE ANNOTATION KEY
- Black bold = primary
- Black = deep primary
- Gray bold = secondary
- Gray = deep secondary

Backward Ball Stretch

The Backward Ball Stretch is a challenging flexibility exercise that targets your thoracic and upper-lumbar spine, along with your core muscles. It will help you increase spinal extension, while stretching your abdominals and latissimus dorsi muscle—the broad, flat muscle that covers much of your back on either side. It also helps you to develop balance and coordination.

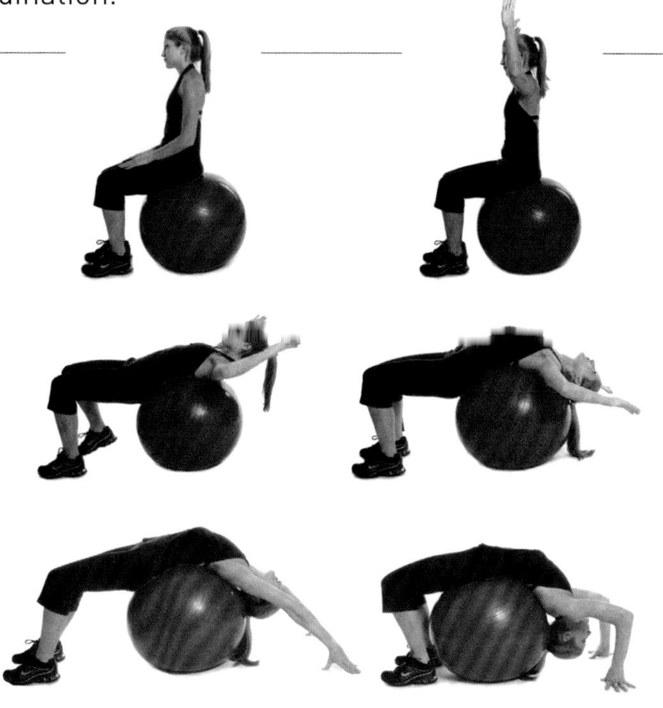

- Sit on a Swiss ball in a well-balanced, neutral position, with your hips directly over the center of the ball.
- Raise your arms while maintaining good balance, and begin to extend them behind you.
- As you continue to extend your hands backward, walk your feet forward, allowing the ball to roll up your spine.
- As your hands touch the floor, extend your legs as far forward as you comfortably can. Hold this position for a few seconds.
- To deepen the stretch, extend your arms, and walk your legs and hands closer to the ball. Hold this position for a few seconds.
- To release the stretch, bend your knees, drop your hips to the floor, lift your head off the ball, and then walk back to the starting position.

FIND YOUR FORM

Maintain good balance throughout the stretch. Moving slowly and in a controlled manner. Avoid any lateral ball movement, and do not hold the extended position for too long, or until you feel dizzy. Keep your head on the ball until you have dropped your knees all the way down as you release from the stretch.

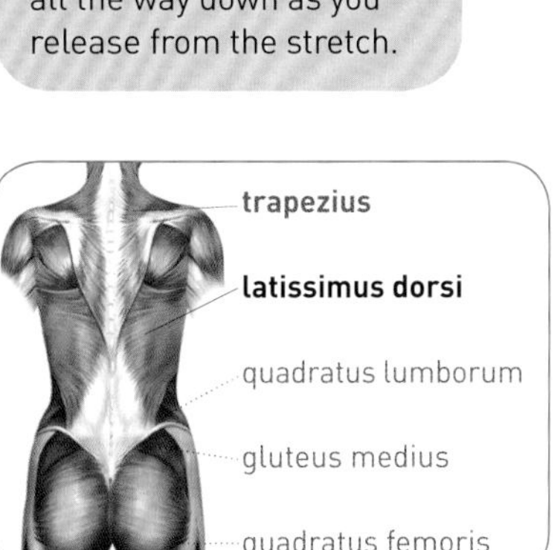

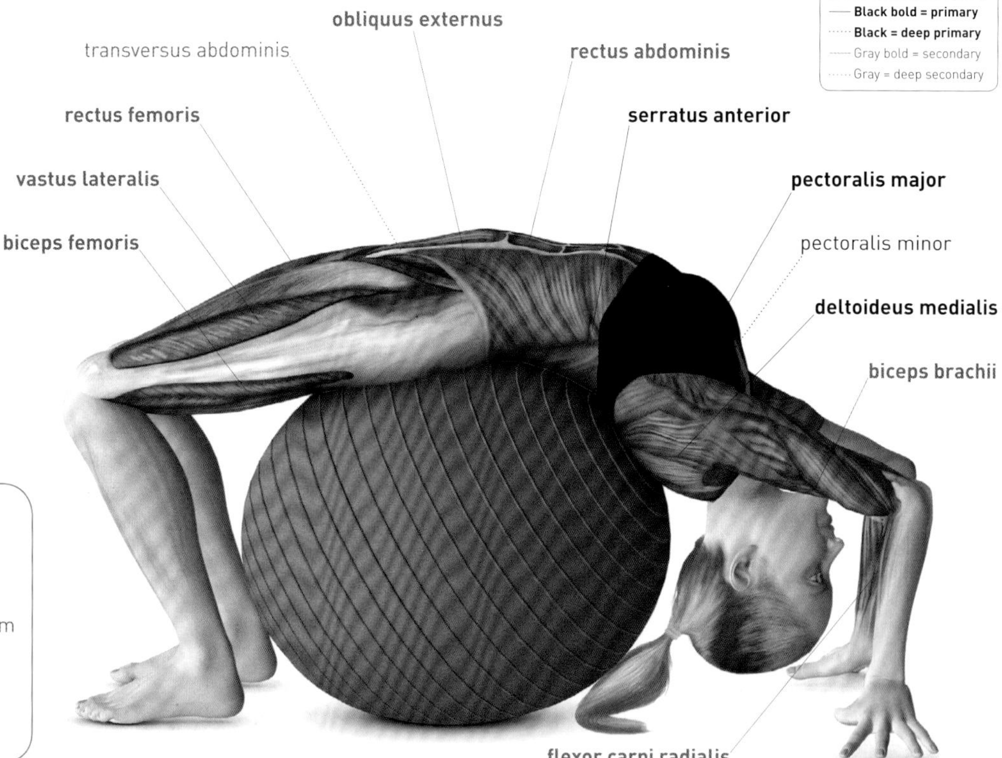

Backward Ball Stretch II

Perform as you would the Backward Ball Stretch (#363), but rather than extend your hands to the floor, roll only to our middle back, and clasp your hands behind your head.

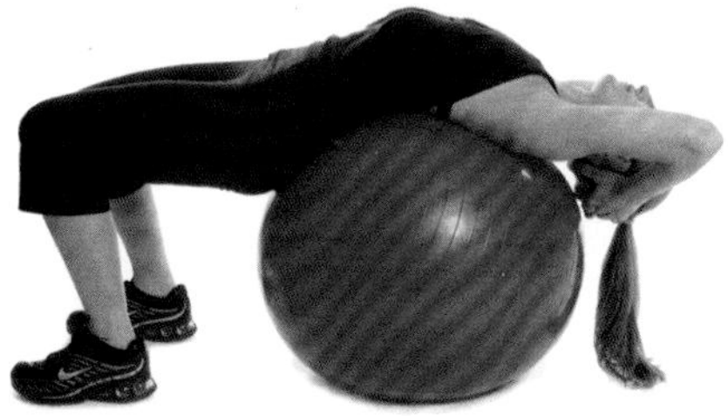

Swiss Ball Bridge with Rotation

Lie on a Swiss ball so that your upper back is on the ball with your hips unsupported. Plant your feet flat on the floor, hip-width apart or wider, and bend your knees to 90 degrees. Grasp a medicine ball with both hands, and position your arms straight up. Rotate your upper body to the left, rolling onto your left shoulder on top of the Swiss ball. Hold briefly, and then slowly roll back to the starting position with the Swiss ball in the center of your shoulders. Repeat the exercise, rotating your torso and rolling your shoulders to the right. Continue rotating from side to side for the desired time or repetitions.

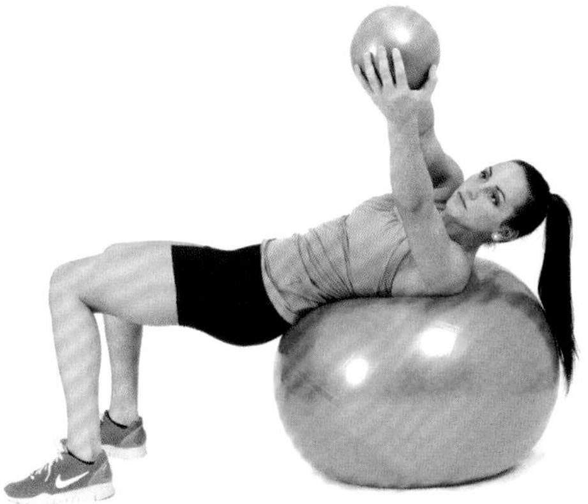

Swiss Ball Bridge Side-to-Side Roll

Lie with your lower back on a Swiss ball and your feet together and your knees bent at 90 degrees. Position your arms out to the sides. Move your upper body across the ball to the left, rolling the ball under your shoulders and toward your left shoulder. Hold for 5 seconds, and then slowly roll the ball back to the center of your shoulders. Return to the starting position, and then roll to the right.

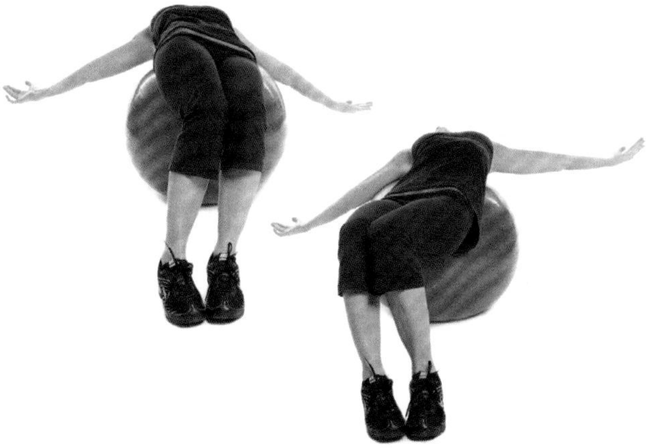

Standing Backbend

Stand tall with you feet placed at a comfortable width apart, your toes pointed forward or canted to the sides. Place your arms over your head, making sure that they are straight and tight with your hands flat, palms up, and fingers pointing behind you. Slowly arch backward, and look downward for the floor. Keep your arms locked as you move closer to the floor. Place your hands on the floor, and keep your feet firmly planted. Your head should look back toward the floor while you hold the position. To safely practice this move, you can stand about a foot from a wall, facing away, and use the wall to walk your hands down until they reach the floor. You can also practice in front of a bench or other platform, and arch back only as far as the elevated surface.

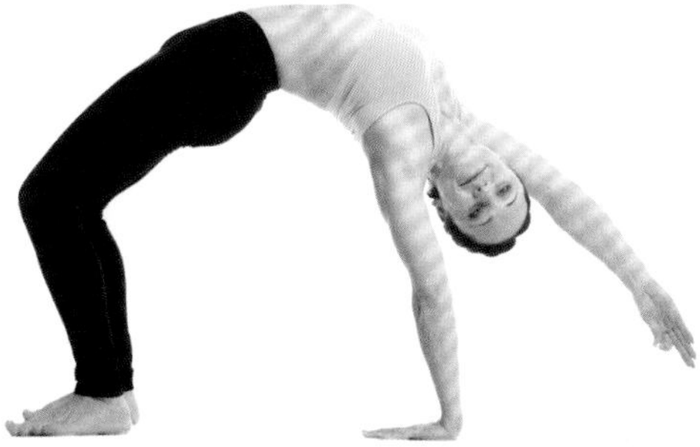

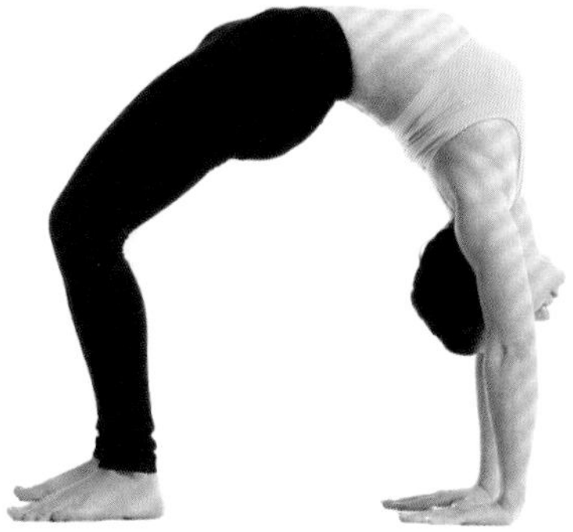

Swiss Ball Leg Bridge

The Swiss Ball Leg Bridge is low-intensity move that packs a lot of punch, effectively toning and strengthening your abdominals and glutes. You can amp up this basic move by adding leg lifts and curls to further increase its benefits.

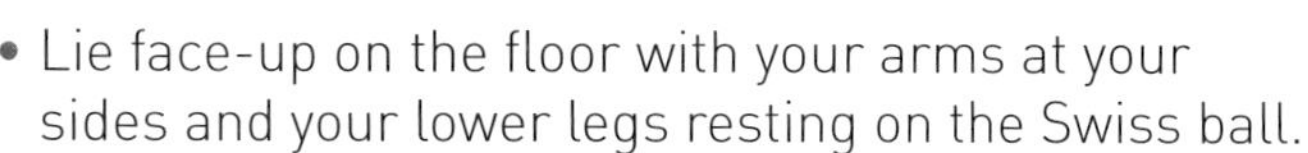

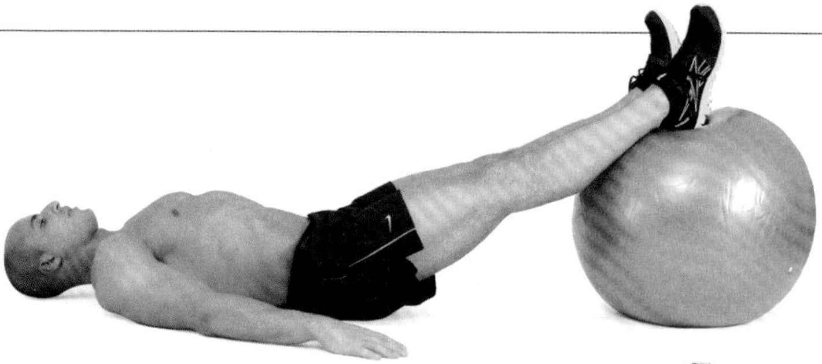

- Lie face-up on the floor with your arms at your sides and your lower legs resting on the Swiss ball.
- Press your palms into the floor and engage your abdominal muscles as you lift your upper body off the floor. Your body should form a diagonal line. If desired, hold for a few seconds.
- Slowly and with control, lower back to starting position. Repeat for the desired repetitions.

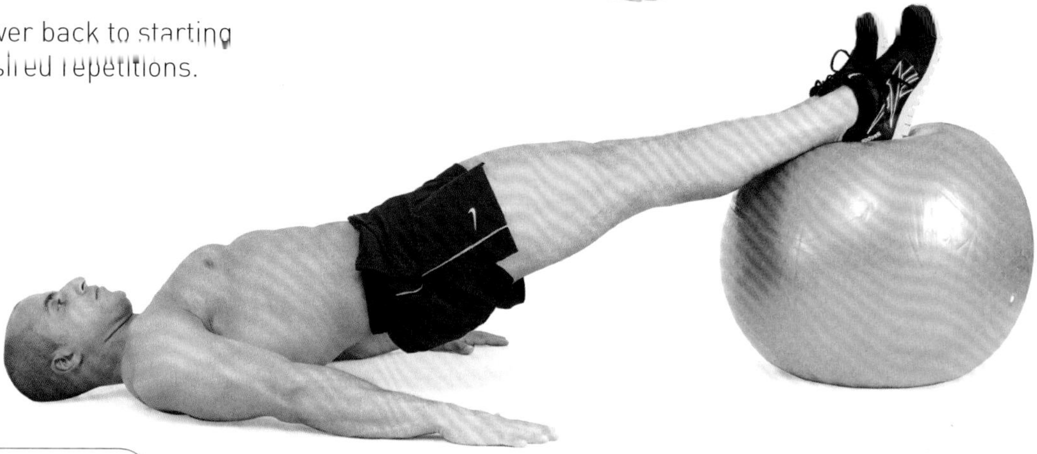

➔ FIND YOUR FORM

Keep your abs fully engaged to keep your body in a stable line from feet to shoulders.

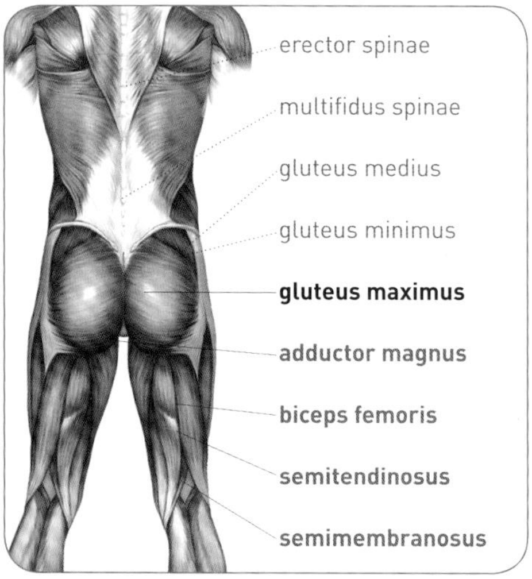

erector spinae
multifidus spinae
gluteus medius
gluteus minimus
gluteus maximus
adductor magnus
biceps femoris
semitendinosus
semimembranosus

MUSCLE ANNOTATION KEY
Black bold = primary
Black = deep primary
Gray bold = secondary
Gray = deep secondary

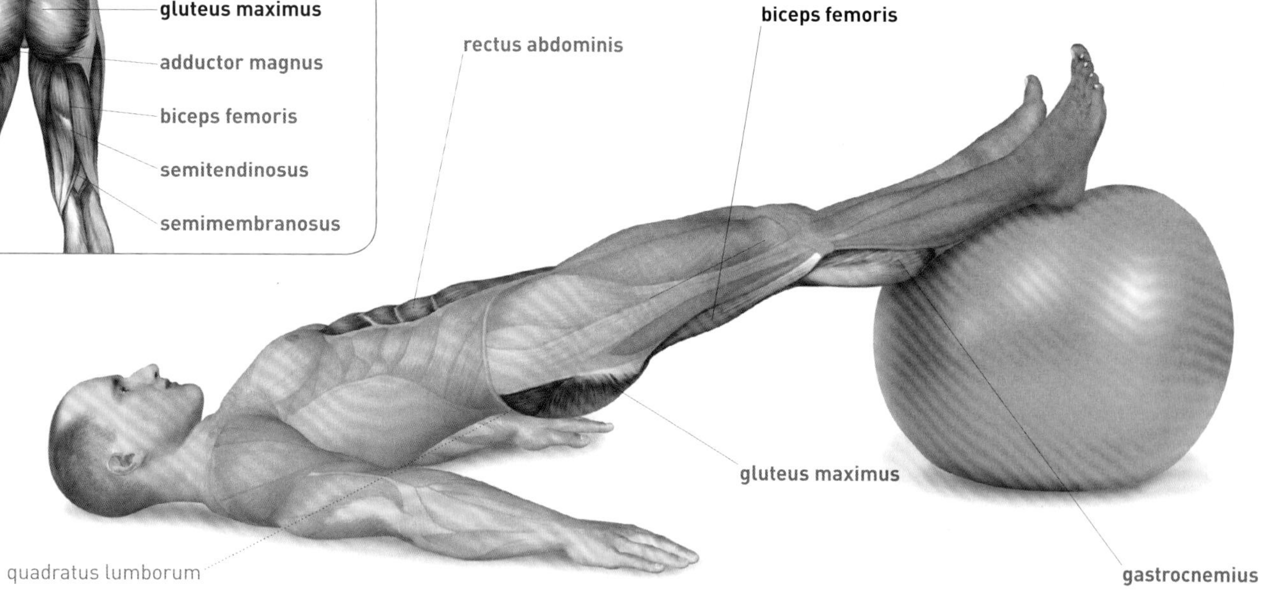

biceps femoris
rectus abdominis
gluteus maximus
quadratus lumborum
gastrocnemius

369 Swiss Ball Bridge with Leg Raises

Perform as you would the Swiss Ball leg Bridge (#368), and then in the raised position, lift one leg off the ball, extending it upward while maintaining your form. Return to starting position. Repeat on the other side, keeping both legs straight and your back neutral as you move. continue for the desired repetitions.

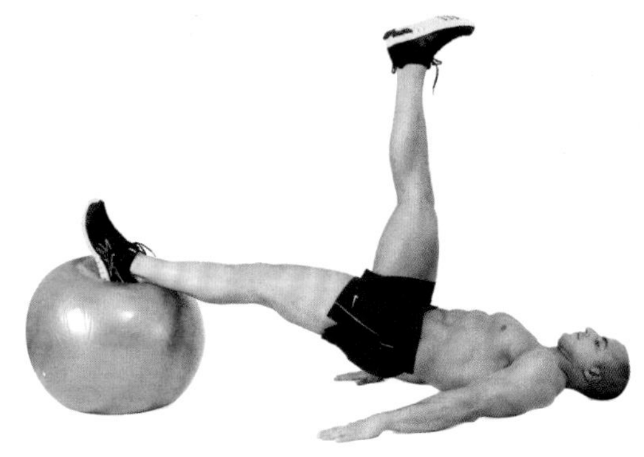

370 Swiss Ball Bridge with Leg Curl

Lie on the floor with your arms out to the sides at shoulder height or extended along your sides, palms down, and perform as you would the Swiss Ball Leg Bridge (#368). From the raised position, pull your heels toward you and roll the ball as close to your butt as possible. Pause, then roll back to the Bridge position, lower your hips to the floor, and continue for the desired repetitions.

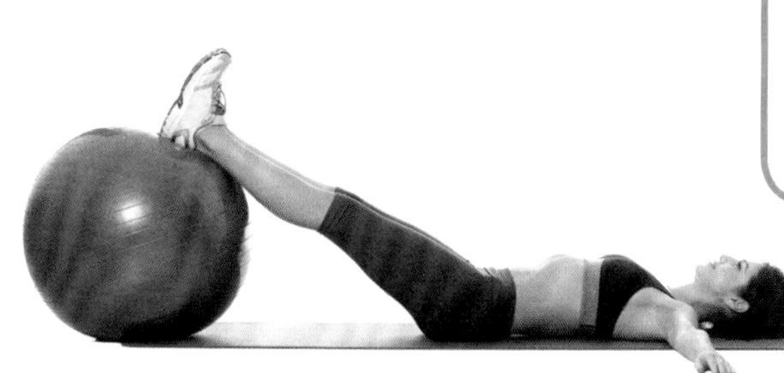

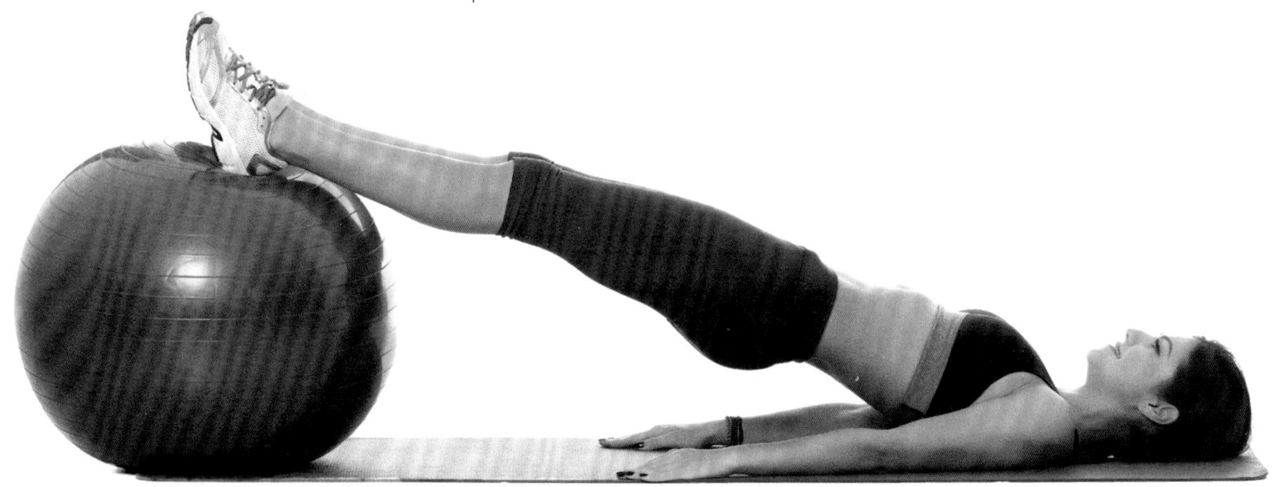

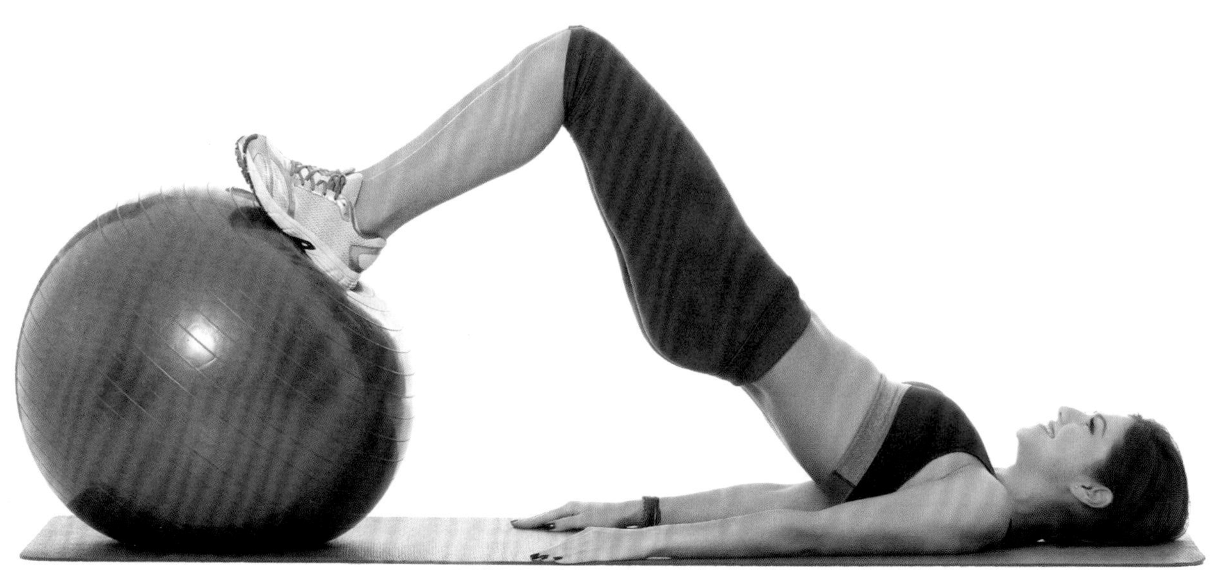

Bird Dog

High-intensity workouts can be hard on your lower back, so including exercises that support the muscles of your spine—especially the lumbar region—can help you stave off discomfort and keep you ready to work hard. The Bird Dog, also called the Quadruped Arm/Leg Raise, targets a group of deep muscles that run along your spinal column called the erector spinae muscles, which work to extend your torso. As well as being an effective lower-back move, the Bird Dog is a classic that will help you hone your balance, stability, and coordination.

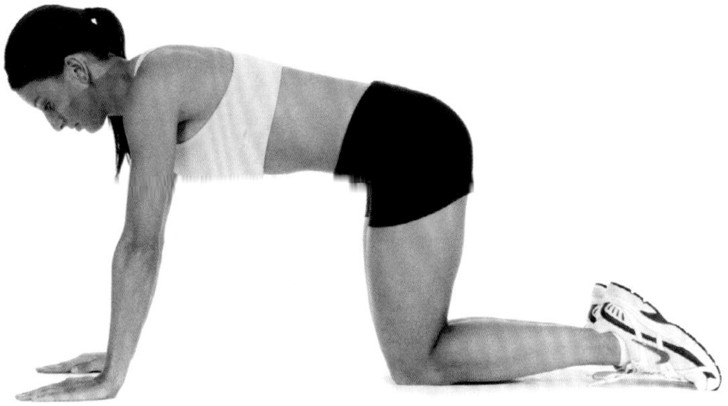

- Kneel on all fours with your hands under your shoulders and knees under your hips, while keeping your head, neck, and back straight. Engage your abdominals by drawing your navel up toward your spine.
- Raise your right arm and reach it forward until it is in line with your torso. At the same time, kick your left leg upward until it is parallel to the floor, while keeping your torso still.
- Bring your arm and leg back to the starting position, and then repeat sequence on the other side, alternating for the desired time or repetitions.

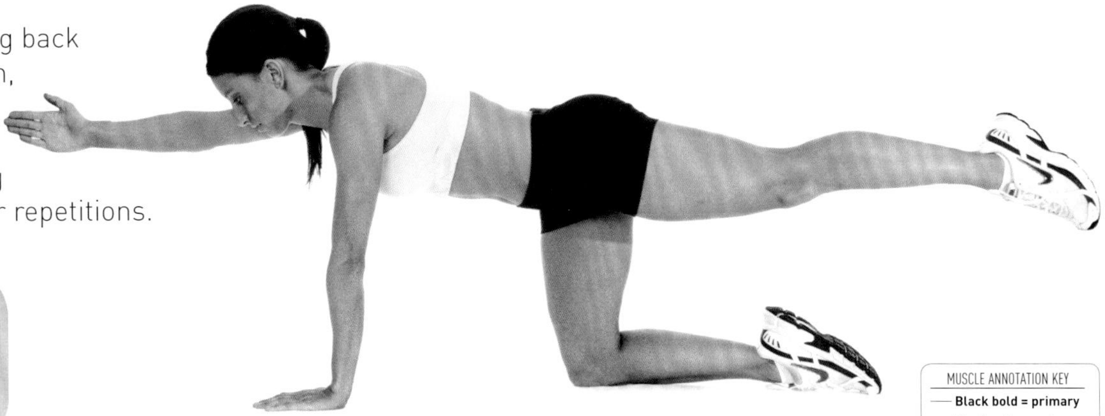

➔ FIND YOUR FORM
Do not allow your pelvis to bend or rotate as you extend your arm and leg.

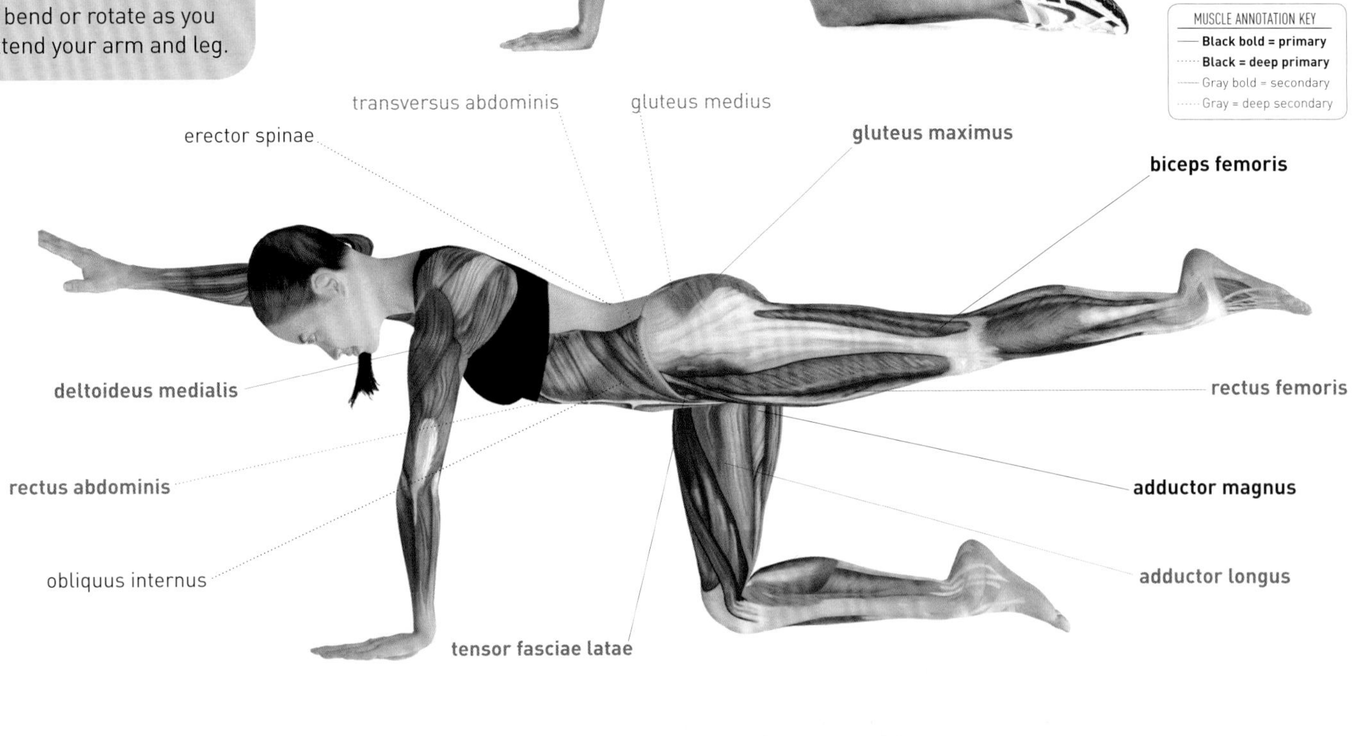

MUSCLE ANNOTATION KEY
Black bold = primary
Black = deep primary
Gray bold = secondary
Gray = deep secondary

transversus abdominis
gluteus medius
erector spinae
gluteus maximus
biceps femoris
deltoideus medialis
rectus femoris
rectus abdominis
adductor magnus
obliquus internus
adductor longus
tensor fasciae latae

Pointer

Assume the drop position, and then extend your left arm straight forward while raising your right leg until your body forms a straight line from toe to shoulder. Pause at the top of the movement, and then lower back to the drop position. Repeat on the opposite side.

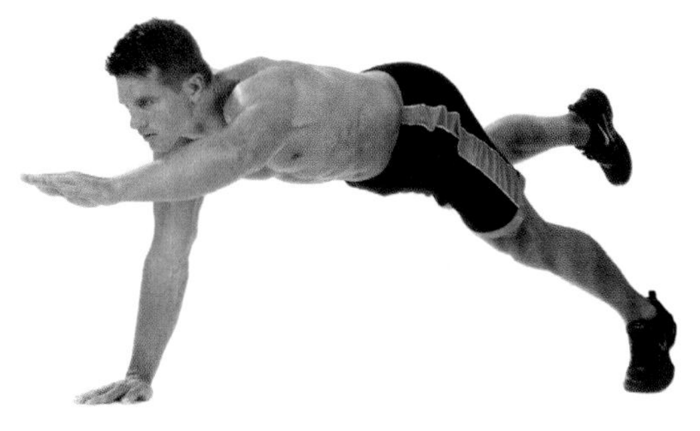

Roller Quadruped Knee Pull-In

Place the foam roller on the floor. Kneel on the roller with your hands placed on the floor in front of you. Your hands should be slightly in front of your torso, and your hips should be lifted off your heels. Round out your torso as you pull your knees toward your hands, allowing the roller to move toward your feet. Repeat for the desired reps and sets.

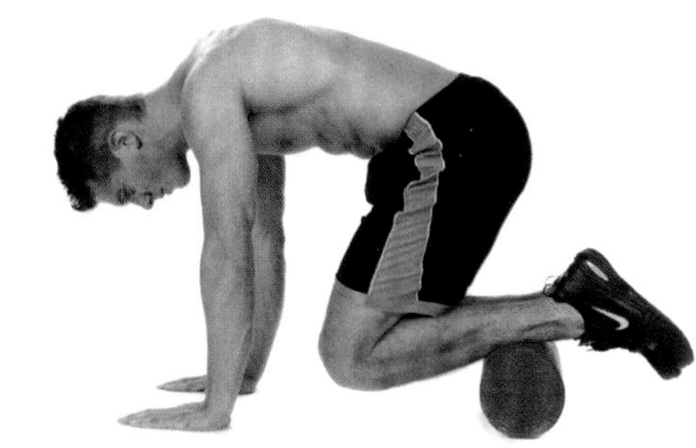

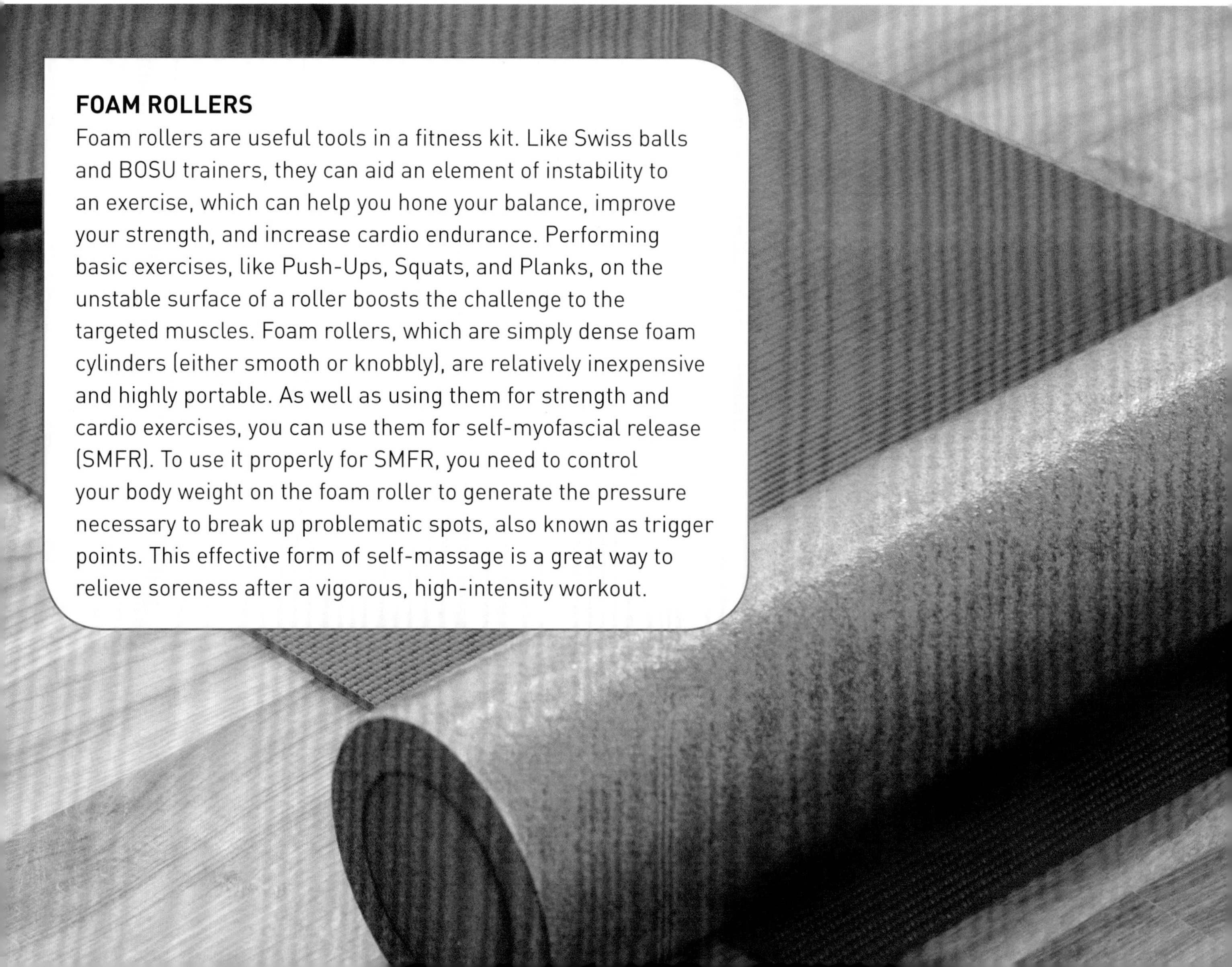

FOAM ROLLERS

Foam rollers are useful tools in a fitness kit. Like Swiss balls and BOSU trainers, they can aid an element of instability to an exercise, which can help you hone your balance, improve your strength, and increase cardio endurance. Performing basic exercises, like Push-Ups, Squats, and Planks, on the unstable surface of a roller boosts the challenge to the targeted muscles. Foam rollers, which are simply dense foam cylinders (either smooth or knobbly), are relatively inexpensive and highly portable. As well as using them for strength and cardio exercises, you can use them for self-myofascial release (SMFR). To use it properly for SMFR, you need to control your body weight on the foam roller to generate the pressure necessary to break up problematic spots, also known as trigger points. This effective form of self-massage is a great way to relieve soreness after a vigorous, high-intensity workout.

Fire Hydrant

The Fire Hydrant, also known as the Quadruped Left Lift, is a multifaceted move that targets your core, pelvic stabilizers, and abductor leg muscles. It can improve your pelvis stability and strengthen your hips and legs.

- Kneel on your hands and knees, your spine in neutral position.
- Keep your weight centered and raise your right knee—still bent—out to the side.
- Raise and lower your leg without moving your hips. Repeat for the desired reps, and then switch legs.

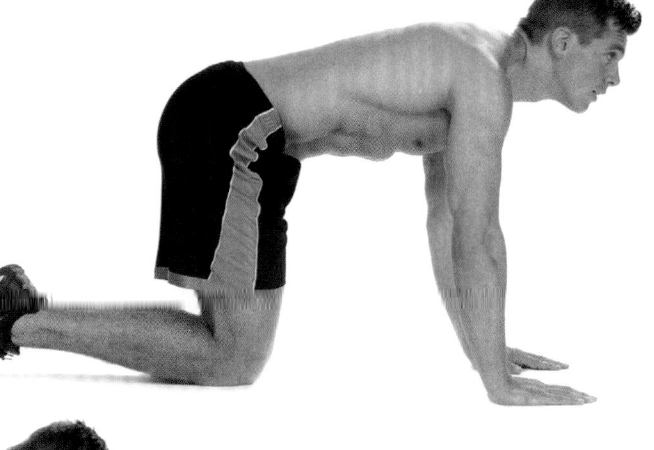

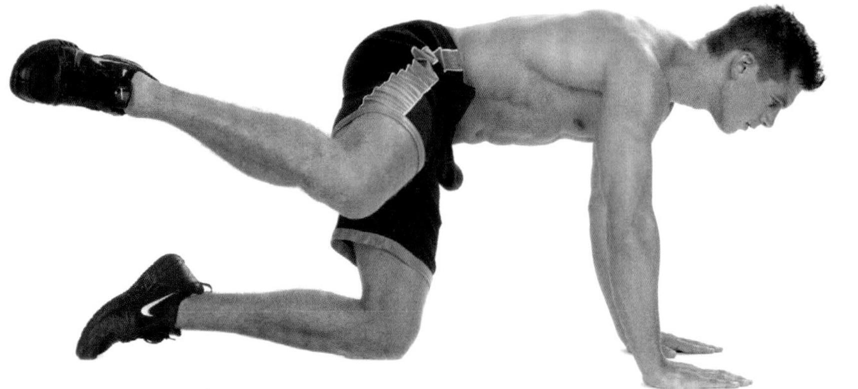

FIND YOUR FORM

Maintain a neutral spine to prevent your lower back from sagging. Keep your chin tucked, and press your hands into the floor to keep the shoulders from sinking near the ears. Avoid lifting your hip as you lift your leg.

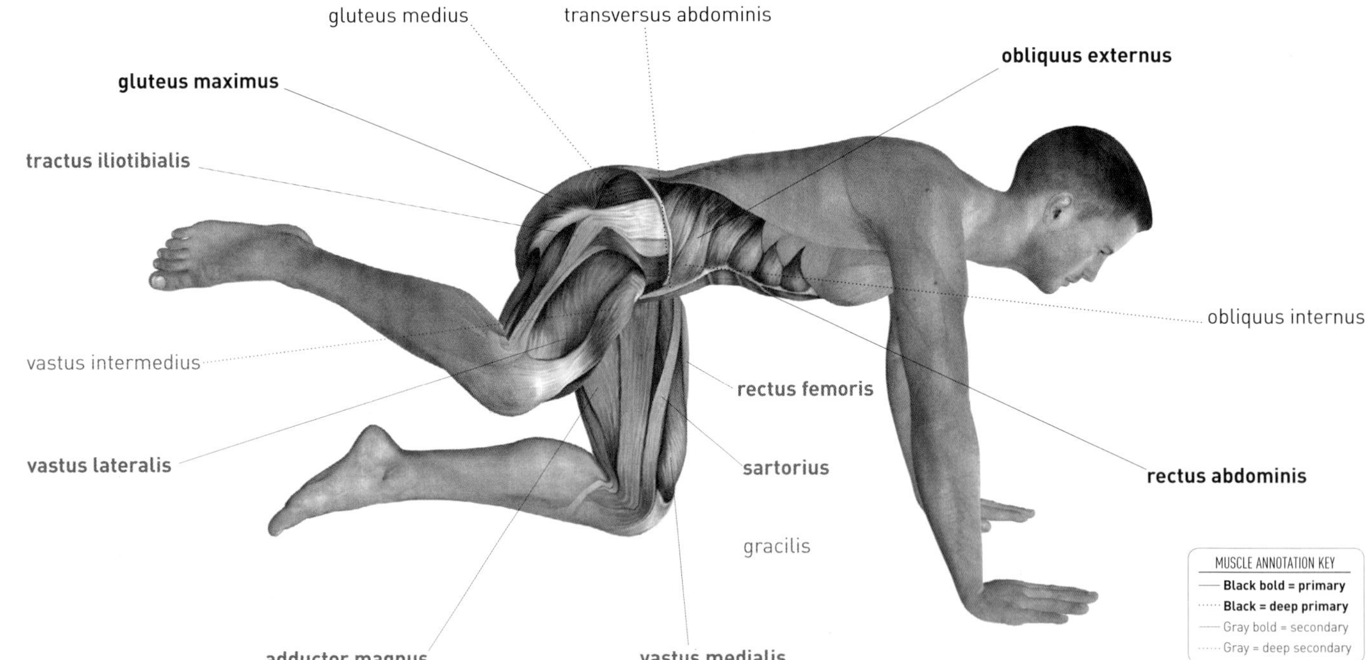

Straight-Leg Fire Hydrant

Kneel on your hands and knees, and then lift one leg straight up until it is parallel to the floor, making sure to keep it in line with your hip. Return to the starting position, and repeat with the opposite leg. Continue to alternate for the desired repetitions.

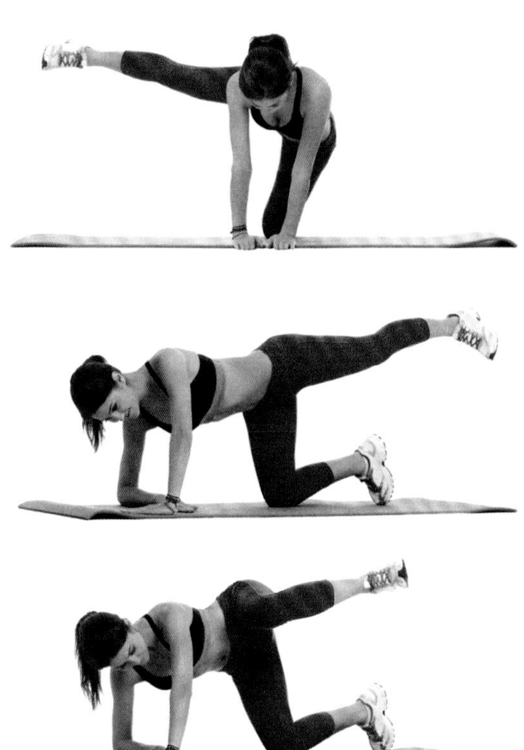

Fire Hydrant In-Out

Kneel on your hands and knees, resting your right arm on your forearm, palms down, and your left lined up under your shoulder. Your spine should be in a neutral position. Keeping your left leg bent at a 90-degree angle, raise it to the side, and then straighten it until it is fully extended behind you so that it is in line with your torso. Continue for the desired repetitions, and then repeat on the other side.

377 Clamshell Series

The Clamshell Series takes you through a sequence of movements that will work both your inner and outer thighs while challenging your coordination.

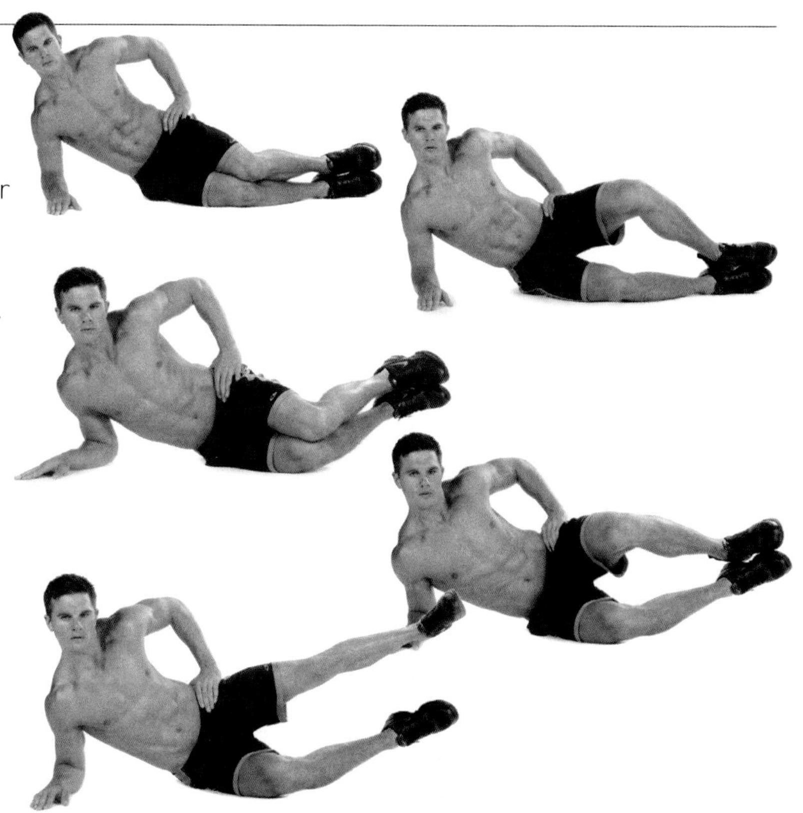

- Lie on your right side with knees bent and stacked on top of each other. Bend your left elbow, placing it directly underneath your shoulder so that your forearm is supporting your upper body. Place your left hand on your hip.
- Without moving your hips, open your left knee upward, and then return to the starting position. Repeat for the desired repetitions.
- Lift both ankles off the floor, making sure to maintain a straight line with the torso.
- While your ankles are still lifted, lift and lower your left knee to open and close your legs. Repeat for the desired repetitions.
- The final part of this series begins with both ankles elevated. Lift your left knee to separate your legs, and then straighten your left leg, being careful not to move the position of your thigh. Bend your knee and return to the starting position. Repeat for the desired repetitions, and then repeat all steps on the opposite side.

Squat Thrust

The Squat Thrust is a powerhouse of an exercise, combining the strength-training benefits of a squat or push-up move with high-intensity cardio. On its own, this exercise is challenging, but it is also the main component of the classic Burpee.

- Stand with your feet hip-width apart and your arms above your head.
- Drop into a squat position, placing your hands on the floor.
- In one quick, explosive motion, kick your feet back to assume a drop position.
- In another quick motion, push through both feet to return to the squat position.
- Continue performing for the desired time or repetitions.

FIND YOUR FORM

Make sure you keep your back flat during as you perform the drop position portion of this exercise.

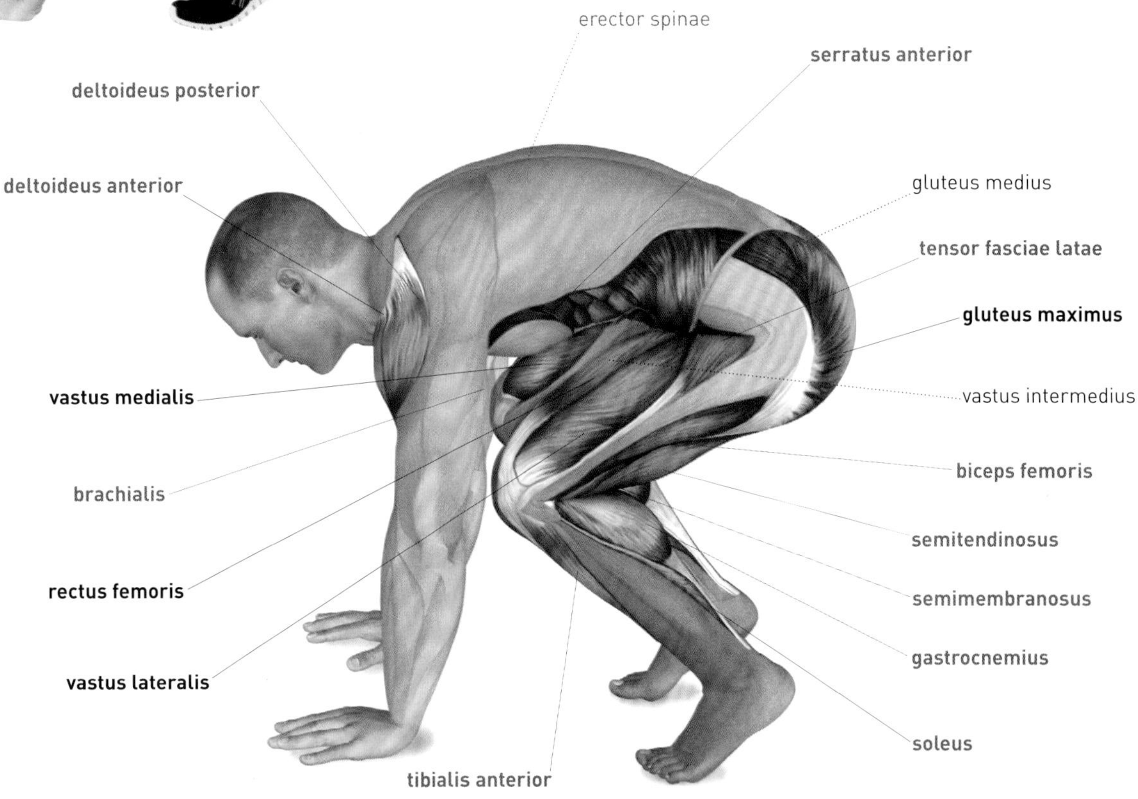

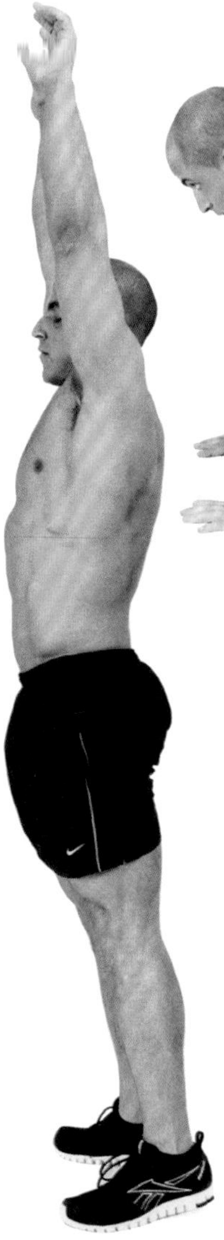

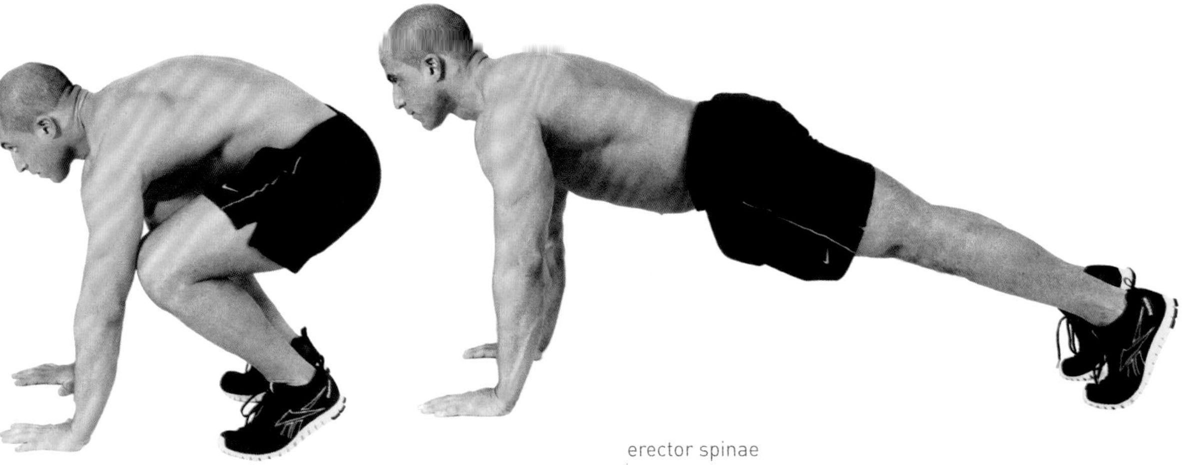

erector spinae

serratus anterior

deltoideus posterior

deltoideus anterior

gluteus medius

tensor fasciae latae

gluteus maximus

vastus medialis

vastus intermedius

brachialis

biceps femoris

semitendinosus

rectus femoris

semimembranosus

gastrocnemius

vastus lateralis

soleus

tibialis anterior

MUSCLE ANNOTATION KEY
— Black bold = primary
······ Black = deep primary
— Gray bold = secondary
······ Gray = deep secondary

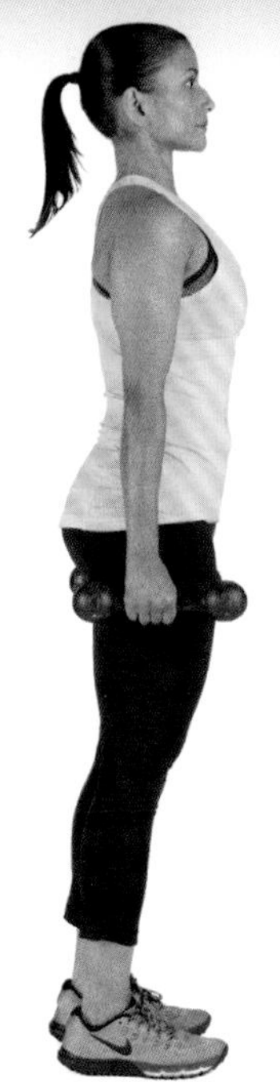
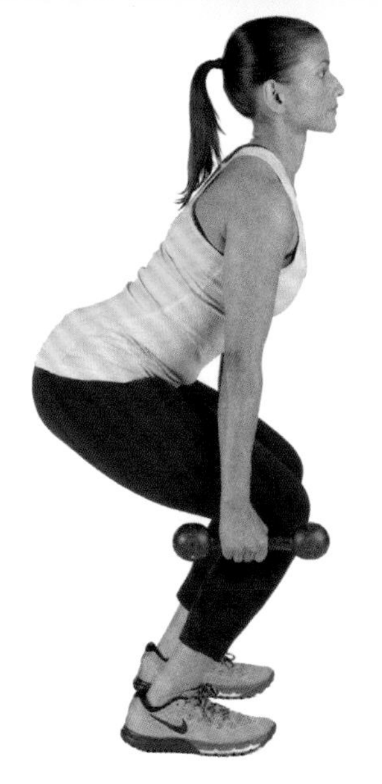
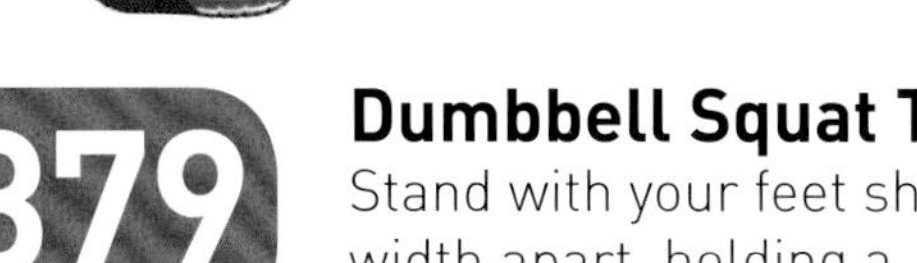
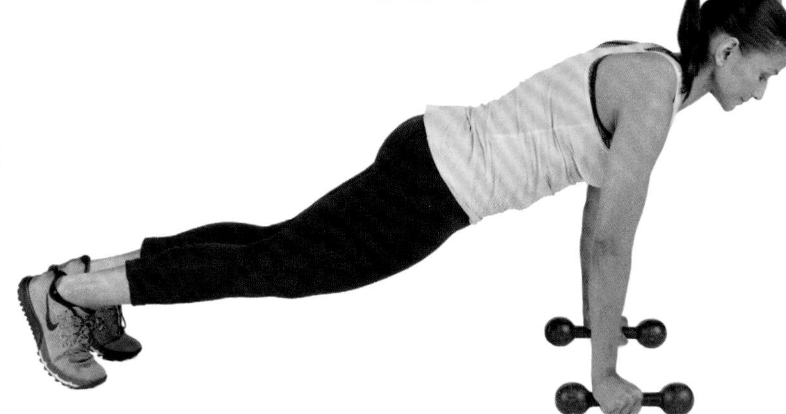

379 Dumbbell Squat Thrust

Stand with your feet shoulder width apart, holding a dumbbell in each hand. Perform as you would a Squat Thrust (#378). Repeat for the desired time or repetitions.

380 Burpee

The names Burpee and Squat Thrust are often used interchangeably, but there is an important difference: a Burpee takes you through the same moves as a Squat Thrust but adds a jump at the end. This plyometric boost takes this already powerful calisthenic exercise to the next level, amping up its cardio and strength benefits. Challenge yourself with one of this versatile exercise's many variations; for example, you can add different kinds of jumps or perform it on one leg.

- Stand with your feet hip-width apart and your arms above your head.
- Drop into a squat position, placing your hands on the floor.
- In one quick, explosive motion, kick your feet back to assume a drop position to perform a Basic Push-Up (#226).
- In another quick motion, jump into the air, and return to the starting position.
- Continue performing for the desired time or repetitions.

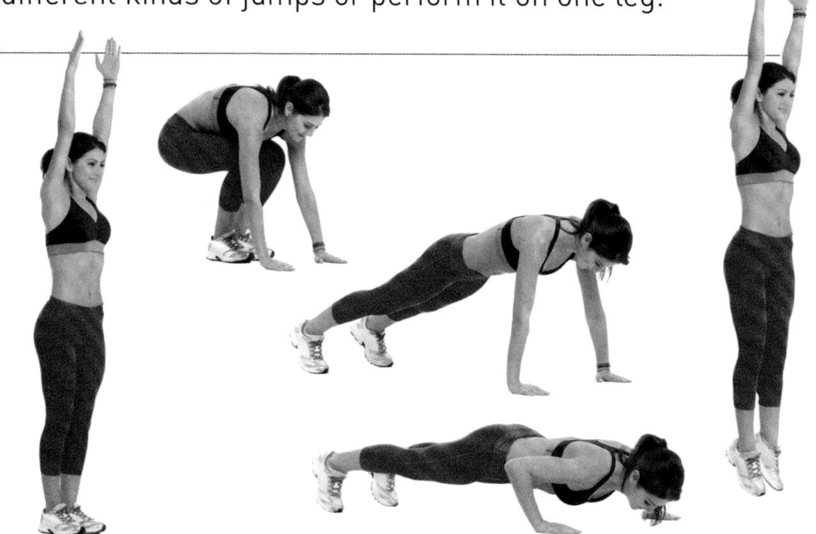

381 Burpee with Pull-Up

Stand with your shoulders positioned under a pull-up bar. Perform a Burpee (#380), and then return to the drop position. From there, jump up to reach for the bar with your arms fully extended, grasping the bar with an overhand grip. In a smooth motion, pull your body up, and then lower it until your arms are again fully extended. Return to the standing position, and then continue performing all steps for the desired time or repetitions.

382 Side Burpee

Perform as you would a Burpee (#380), but instead of jumping your feet straight out into the drop position, jump your legs out to the side so your body is at a diagonal. Alternate jumping to the right and left as you continue for the desired time or repetitions.

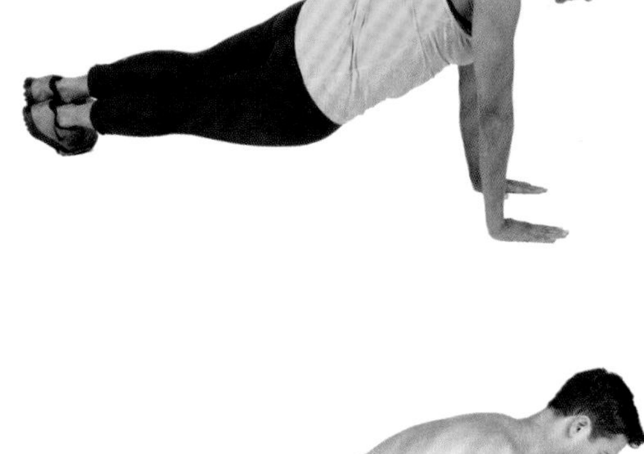

383 Renegade Burpee

Stand with your feet hip-width apart, holding a kettlebell or dumbbell in each hand and Drop into a squat position, and place the weights on the floor. Kick your feet back into the drop position with your hands still on top of the weights and shoulder-width apart. Holding the drop position, bend your right elbow and raise the dumbbell until your elbow passes your torso, while pressing into your left arm for balance. Lower your right arm, and perform the same row action with your left arm. Return your feet back to the squat position, under your hips, and then stand up. Alternate right and left rows as you continue for the desired time or repetitions.

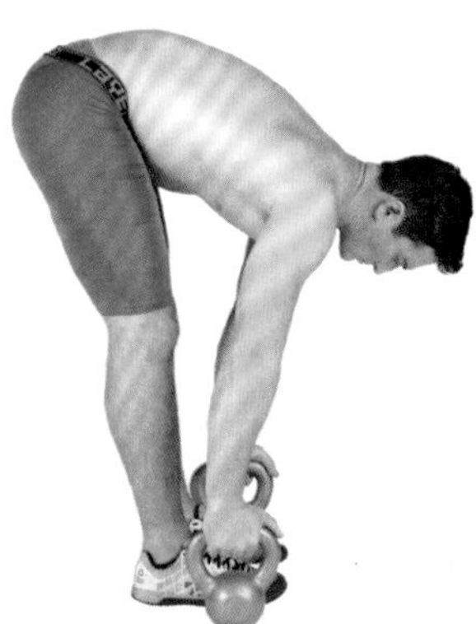

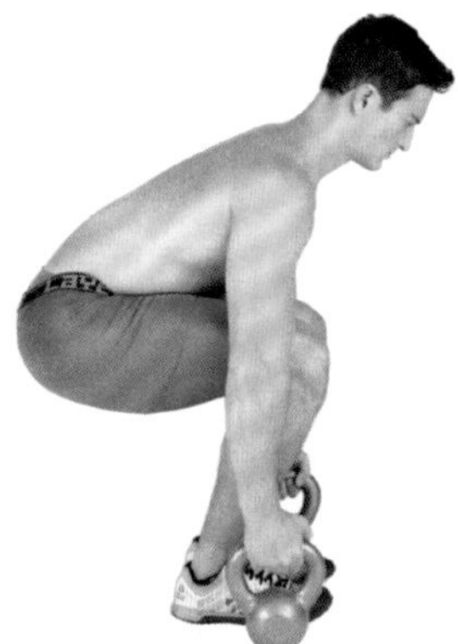

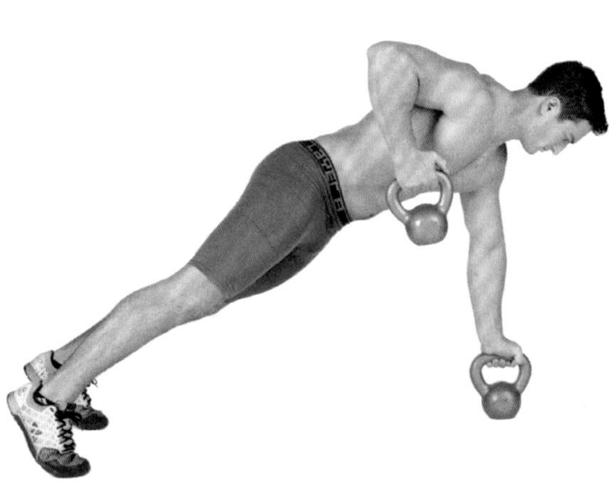

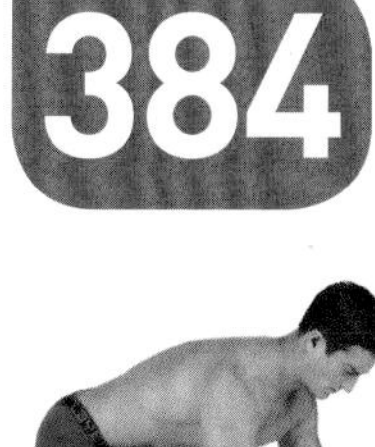

Burpee with Push-Up to Clap

Perform as you would a Burpee (#380), and then from the Push-Up, explode upward and clap your hands. Land with soft, bent elbows, and then continue for the desired time or repetitions.

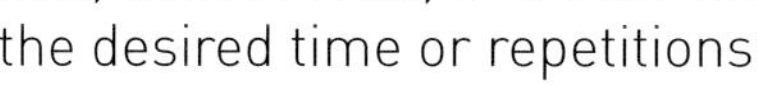

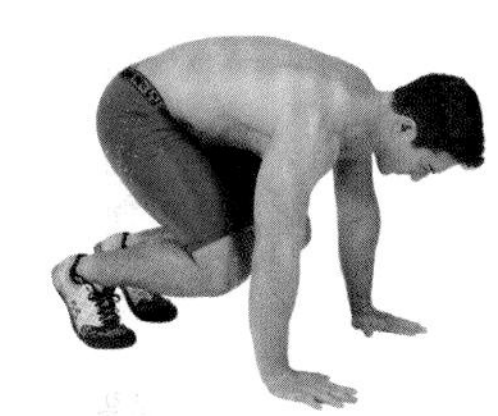

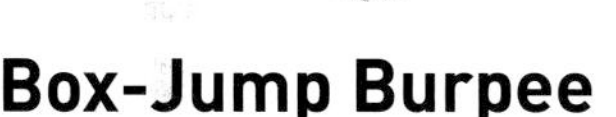

385 Box-Jump Burpee

Stand in front of a high aerobic step or low box. Perform as you would a Burpee (#380), but jump up onto the step when you come up rather than jumping straight up in place. Continue for the desired time or repetitions.

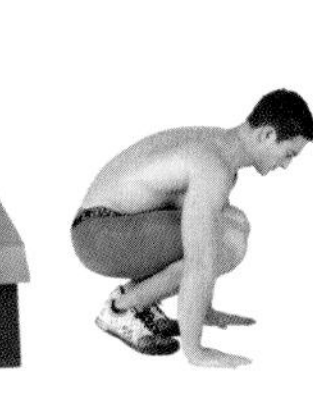

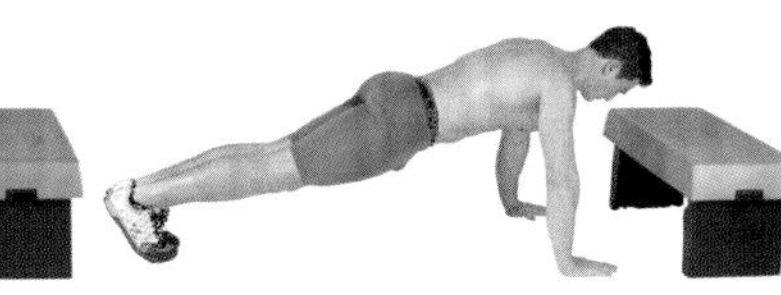

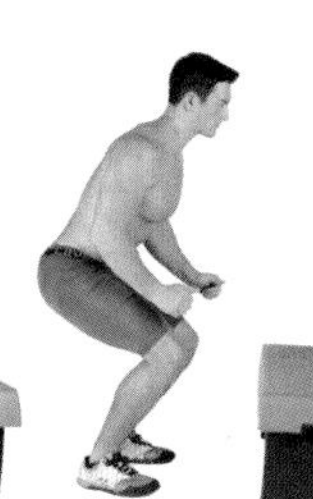

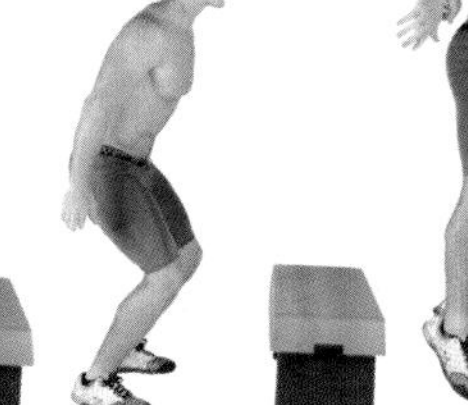

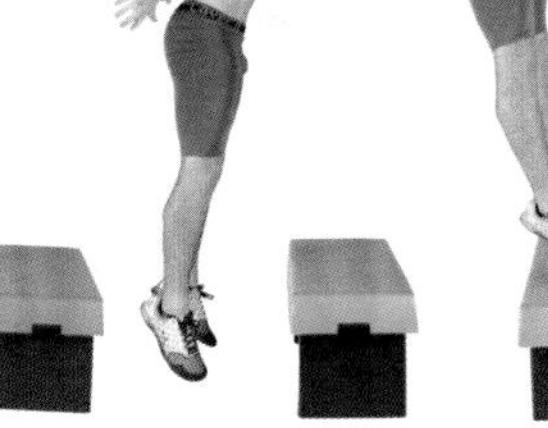

Burpee Broad Jump

Assume a squat position with your heels outside of shoulders and your toes slightly pointed outward. Propel yourself into a jump off both feet, jumping as far forward as far as possible. As you land, bend your hips and knees while leaning forward until your hands touch the floor. Immediately jump both feet backward into the drop position. From the drop position, reverse the process.

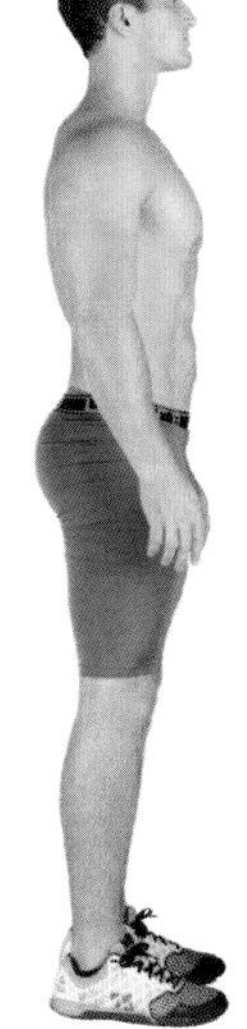

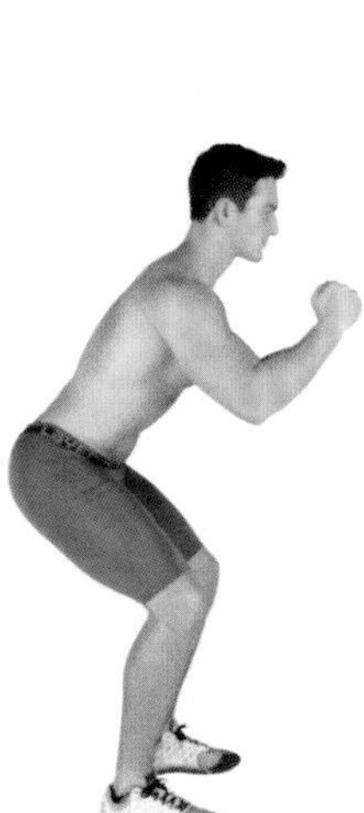

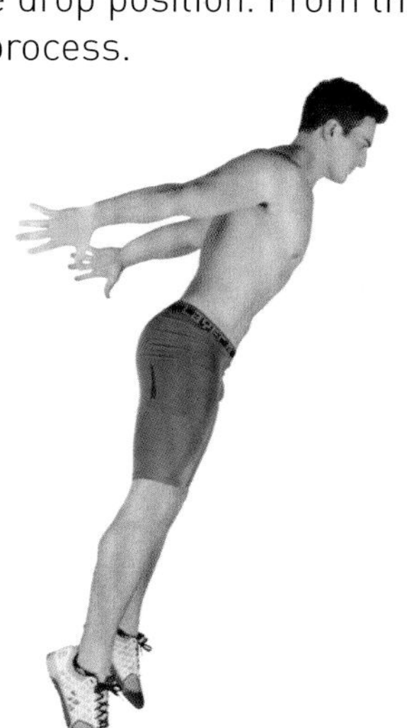

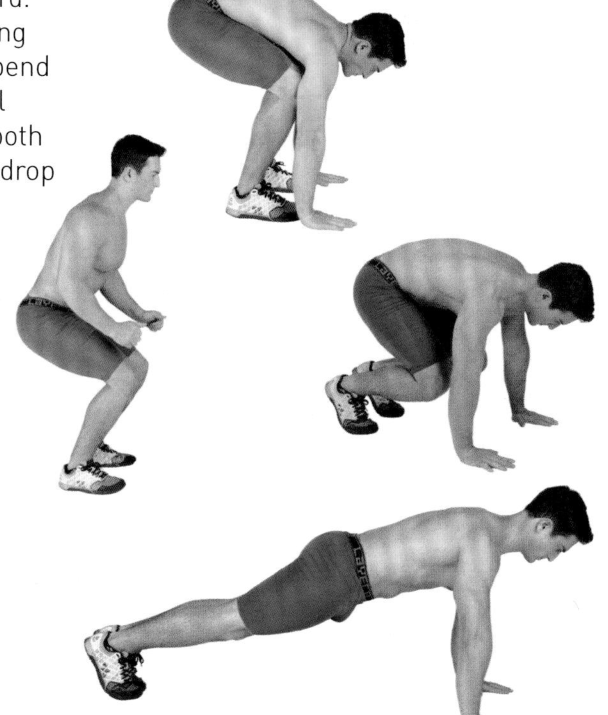

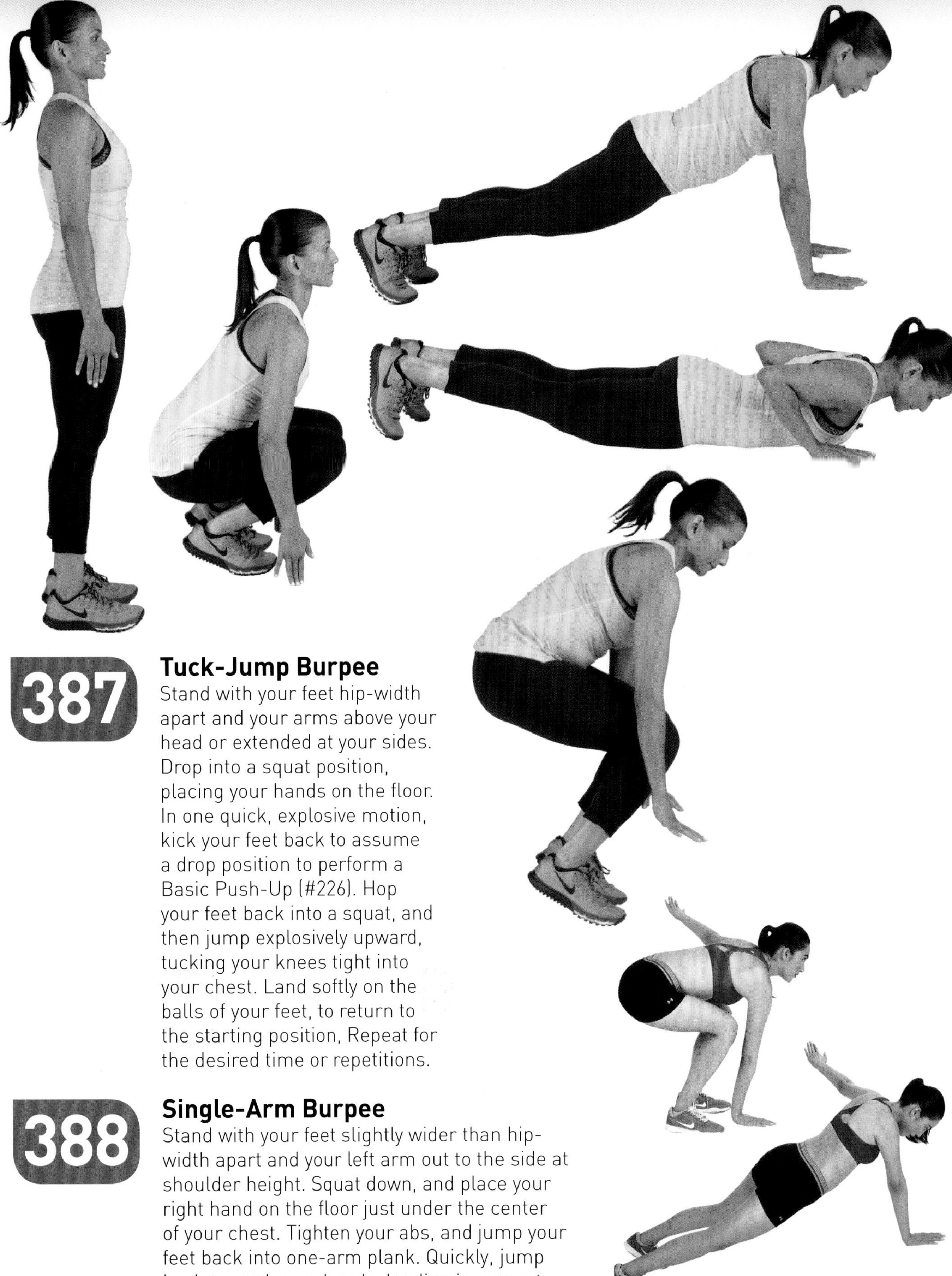

387 Tuck-Jump Burpee

Stand with your feet hip-width apart and your arms above your head or extended at your sides. Drop into a squat position, placing your hands on the floor. In one quick, explosive motion, kick your feet back to assume a drop position to perform a Basic Push-Up (#226). Hop your feet back into a squat, and then jump explosively upward, tucking your knees tight into your chest. Land softly on the balls of your feet, to return to the starting position, Repeat for the desired time or repetitions.

388 Single-Arm Burpee

Stand with your feet slightly wider than hip-width apart and your left arm out to the side at shoulder height. Squat down, and place your right hand on the floor just under the center of your chest. Tighten your abs, and jump your feet back into one-arm plank. Quickly, jump back toward your hands, landing in a squat. Repeat for the desired time or repetitions.

389 Single-Leg Burpee

Stand with your weight entirely on one leg, and bend your opposite knee to lift your foot from the floor. Bend your standing leg and squat, placing your hands on the floor under your shoulders. Jump your leg behind you to bring your body into a straight line, then immediately hop it back towards your hands and explode upwards into the air. Continue, switching legs with each repetition.

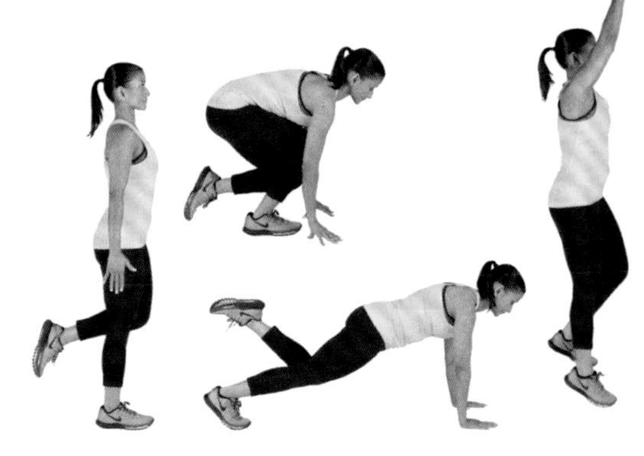

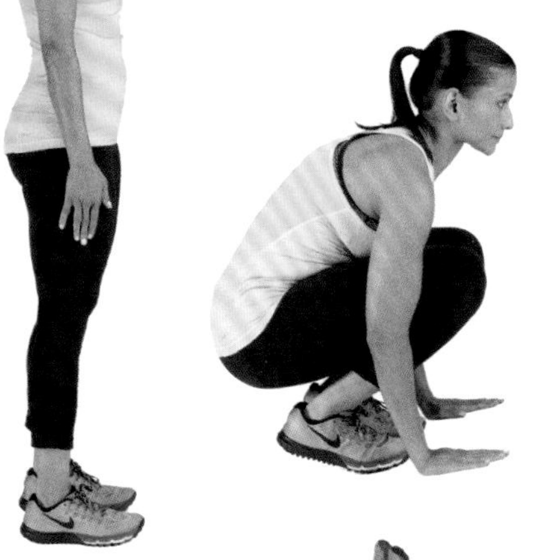

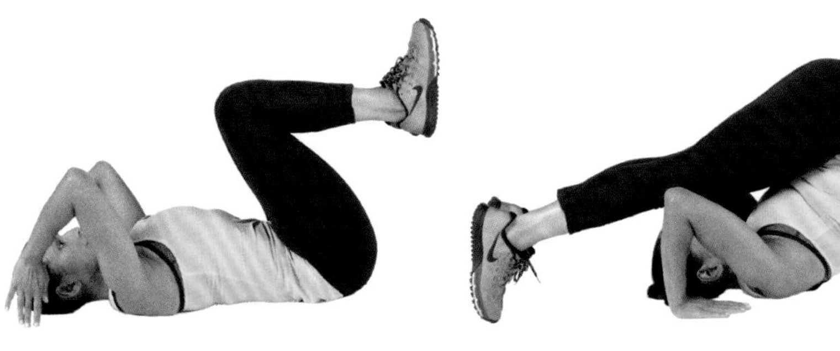

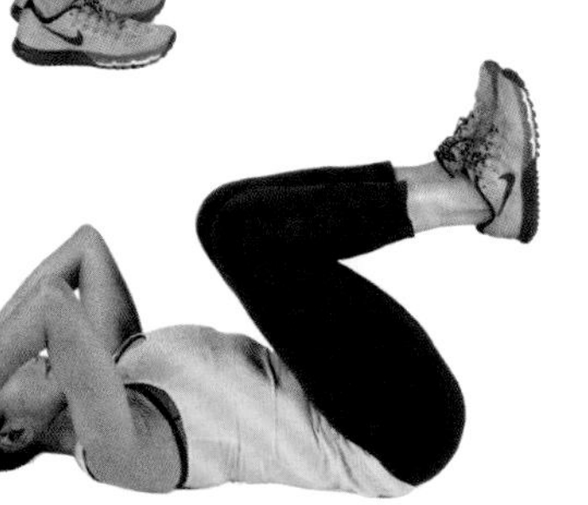

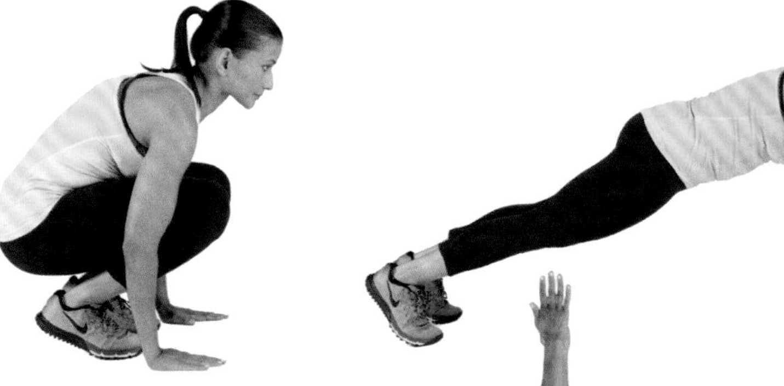

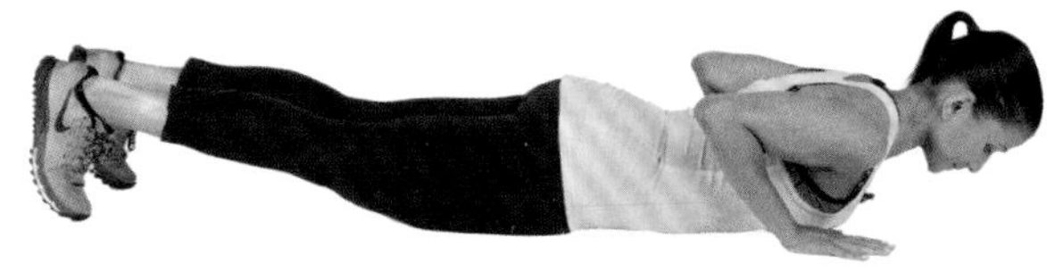

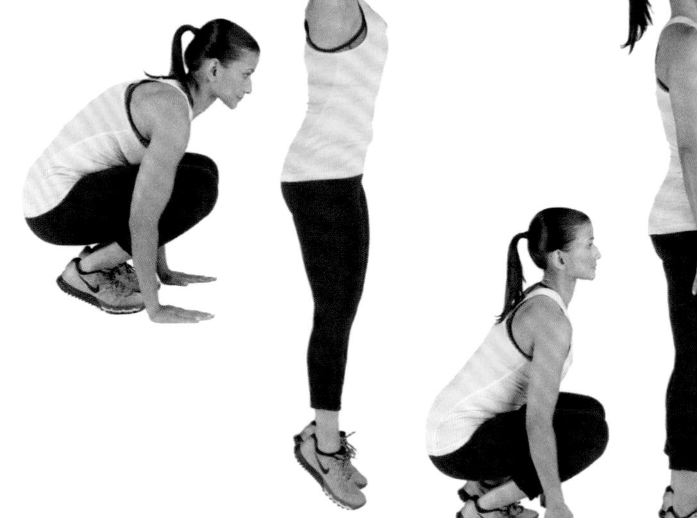

390 Burpee Deck Squats

Place a mat on the floor and stand in front of it with your back to it. Squat down to your toes, roll back on the mat bringing your legs as far back as you can, and then roll back up. As soon as you stand up, perform a Burpee (#380. Repeat for the desired time or repetitions.

Scissors

The Scissors exercise, taken from the demanding discipline of Pilates, improves core stability and increases abdominal strength and endurance. It can be modified by performing all the repetitions on one leg before switching to the other.

- Lie supine on the floor, your arms by your sides and your legs raised in a tabletop position. Inhale, drawing in your abdominals.
- Reach your legs straight upward, and lift your head and shoulders off the floor. Hold the position while lengthening your legs.
- Stretching your right leg away from your body, raise your left leg toward your trunk. Hold your left calf with your hands, pulsing twice while keeping your shoulders down.
- Switch your legs in the air, reaching for your right leg. Stabilize your pelvis and spine. Repeat sequence for the desired repetitions on each leg.

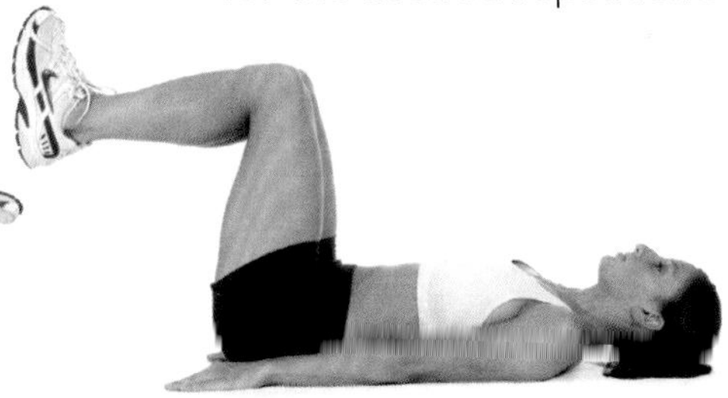

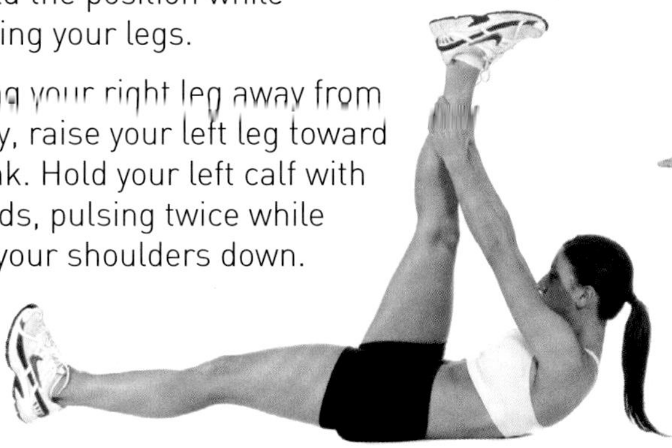

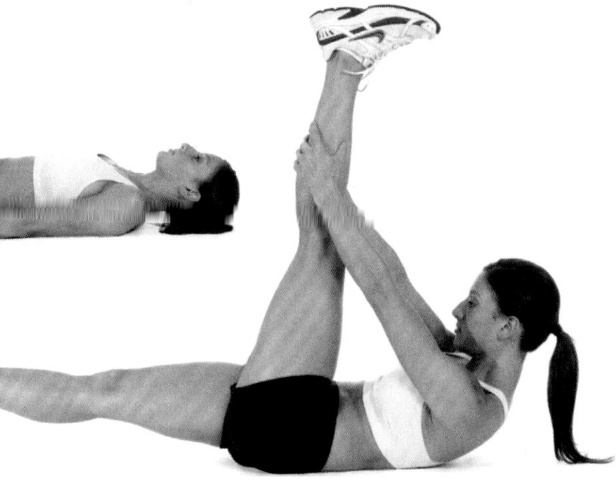

FIND YOUR FORM

Keep your abdominals tight and your lower back well grounded into the floor.

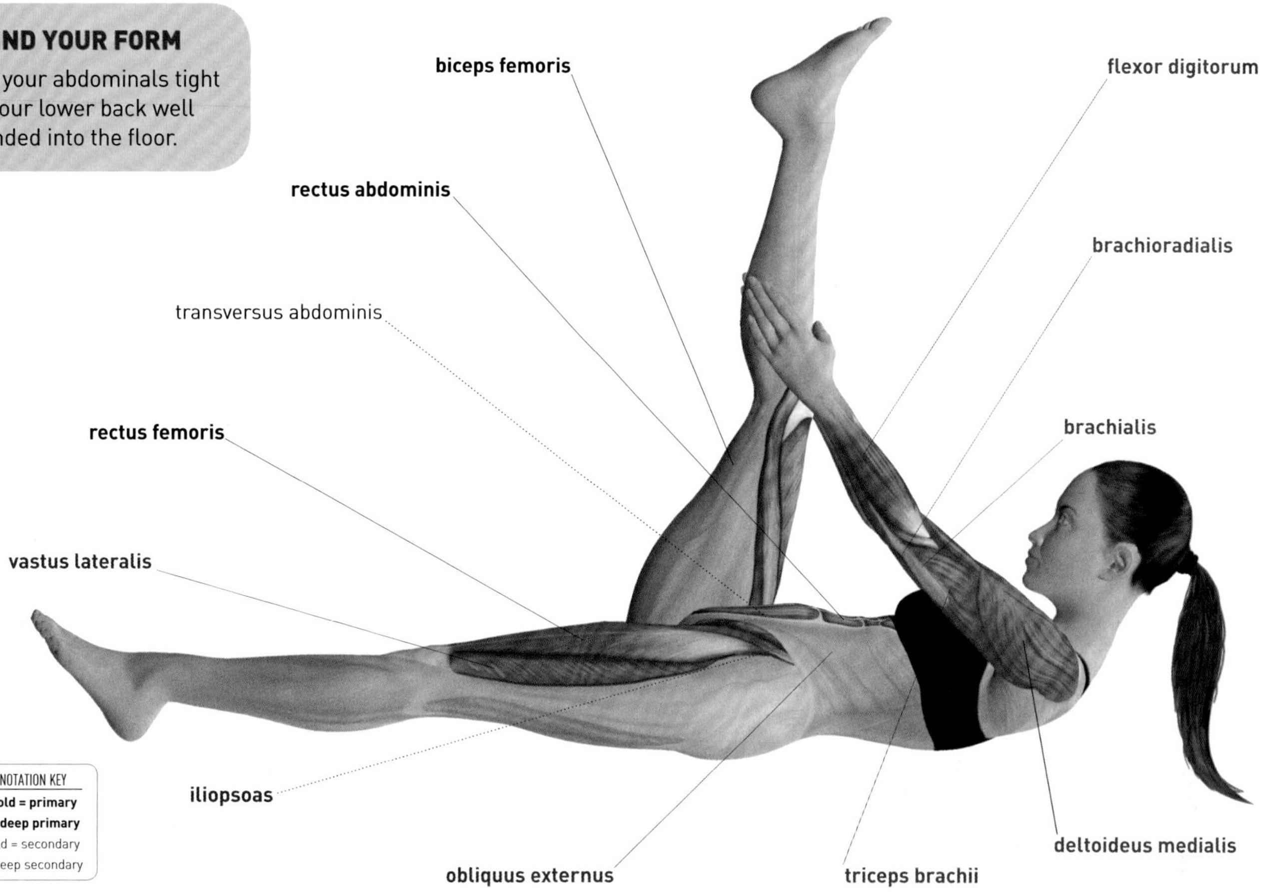

biceps femoris
flexor digitorum
rectus abdominis
brachioradialis
transversus abdominis
rectus femoris
brachialis
vastus lateralis
iliopsoas
deltoideus medialis
obliquus externus
triceps brachii

MUSCLE ANNOTATION KEY
— Black bold = primary
······ Black = deep primary
— Gray bold = secondary
······ Gray = deep secondary

392 Single-Leg Circles

Lie flat on the floor, with both legs and arms extended. Bend your right knee toward your chest, and then straighten your leg upward. Anchor the rest of your body to the floor, straightening both knees and pressing your shoulders back and down. Cross your raised leg up and over your body, aiming for your left shoulder. Continue making a circle with the raised leg, returning to the center. Switch directions so that you aim your leg away from your body. Repeat with the other leg.

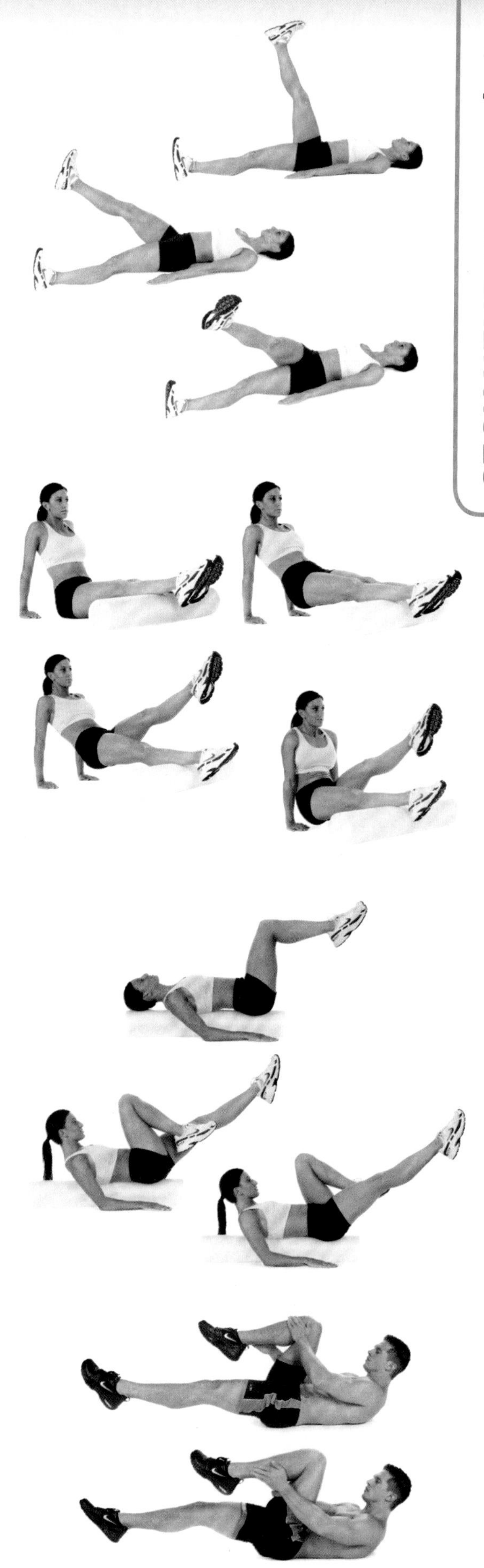

393 Single-Leg Calf Press

Sit with your legs outstretched in front of you, with a foam roller placed under your knees. Place your hands on the floor to support your torso, your fingers pointing forward. Press into the floor to lift your hips, keeping your legs firm. Lift one leg off the roller and hold it steady, making sure not to drop your hips. Keep your leg elevated, and press your opposite leg into the roller, drawing your hips back toward your hands. Return to the starting position, rolling your calf muscle along the roller and keeping your lifted leg straight in the air. Repeat with the other leg.

394 Foam Roller Bicycle

Lie supine with a roller placed lengthwise under your spine, your buttocks and shoulders resting on the roller. Place your forearms on the floor on either side of the roller to balance yourself. Draw your knees up to a tabletop position, and them keeping your back flat, lift your head, neck, and shoulders off the roller. Straighten your right leg. and pull your left knee toward your chest, keeping your head, neck, and shoulders lifted. Switch legs while maintaining your balance, imitating the pedaling of a bicycle. Repeat on the other side.

395 Abdominal Kicks

Lie in supine position with your legs extended. Lift from the shoulders as you pull your right knee toward your chest and straighten your left leg, raising it about 45 degrees from the floor. Place your right hand on your right ankle, and your left hand on your right knee. Keep switching your hand and leg placement for the desired repetitions.

396 Supine Marches

Lie lengthwise on a foam roller. Place your arms on the floor by your sides, bending your knees so that your feet rest flat on the floor. Pointing your toes, and keeping the hips from lifting or shifting, raise one knee toward your chest, being careful to keep your hips stationary. Continue alternating legs as you establish a smooth "marching" rhythm.

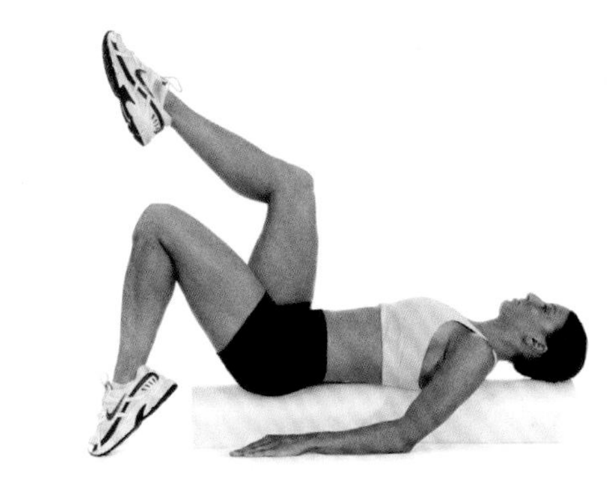

397 Tiny Steps

Lie supine with your knees bent and feet flat on the floor. Place your hands on your hip bones. Raise your right knee to your chest while pulling your navel toward your spine. Hold the position at the top. As you continue to pull your navel toward your spine, lower your right leg onto the floor while controlling any movement in your hips. Alternate legs to complete the full movement. Continue for the desired repetitions.

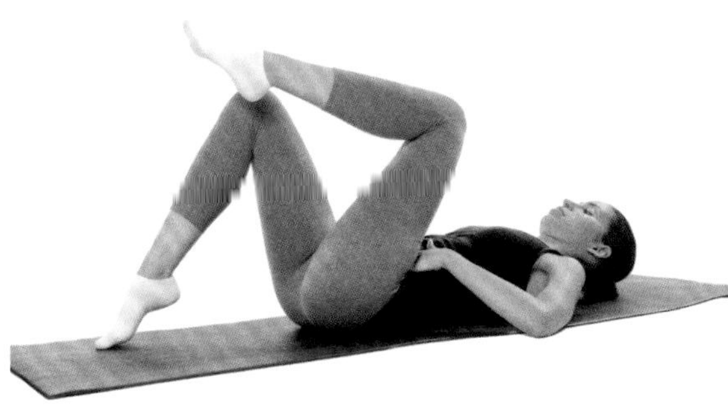

398 Double Leg Raise

The Double Leg Raise looks like a simply move—and it is in theory. But in practice, this exercise presents a strong challenge to your abdominals and hip flexors. Mastering this intense Pilates staple can result in a strong, stable core.

- Lie on your back with your arms along your sides, and extend your legs straight up toward the ceiling. Rotate your legs out slightly, keeping the heels together and inner legs pulled in the center line, and your toes pointed.
- Lower your legs so that your feet are just above the floor, and then raise them back to the starting position.

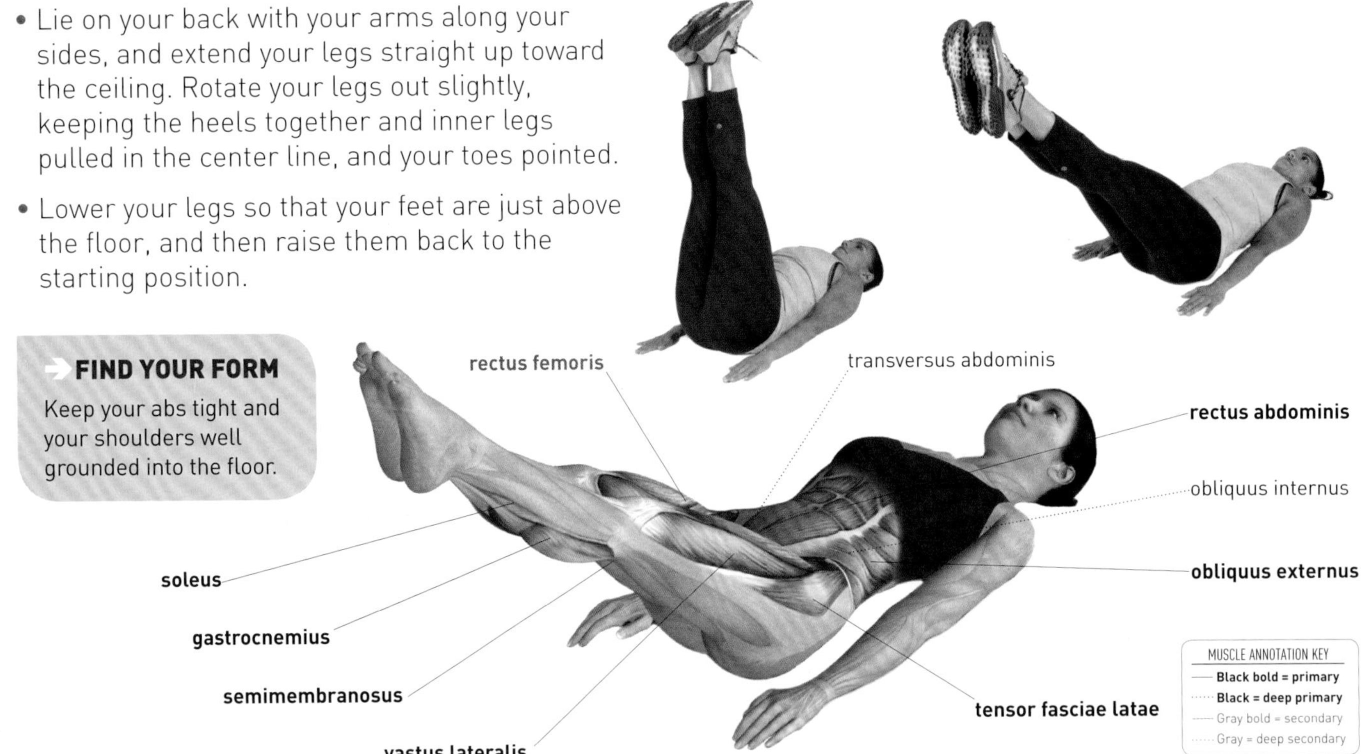

FIND YOUR FORM

Keep your abs tight and your shoulders well grounded into the floor.

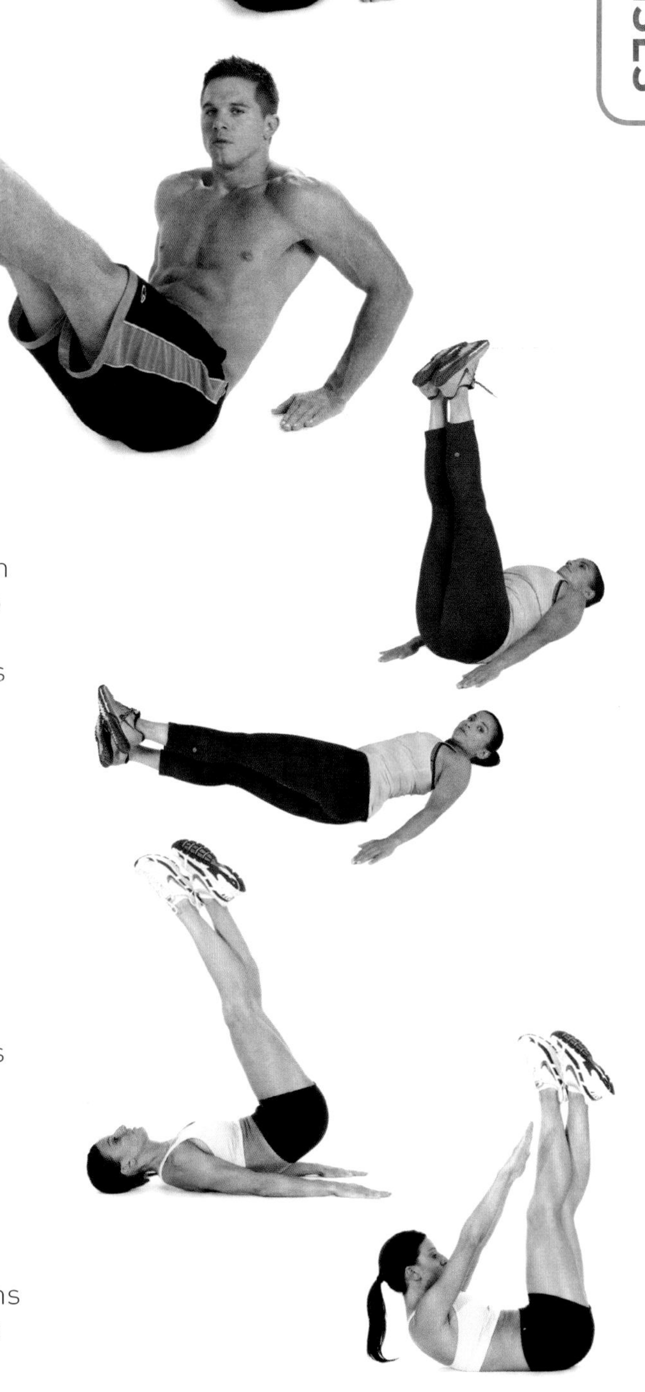

399 Hip Twist

Begin by sitting on the floor with your arms behind your body, supporting your weight. Your legs should be parallel and raised to a high diagonal. Engage your abdominals and shoulders for stabilization. Start to bring both legs across the body to the right. Continue to circle your legs across your body and down as low as pelvic stabilization can be maintained. Return your legs to the starting position. Repeat two to six times in each direction.

400 Corkscrew

Lie supine with your arms along your sides, palms down. Imprint your spine, and lengthen your legs—one at a time—to the ceiling. Keep your legs parallel, firmly pressed together. Stabilize your shoulder blades and your pelvis against the weight of your legs as you inhale and begin circling your legs to the right and down. Continue to circle your legs as you complete the circle on an exhalation. Repeat, "drawing" a circle in the other direction.

401 Abdominal Hip Lift

Lie supine with your arms along your sides, palms down. Lift your legs straight in the air, and cross them at the ankles. Pinching your legs together and squeezing your glutes, press into the back of your arms to lift your hips upward. Slowly return your hips to the floor. Perform for the desired reps, and then switch with the opposite leg crossed in the front.

402 Hip Lift with Arm Reach

Keeping your hips on the floor, raise your arms toward the ceiling. Reach toward your toes as you lift your shoulders off the floor.

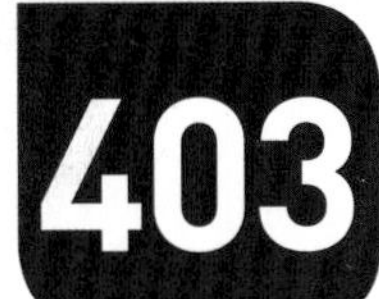

Tabletop Ab Press

The Tabletop Ab Press, also known as the 90-Degree Static Press, demonstrates how an isometric, static exercise can reap high-intensity benefits. It effectively engages your core, and it will also get these muscles ready for a high-energy workout. Its tabletop position is also the base for other dynamic exercises.

- Lie on your back with your knees and feet lifted, your thighs making a 90-degree angle with your upper body. This is the tabletop position.
- Place your hands on the front of your knees, your fingers facing upward, one palm on each leg.
- Flex your feet, and, keeping your elbows bent and pulled into your sides, press your hands into your knees. Create resistance by pushing back against your hands with your knees. Hold for up to a minute, and then repeat for the desired repetitions.

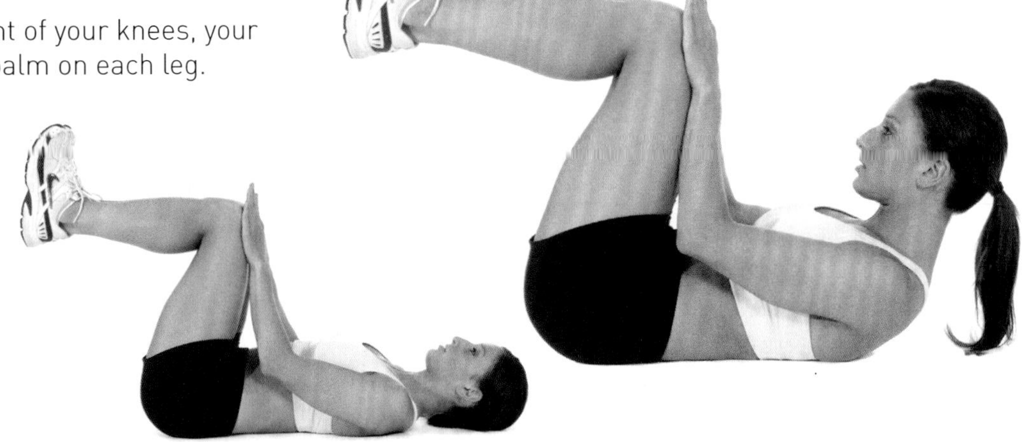

FIND YOUR FORM

To fully engage your core, imagine that you are "zipping" your muscles from your pelvic floor up to your navel.

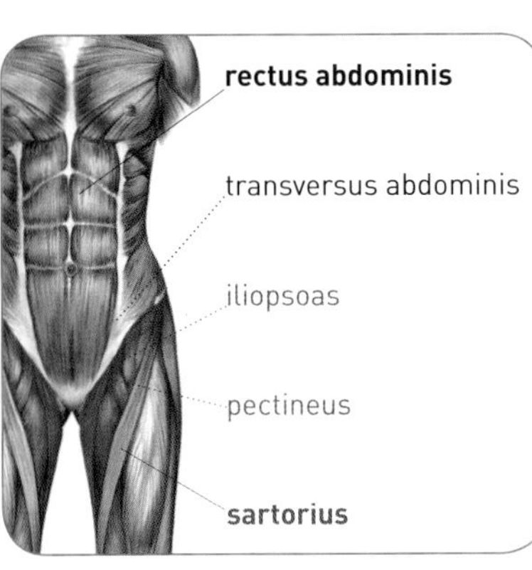

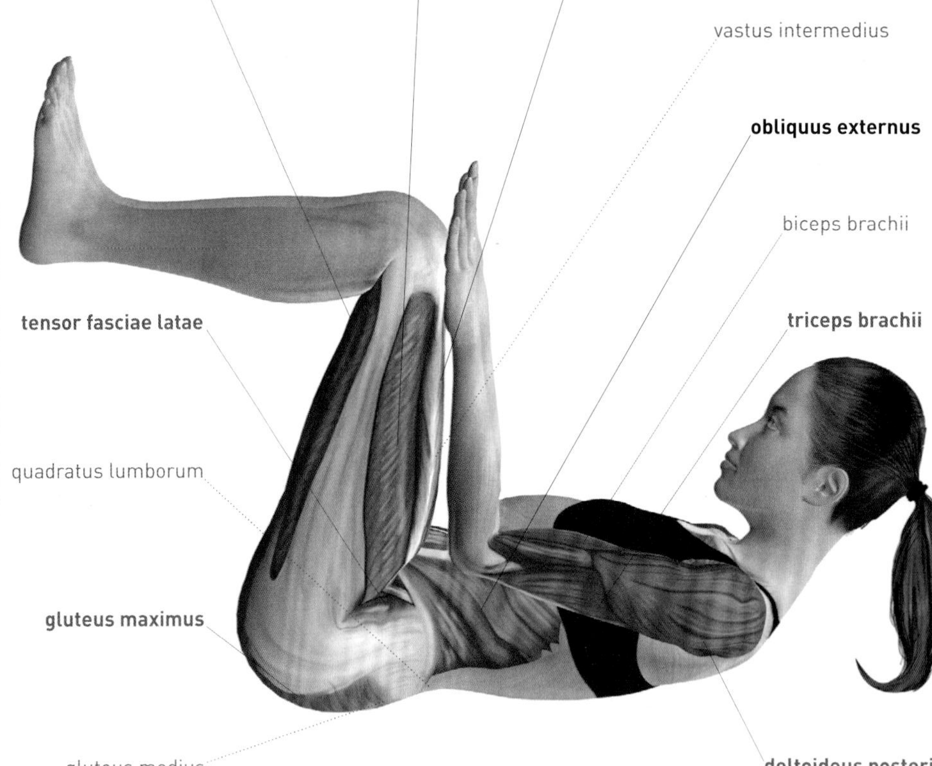

MUSCLE ANNOTATION KEY
- Black bold = primary
- Black = deep primary
- Gray bold = secondary
- Gray = deep secondary

404 The Dead Bug

Lie supine with a foam roller placed lengthwise under your spine, your buttocks and shoulders resting on the roller. Place your hands and forearms flat on the floor for stabilization. Draw your knees up so that your legs form a tabletop position. Lift your head, neck, and shoulders. Press the palms of your hands onto your knees, creating your own resistance as you try to balance. Flex your toes, and keep your elbows pulled in to your sides. Hold for a few seconds, release, and then repeat for the desired repetitions.

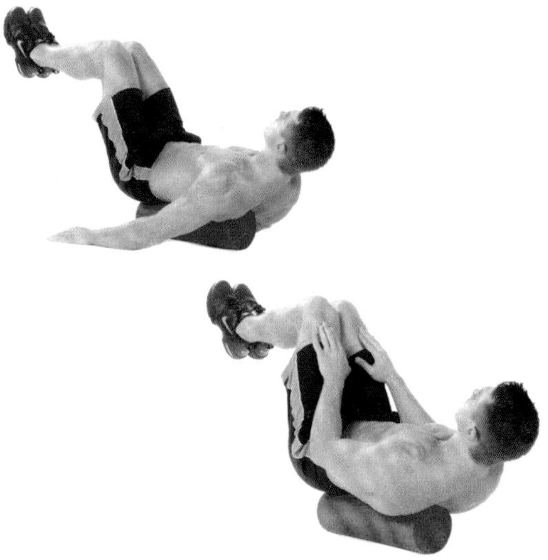

405 Swiss Ball Tabletop Rotation

Lie supine in tabletop position with a Swiss ball between your knees. Press your shoulder blades into the floor, and move your legs and the Swiss ball toward your left. Your hips should roll along with your body, but try to keep the rest of your torso on the floor. Return to the starting position, and then bring the ball toward the left. Continue to alternate sides for the desired repetitions.

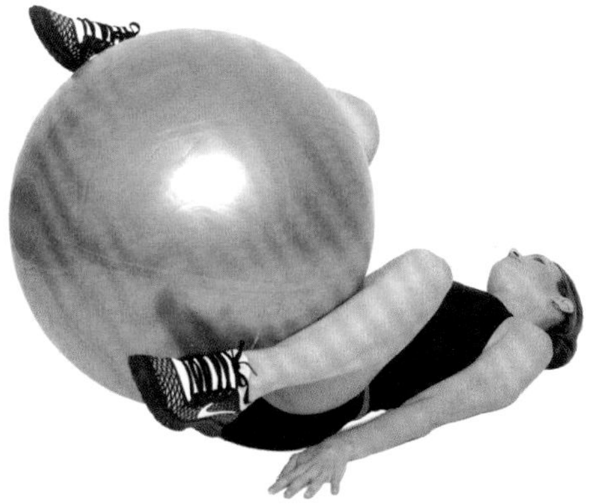

406 Hip Crossover

Lie supine with your knees and feet lifted in tabletop position, your thighs making a 90-degree angle with your upper body. Brace your abdominals, and lower your legs to one side, as close to the floor as you can possibly go without raising your shoulders off the floor. Return to the starting position, and then repeat on the other side. Continue to alternate sides for the desired repetitions.

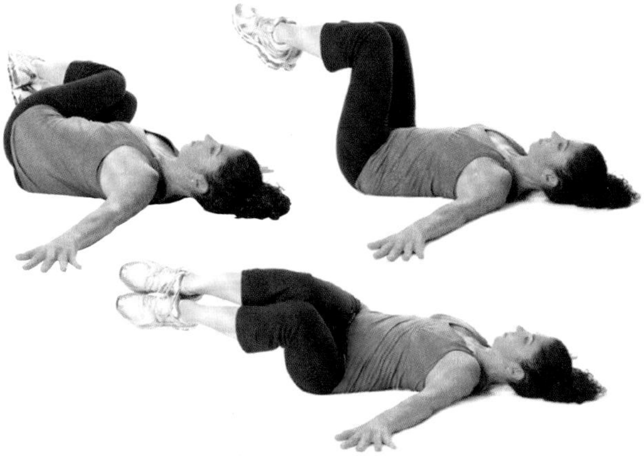

407 Swiss Ball Hip Crossover

Lie on your back, with your arms extended out to your sides. Place your legs on a Swiss ball, with your glutes close to the ball so that your lower body assumes the tabletop position. Perform as you would the Hip Crossover (#405). Continue to alternate sides for the desired repetitions.

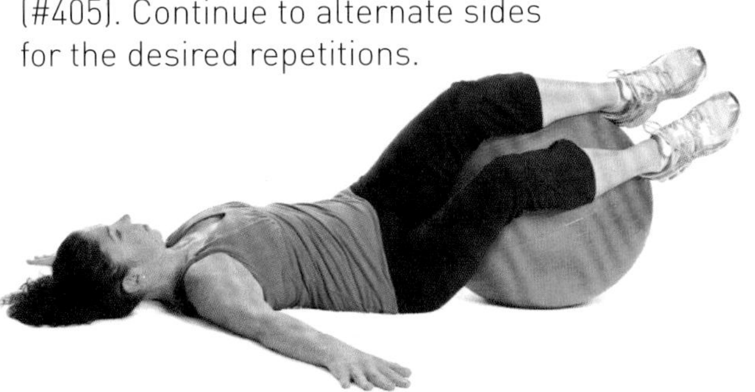

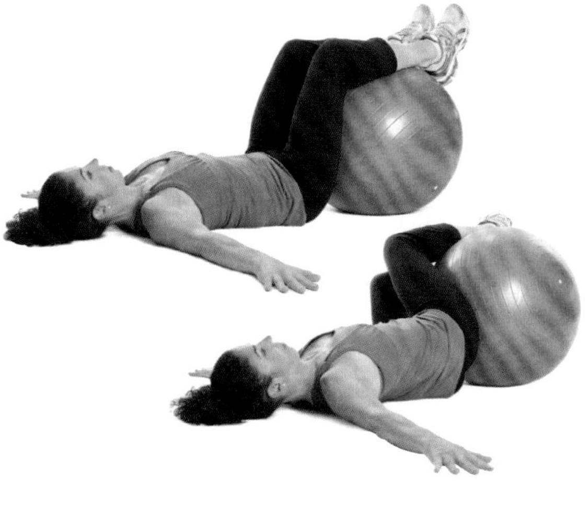

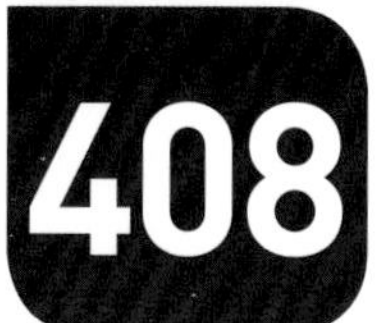

Half Curl-Up

The Half Curl is a simple upper-abdominal exercise that strengthens your core muscles, protecting your back while increasing muscle tone.

- Lie on your back with your knees bent and arms straight by your sides. Squeeze your legs together and keep your feet flat on the floor.
- Using your upper abdominals, curl your upper back and shoulders upward so that your middle back remains pressed to the floor. Keep your arms parallel to the floor and your lower back flat.
- Hold for a few seconds, and then return to the starting position, and repeat for the desired repetitions.

FIND YOUR FORM

Keep your arms parallel to the floor throughout the exercise. Avoid curling your neck too far forward or allowing your feet to lift off the floor.

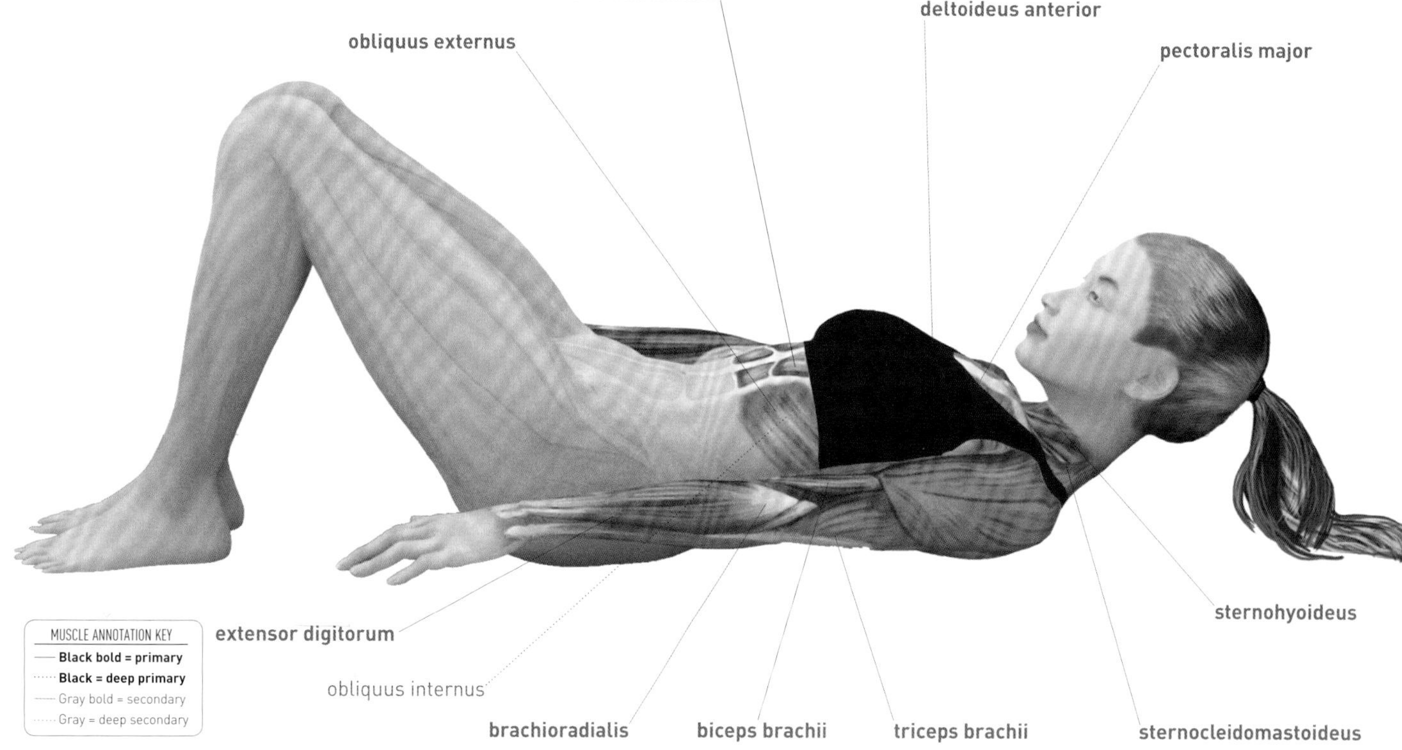

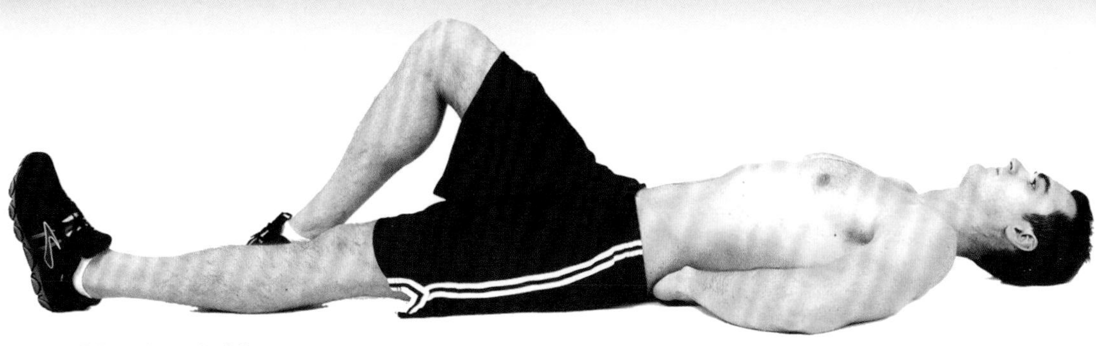

409 McGill Curl-Up

Lie supine with your right leg fully extended and your left leg bent. Place both hands palm-down beneath your lower back. Keeping your abdominal muscles braced, contract them slightly, bringing your head and shoulders off the floor. Hold for a 5-second count. Lower your head, and repeat for the desired repetitions, and then switch legs.

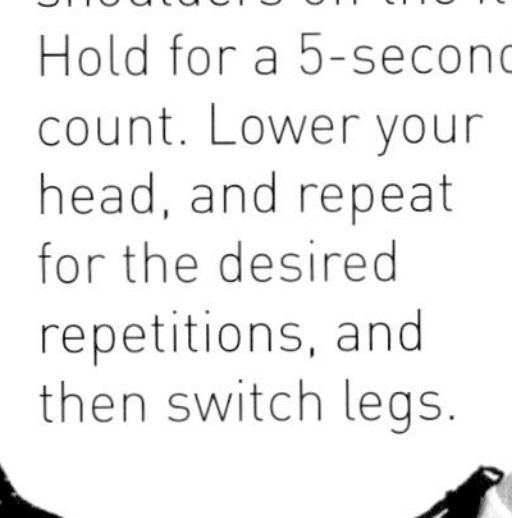

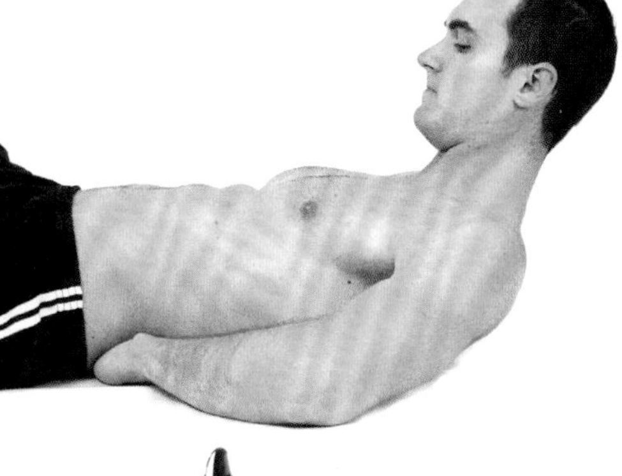

410 Swiss Ball Curl-Up

Lie on your back, with your arms extended by your sides. Place your legs on a Swiss ball, with your glutes close to the ball so that your lower body assumes the tabletop position. Perform as your would a Half Curl-Up (#408). Repeat for the desired repetitions.

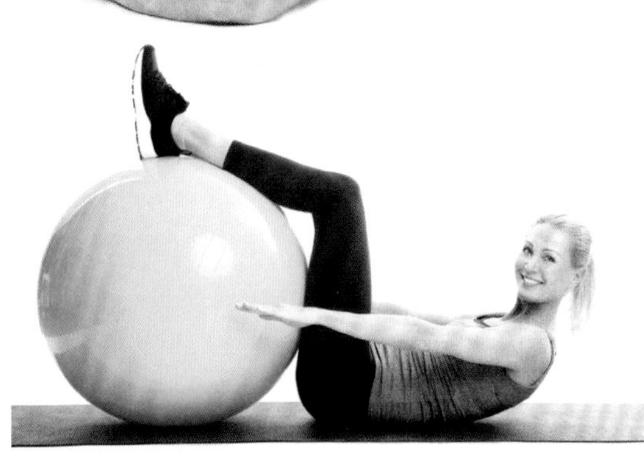

411 Curl-Up

Lie on your back with your knees bent and arms straight by your sides. Squeeze your legs together and keep your feet flat on the floor. Using your upper abdominals, curl your upper back and shoulders upward until your middle back is fully lifted from the floor. Keep your arms parallel to the floor and your lower back flat and pressed into the floor. Hold for a few seconds, and then return to the starting position, and repeat for the desired repetitions.

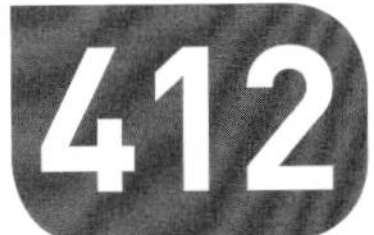

412 Tabletop Curl-Up

Lie on your back with your knees and feet lifted, your thighs making a 90-degree angle with your upper body to assume the tabletop position. Perform as you would the Curl-Up (#411). Repeat for the desired repetitions.

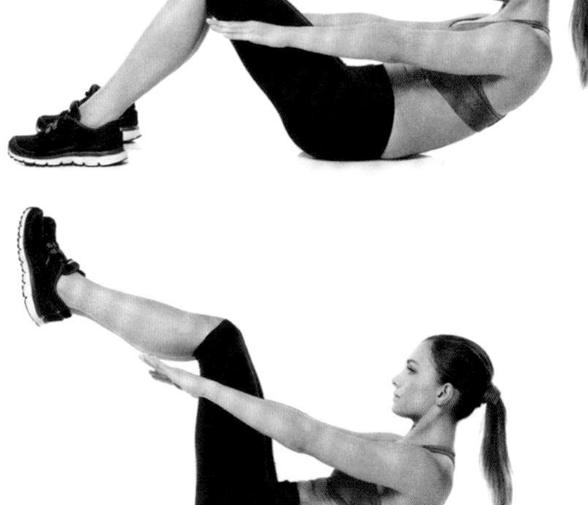

413 Crunch

Long the go-to strength move for toning the abdominals, the Crunch works the pectorals major, rectus abdominals, external obliques, internal obliques, and transverse abdominals. With its many variations, however, this strength-training move can be incorporated into a high-intensity regimen. Form is essential, so mastering the basic move can help you work in its more demanding versions.

- Lie supine on the floor with your knees bent, and clasp your hands behind your head.
- Keeping your elbows wide, engage the abdominals, and lift your upper torso to achieve a crunching movement.
- Moving with control, return to the starting position. Continue at a quick, but controlled pace.

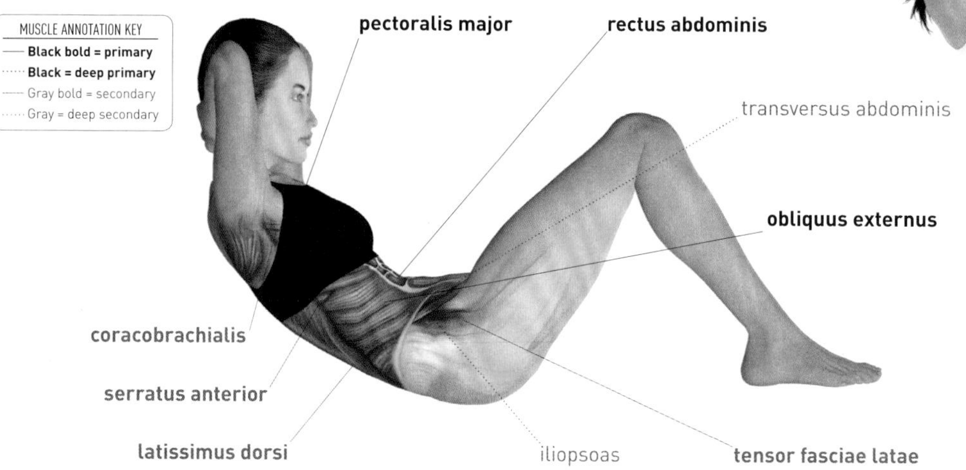

FIND YOUR FORM

Fully engage your abs; this tension will help ensure that you do not overarch your back. Be sure the movement originates with your core—avoid pulling on your neck or drawing your elbows in, which may strain your neck muscles and vertebrae.

414 Reverse Crunch

Lie supine on the floor, and extend your arms at your sides. Raise your knees and feet so that they create a 90-degree angle. Contract your abdominals, and exhale as you lift your hips off the floor; your knees will move toward your head. Inhale, and slowly lower.

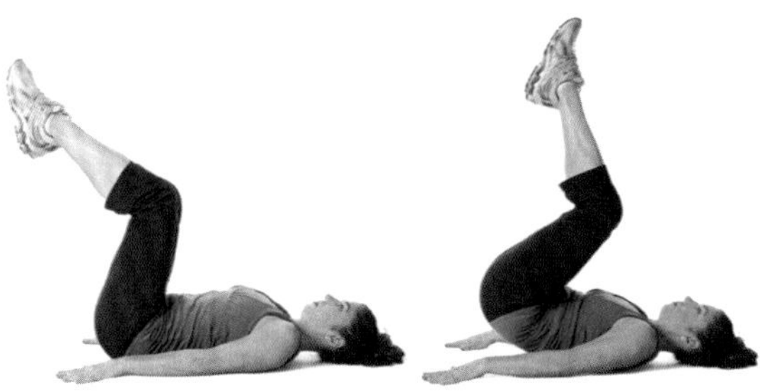

415 Cable Crunch

Kneel in front of a cable station with a rope attachment connected to the top pulley. Grip the rope, resting your wrists against your forehead. Flex your hips slightly to take the weight and to hyperextend your lower back. Keeping your hips stationary, bend at the waist so that your elbows move down toward the middle of your thighs. Hold for one count, and return to the starting position.

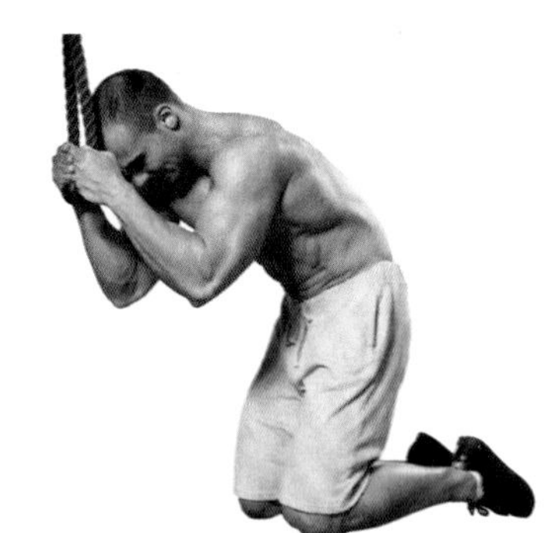

416 Lemon Squeezer

Lie supine on the floor. Lift your legs, head, neck, and shoulders slightly off the floor. Raise your arms until they are parallel to the floor. Pulling your knees in toward your chest, reach your arms toward your ankles, so that your torso lifts completely off the floor. Slowly open up, lengthening your legs and lowering back to the starting position. Repeat the motion without completely lying down. Repeat for the desired repetitions.

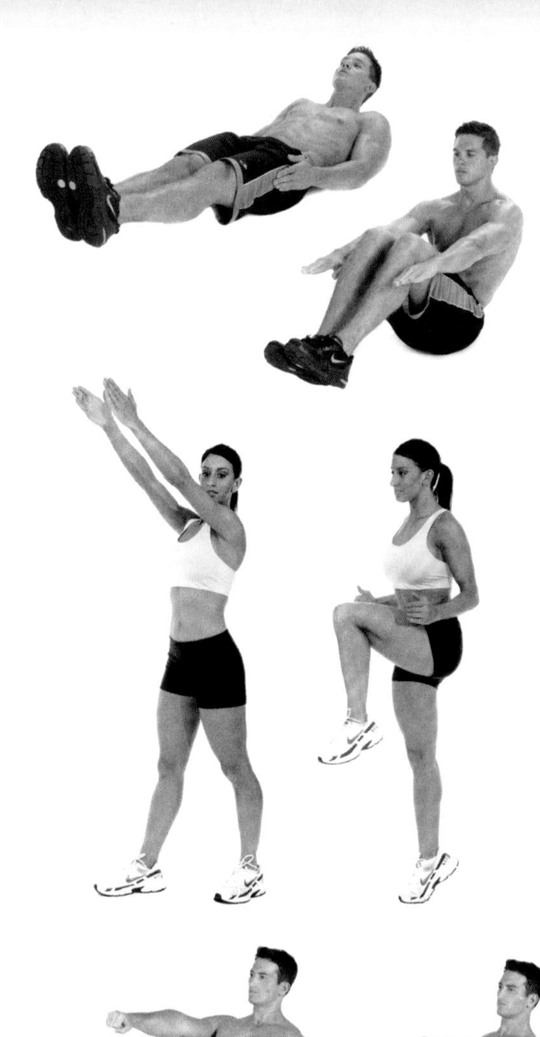

417 Standing Knee Crunch

Standing tall with your left leg in front of your right, extend your hands toward the ceiling, your arms straight. Shift your weight onto your left foot, and raise your right knee to hip height. Simultaneously rise on the toes of your left foot while pulling your elbows down by your sides, your hands making fists to create the crunch. Pause at the top of the movement, and then return to the starting position. Repeat the sequence with your right leg as the standing leg.

418 Punching Abs

Sit with your legs extended and feet together, knees slightly bent. Brace your core and lean back slightly, with your fists at each side of your chest, elbows bent. Punch your right fist forward at shoulder height, and then quickly return to the starting position, and repeat on the other side. Continue alternating punching right and left for the desired repetitions.

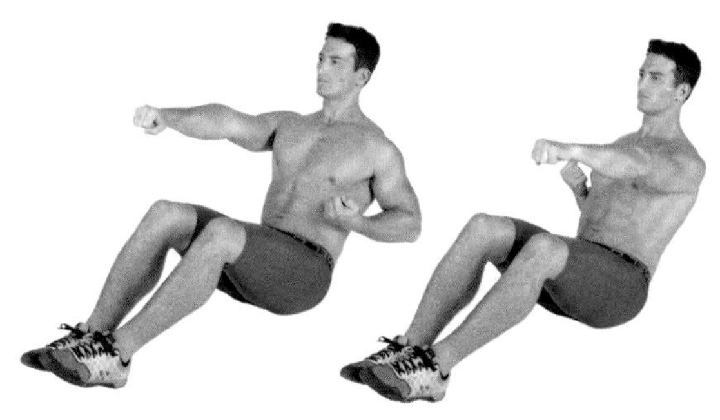

419 Forearm Side Plank Crunch

Get into the Forearm Side Plank position (#325). Bend your top elbow, while at the same time bending your top knee and bringing it toward your elbow to create the crunch. Perform the desired repetitions, and then repeat on the other side.

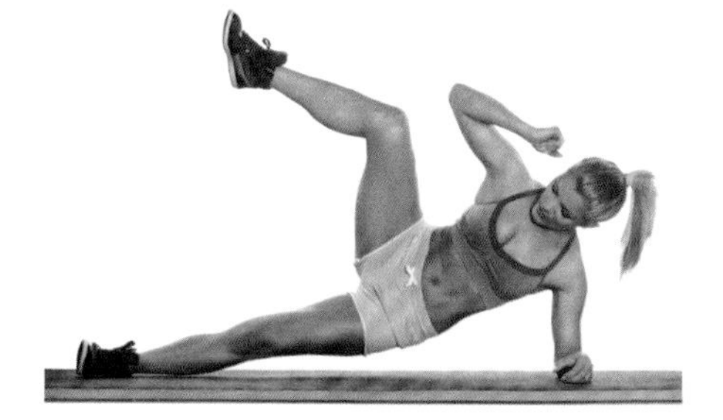

420 Foam Roller Diagonal Crunch

Lie lengthwise on a foam roller. With your legs straight and your feet pressed into the floor, extend your arms over your head. As you raise your head, neck, and shoulders, leave your right leg and left arm on the floor, using your hand for support. Raise your left leg and right arm, and reach for your ankle. Return to the starting position, and repeat on the other side.

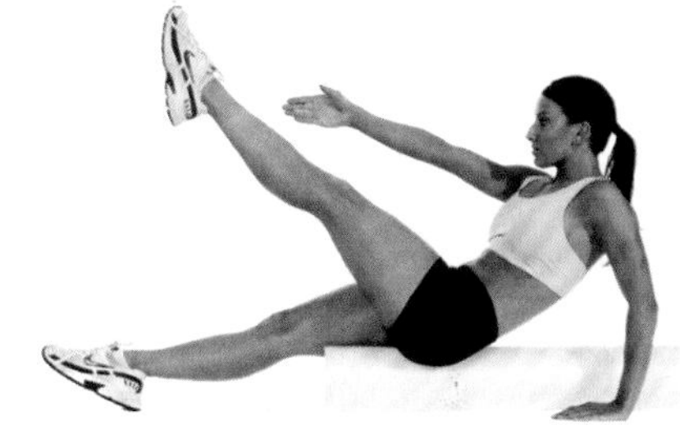

421

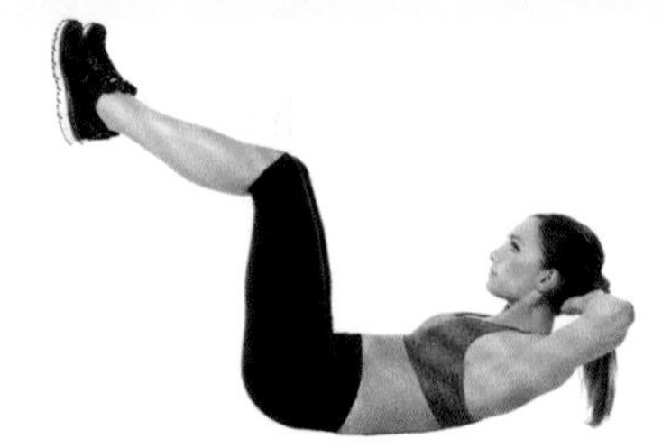

Tabletop Crunch

Get into the top position with your knees bent so that your shins are parallel to the floor, and then perform as you would a Crunch (#413). Repeat for the desired repetitions.

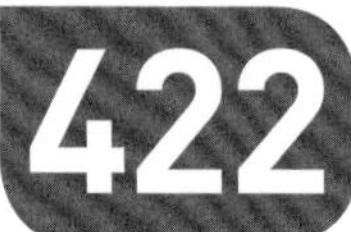

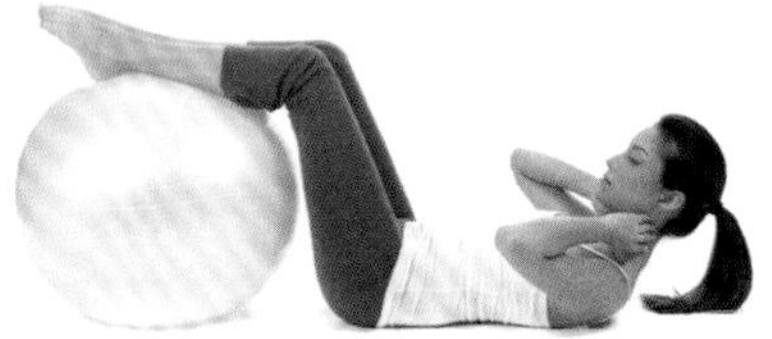

Swiss Ball Tabletop Crunch

Lie supine in the tabletop position with the back of your calves resting on a Swiss Ball. Perform as you would a Crunch (#413). Repeat for the desired repetitions.

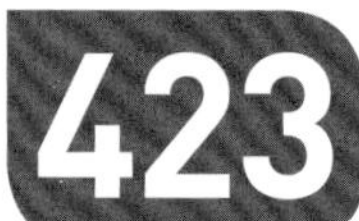

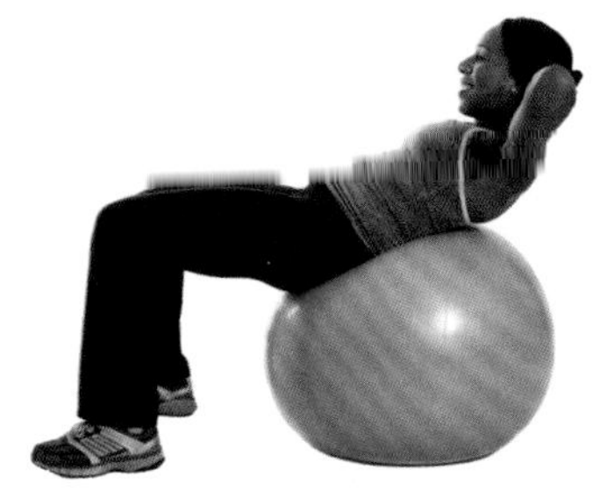

Swiss Ball Crunch

Plant your feet firmly on the floor, and prop your back on a Swiss Ball with your head and neck supported, legs bent, your palms placed on your ears, and your elbows flared outward. Raise your head and shoulders off the ball while contracting your torso toward your waist, keeping your lower back on the ball. Lower, and repeat for the desired repetitions.

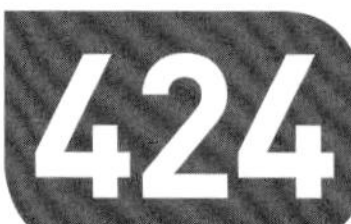

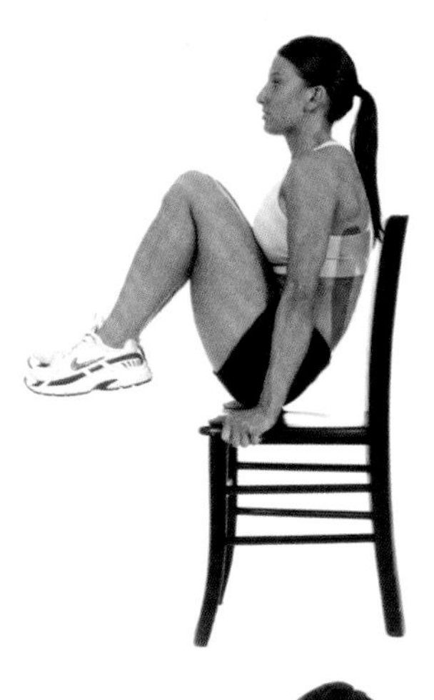

Chair Crunch

Sit on a chair with your hands grasping the sides of the seat and your arms straight. Step forward, bending your knees and lifting your butt off the chair. Your hips and knees should be bent to form 90-degree angles. Tuck your tailbone toward the front of the chair, and bring your knees toward your chest. Bend your elbows simultaneously. At the bottom of the movement, extend your elbows and press through your shoulders. Keeping your head in neutral position, press into the chair and lower your legs to return to the starting position. Repeat for the desired repetitions.

L-Sit

Sit with your legs straight in front of you, your hands placed next to your hips, palms down. Press strongly into the floor to and push yourself up so that your butt and legs rise from the floor. Hold for the desired time period.

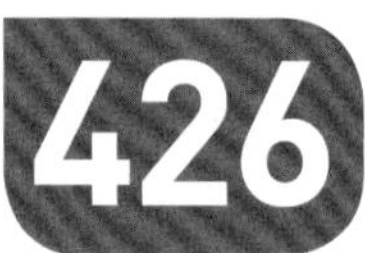

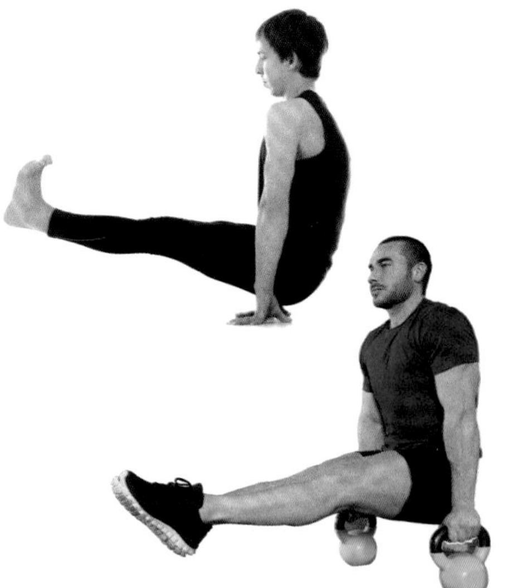

Kettlebell L-Sit

Sit with your legs straight in front of you, your hands grasping the handles of a kettlebell placed next to your hips. Perform as your would an L-Sit (#425). Hold for the desired time period. You can also perform this version on parallel bars.

Crossover Crunch

The Crossover Crunch adds a literal twist to the basic crunch, calling for a greater contribution from the oblique muscles that run along the side of your ribcage. It helps give you a total core workout and can also help stabilize your back —and a strong back is crucial for any high-intensity workout regimen.

- Bring your hands behind your head, lifting your legs off the floor into a tabletop position.
- Roll up with your torso, reaching your right elbow to your left knee and extending the right leg in front of you. Imagine pulling your shoulder blades off the floor and twisting from your ribs and oblique muscles. Continue to alternate sides in a quick, but controlled pace.

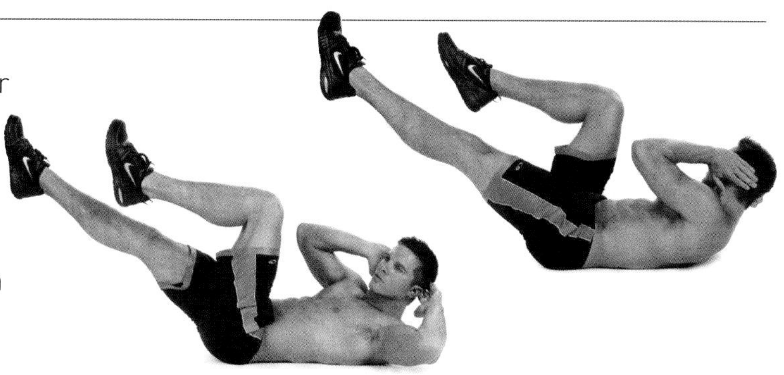

428

Bent-Leg Crossover Crunch

Begin with both feet on the floor. Place the outside of one foot on top of your thigh near your knee. Perform as you would the Crossover Crunch (#418). Repeat for the desired repetitions.

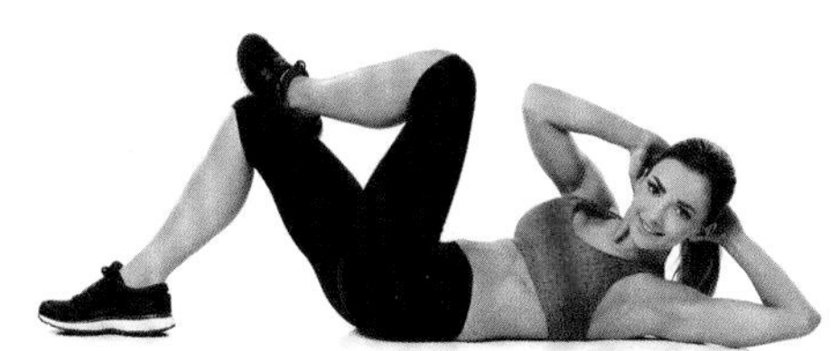

429

Side Raised-Leg Crunch

Lie on your side with your legs slightly bent, your lower hand on your stomach, and the upper behind your head. Raise your head and shoulders off the floor as you lift your legs, keeping your feet together. Lower and repeat for the desired repetitions, and then switch sides.

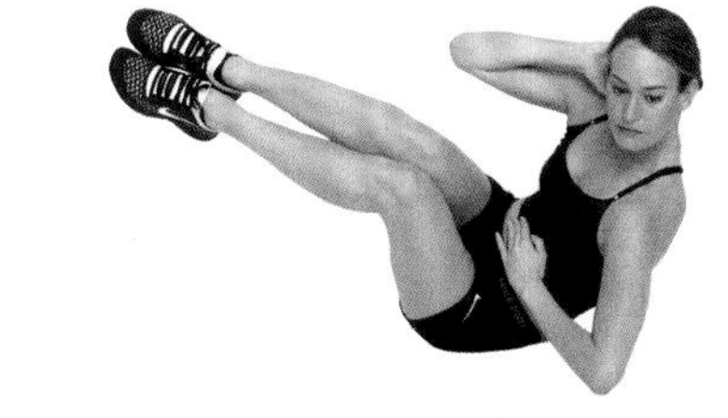

430

Penguin Crunch

Lie supine with your knees bent, your head elevated, and your arms straight at your sides and raised off the floor. Holding your torso in a flexed position, lean to the right, and reach your right hand forward. Hold for one count, and then pull it back Repeat on your left side. Continue to alternate sides for the desired repetitions.

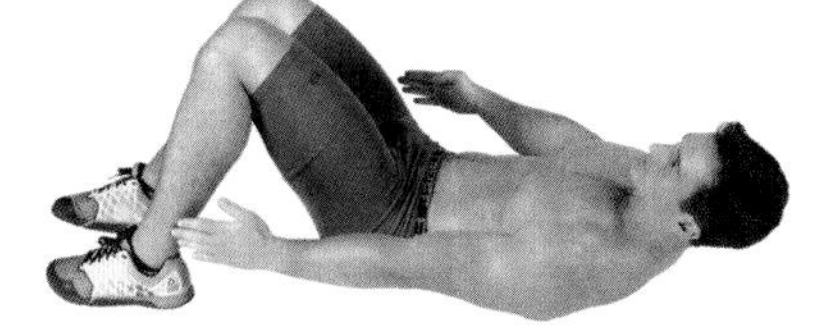

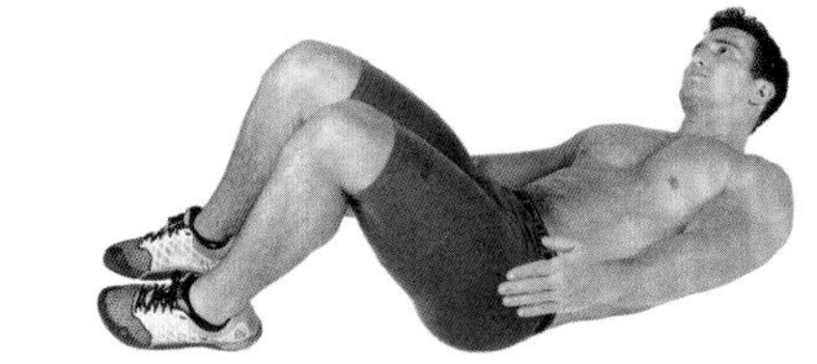

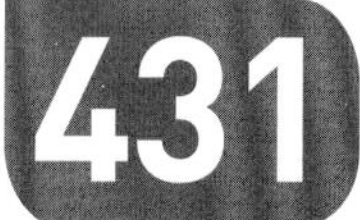

Alternating Crunch

Lie supine with your legs bent. Place your palms behind your ears, flaring your elbows outward. Raise your head and shoulders off the floor while contracting your trunk toward your waist as you rotate your elbow toward the opposite knee. Lower, and repeat on the other side. Continue to alternate sides for the desired repetitions.

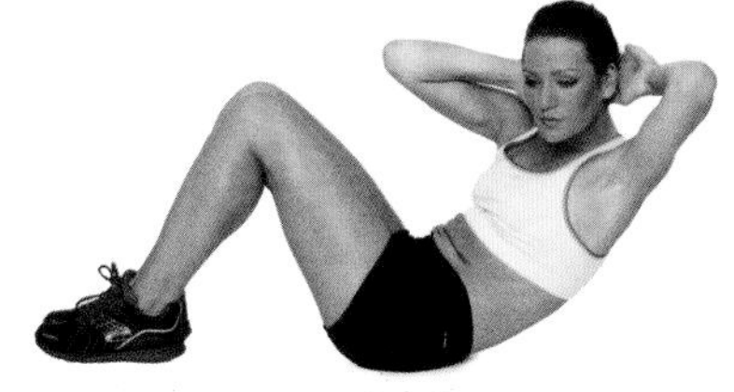

432 Straight-Leg Hanging Knee Raise

Grab a pull-up bar with your palms facing forward. Your feet should not be contacting the ground. Pull on the bar so that your shoulders are down and away from your ears, keeping your legs straight and your knees and ankles taut. Keeping your lower back flat, kick forward to bring both legs up to horizontal. Slowly allow your legs to drop in a controlled manner until they are directly beneath you and back to the starting position. Repeat for the desired repetitions.

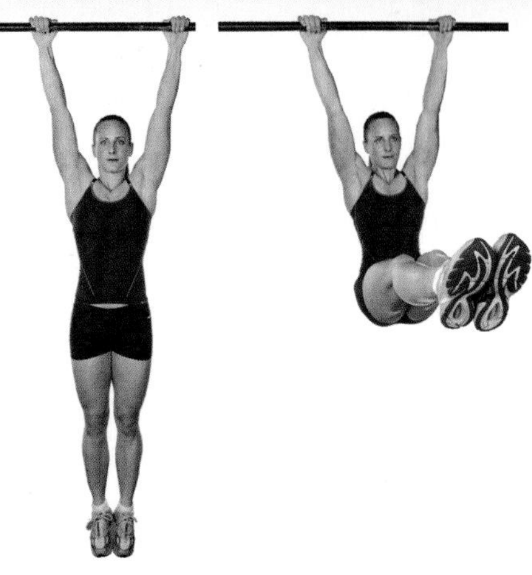

433 Bent-Knee Hanging Knee Raise with Medicine Ball

Hang with your upper arms in ab straps attached to a pull-up bar, clasping a medicine ball between your knees. Grasp the top of the stirrups with your hands, pull your upper arms and elbows downward and your upper legs and knees upward toward your elbows, flexing at the hips. Return to the starting position in a slow and controlled manner. Repeat for the desired repetitions.

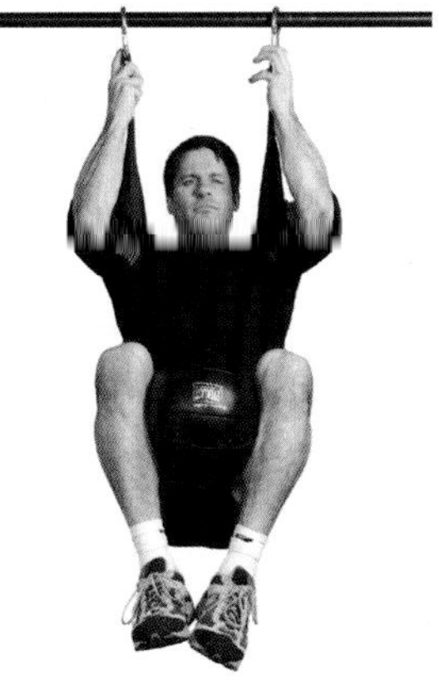

434 Hanging Knee Raise with Rotation

Hang with your upper arms in ab straps attached to a pull-up bar, with your elbows bent at 90-degree angles, pointing forward just above shoulder height. Grasp the straps with your hands, and pull your upper arms and elbows downward while rotating your upper legs and knees upward toward your elbow, flexing at the hips. Tuck your hips forward and bring your chest forward slightly. Return to the starting position in a slow and controlled manner. Repeat for the desired repetitions.

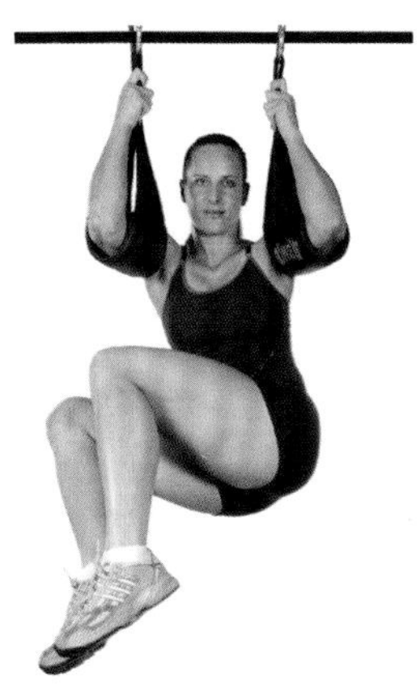

435 Layout on Rings

With body rigid and at a 45-degree angle to the floor, grasp gymnastic rings directly under your shoulder with a palms-down grip, so that rings are parallel and directly beneath your chest, your legs, hips, and spine forming a straight line. With your arms straight, push your hands forward and outward, using your toes as a fulcrum and allowing your entire body to descend in a controlled manner until your arms are in a horizontal position. Return by pulling your arms back toward the floor until your body returns to start position. Repeat for the desired repetitions.

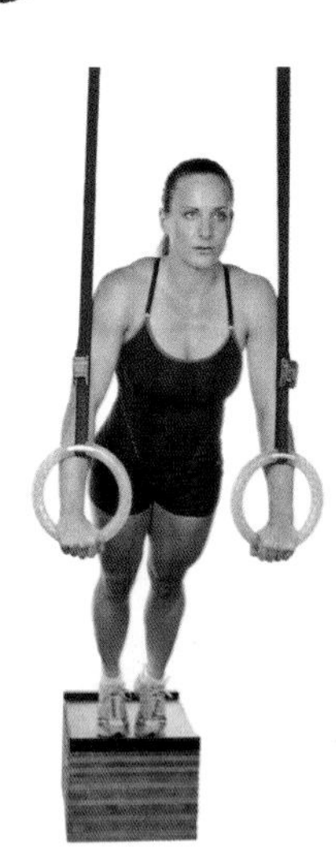

436 Turkish Get-Up

The Turkish Get-Up is a simple but comprehensive exercise that targets a wide range of muscles, including those in the shoulders, core, thighs, back, glutes, and arms. It increases stability in the hips and aids balance throughout the body. Make it more of a challenge by holding a dumbbell or kettlebell in your raised hand.

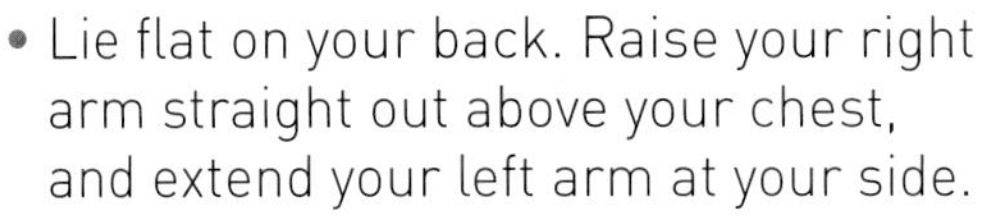

- Lie flat on your back. Raise your right arm straight out above your chest, and extend your left arm at your side.
- Flex your right knee, and place your right foot flat on the floor.
- Rotate your core slightly to the left, and lift your shoulders off the floor, supporting your weight on your left forearm. Next, plant your left hand on the floor and lift yourself up to a sitting position.
- Lift your hips upward, and tuck your left leg under your body to support yourself on your left knee.

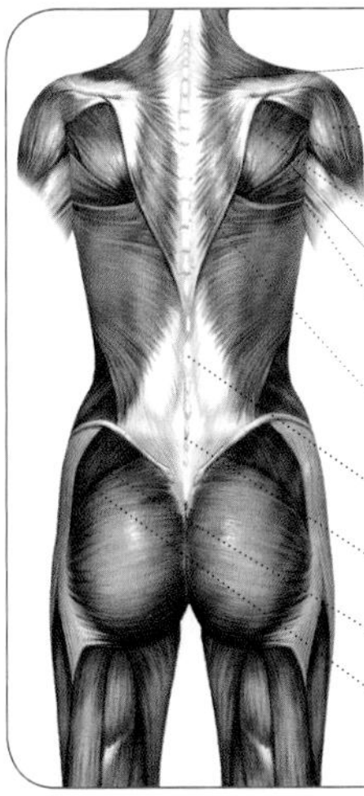

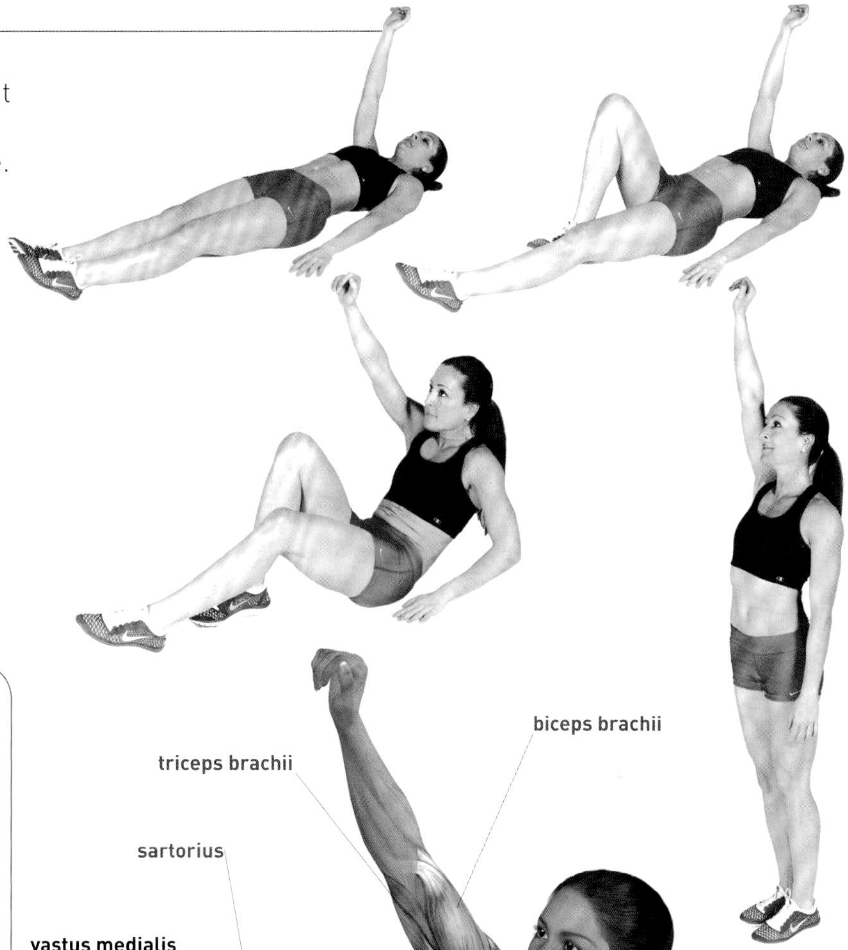

trapezius
deltoideus posterior
infraspinatus
supraspinatus
teres minor
subscapularis
rhomboideus
erector spinae
multifidus spinae
gluteus minimus
gluteus medius

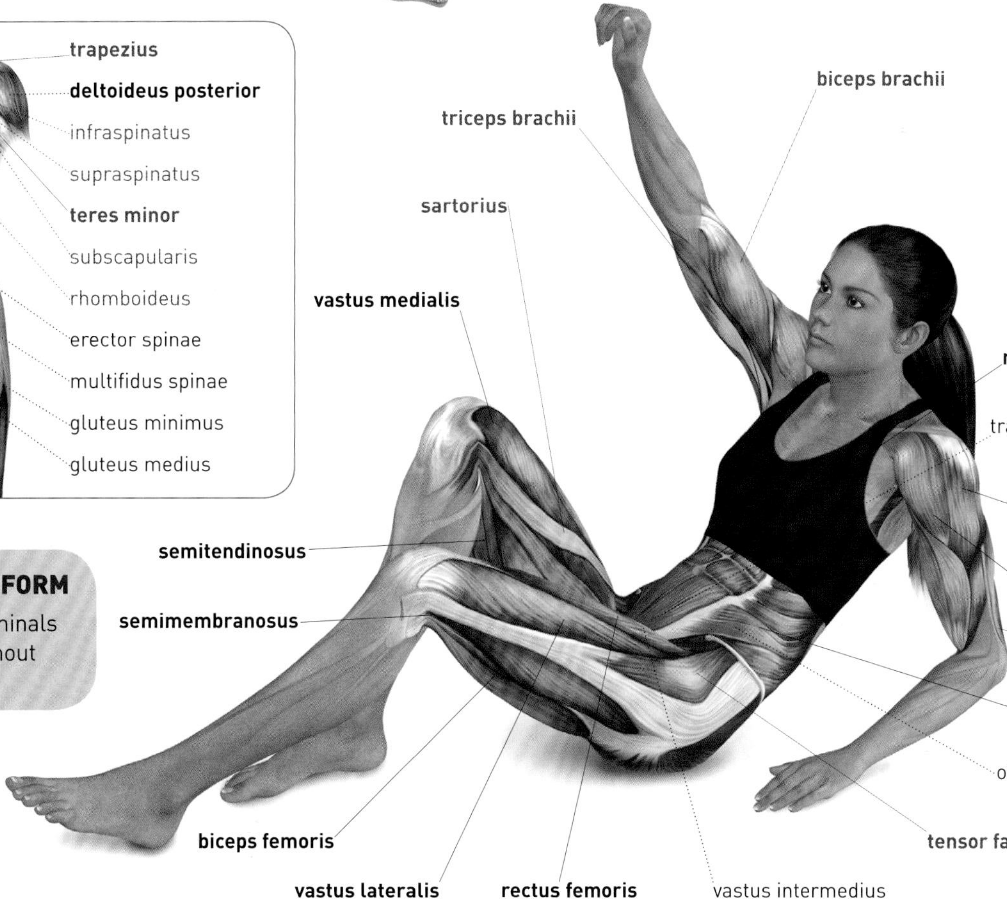

FIND YOUR FORM
Keep your abdominals engaged throughout the movement.

MUSCLE ANNOTATION KEY
Black bold = primary
Black = deep primary
Gray bold = secondary
Gray = deep secondary

biceps brachii
triceps brachii
sartorius
vastus medialis
rectus abdominis
transversus abdominis
deltoideus medialis
semitendinosus
deltoideus anterior
semimembranosus
brachialis
obliquus externus
obliquus internus
biceps femoris
tensor fasciae latae
vastus lateralis
rectus femoris
vastus intermedius

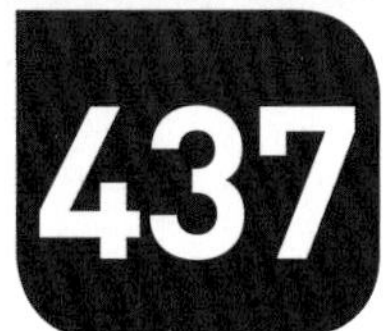

437 Sit-Up

The sit-up is to the abdominals what the bench press is to the pectorals: a highly effective exercise. The iconic sit-up is widely used on a daily basis and for good reason: it's the perfect exercise for the rectus abdominis. It is similar to a crunch, but sit-ups have a fuller range of motion and condition additional muscles.

- Lie supine with your legs bent and your hands clasped behind your head.
- Start by pushing through your heels for support and raising your trunk off the ground, contracting your abdominals while lifting up toward your knees.
- Lower, and repeat for the desired repetitions.

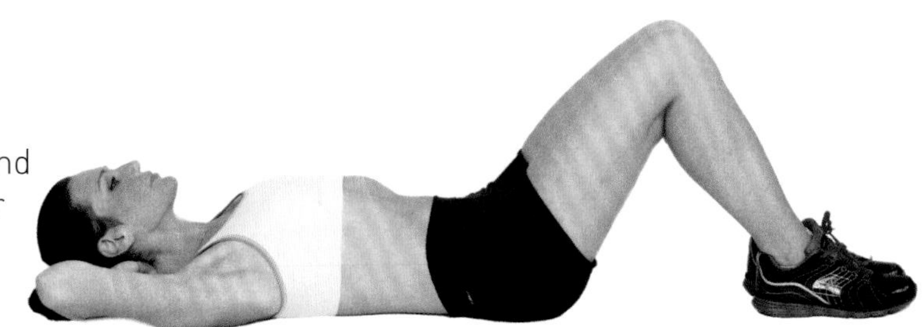

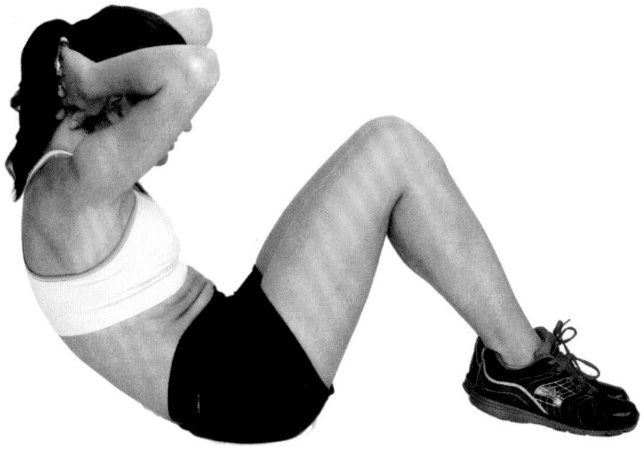

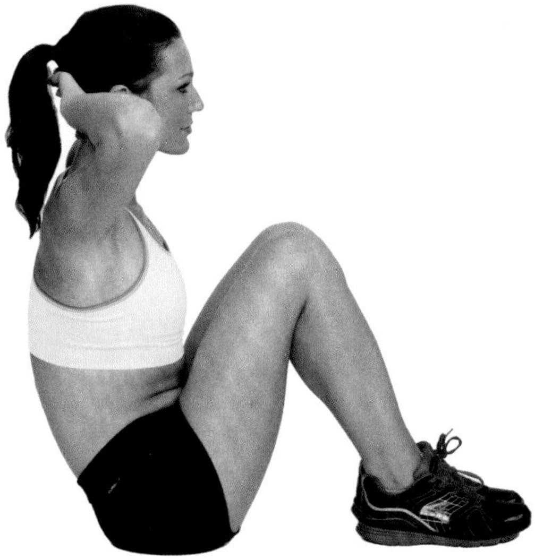

➔ FIND YOUR FORM

Lead from your navel, employing a precise range of motion and avoiding wildly swinging upward. Lower with control, and avoid overusing your neck or stressing your lower back.

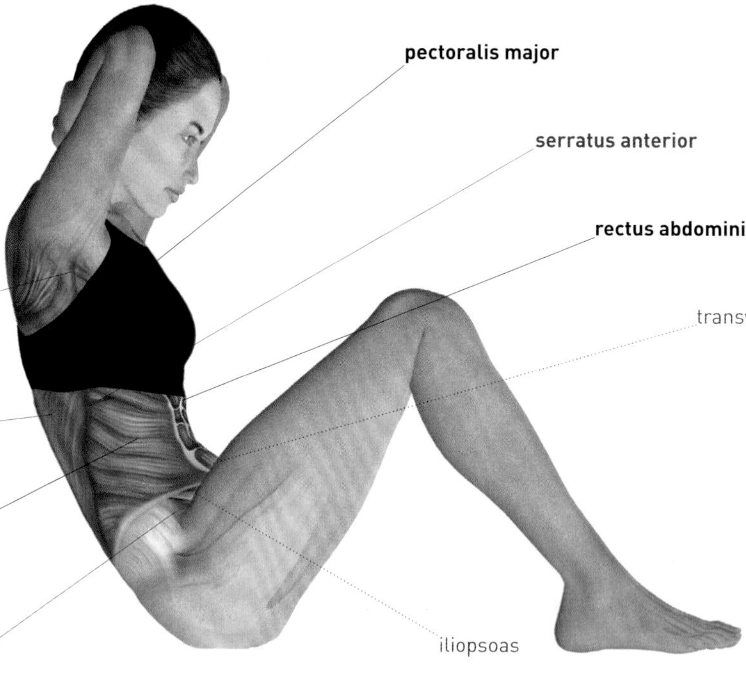

pectoralis major

serratus anterior

rectus abdominis

transversus abdominis

coracobrachialis

latissimus dorsi

obliquus externus

tensor fasciae latae

iliopsoas

MUSCLE ANNOTATION KEY
- **Black bold = primary**
- Black = deep primary
- Gray bold = secondary
- Gray = deep secondary

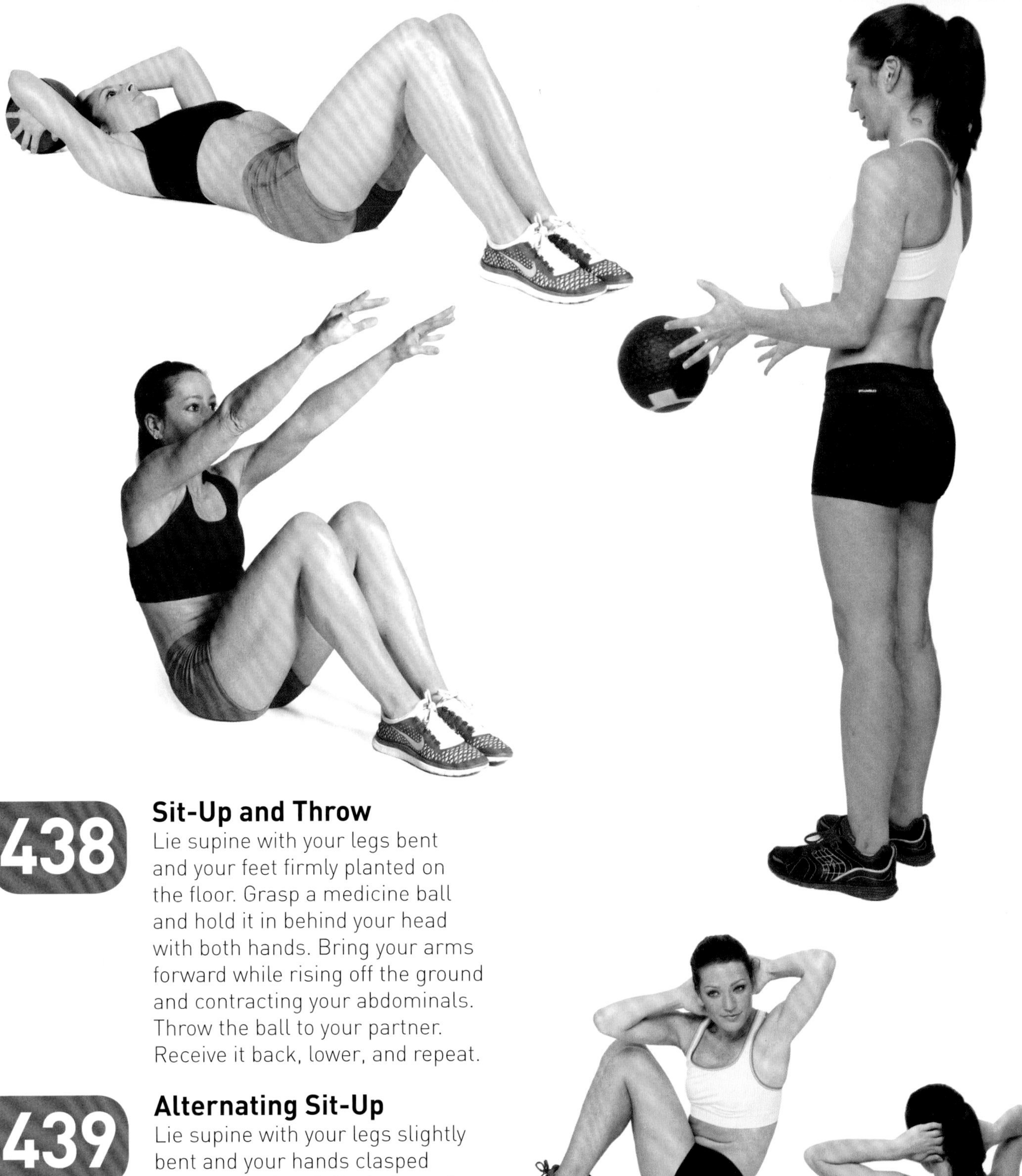

438 **Sit-Up and Throw**

Lie supine with your legs bent and your feet firmly planted on the floor. Grasp a medicine ball and hold it in behind your head with both hands. Bring your arms forward while rising off the ground and contracting your abdominals. Throw the ball to your partner. Receive it back, lower, and repeat.

439 **Alternating Sit-Up**

Lie supine with your legs slightly bent and your hands clasped behind your head. Push through your heels for support and raise your trunk off the floor. Rotate to the left so your elbow touches your opposite knee, and contract your abdominals. Lower and repeat, rotating to the other side. Continue alternating sides for the desired repetitions.

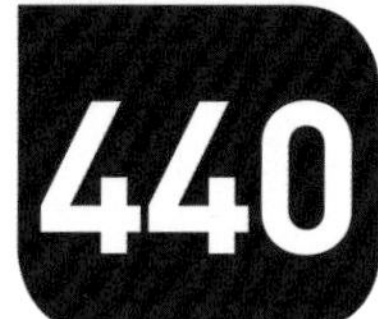

V-Up

The V-Up, also known as a Pike Crunch or Jackknife, is a challenging core movement. It has multiple benefits, including strengthening your abdominal muscles and increasing your overall flexibility and coordination. Performing V-Ups is also an efficient way to strengthen your lower-back muscles and tighten your quadriceps.

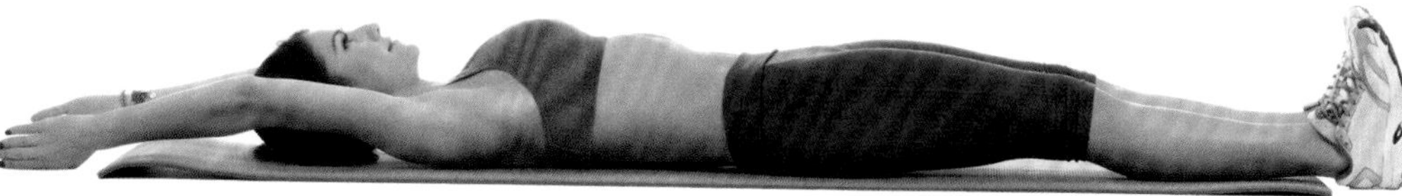

- Lie on your back with your legs extended and your arms raised overhead, your palms facing each other.
- Raise your legs to an angle between 45 and 90 degrees, and then inhale, reaching your arms toward the ceiling as you lift your head and shoulders off the floor.

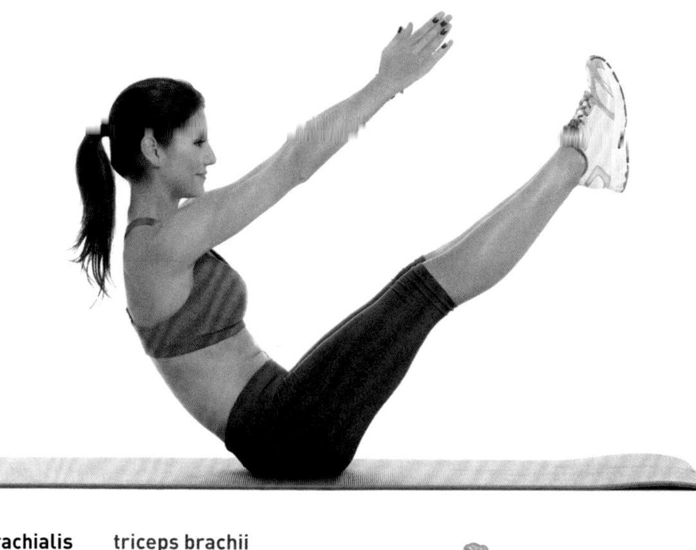

- Exhale, and, while rolling through the spine, lift your rib cage off the floor so that your are balanced on your sit bones.
- Inhale, and reach your arms toward your toes while maintaining a C curve in your back. Exhale, and roll down the spine by articulating one vertebra at a time. Return to the starting position. Repeat for the desired repetitions.

FIND YOUR FORM

Keep your arms and legs straight throughout the movement, and avoid using a jerking motion as your raise or lower your arms and legs.

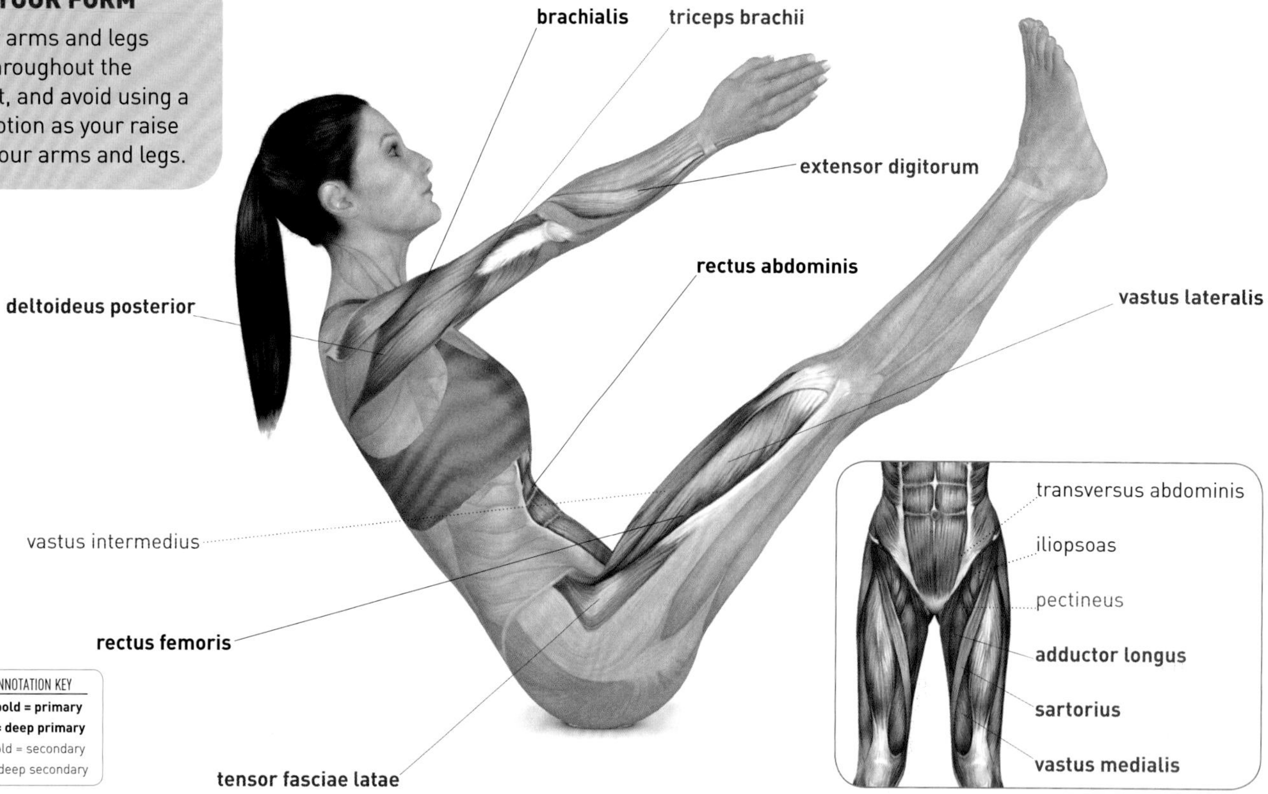

brachialis
triceps brachii
extensor digitorum
rectus abdominis
vastus lateralis
deltoideus posterior
vastus intermedius
rectus femoris
tensor fasciae latae

transversus abdominis
iliopsoas
pectineus
adductor longus
sartorius
vastus medialis

MUSCLE ANNOTATION KEY
Black bold = primary
Black = deep primary
Gray bold = secondary
Gray = deep secondary

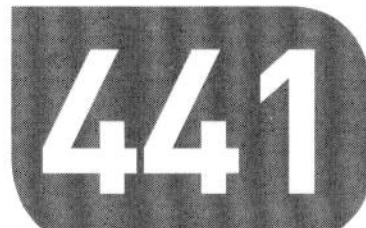

Medicine Ball V-Up

Lie on your back with your legs extended and your arms raised overhead grasping a medicine ball with both hands. Perform as you would a V-Up (#440). Repeat for the desired repetitions.

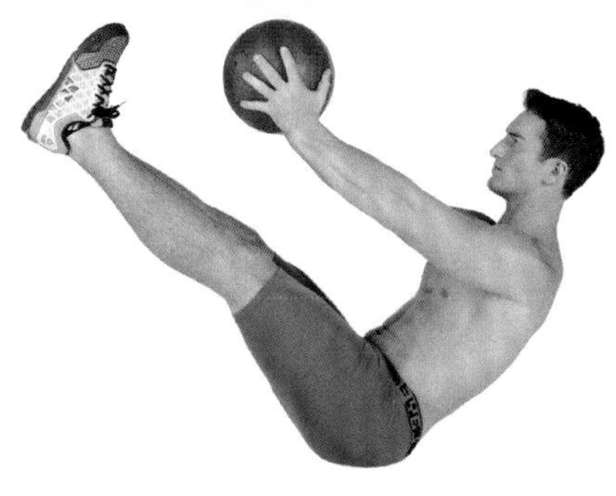

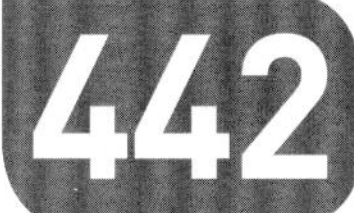

Single-Leg V-Up

Lie on your back with your arms extended over your head, hovering just above the mat behind you, palms up. Bend your knees, and press them together. Anchor your feet into the floor. Extend one leg, straightening it from your hip and out through your foot. Raise your torso to form a 45-degree angle with the floor as you bring your arms up and over your head to reach forward toward your raised foot. With control, curl your spine down to the floor as you bring your arms up overhead and behind you again, keeping your knees pressed together. Repeat for the desired repetitions.

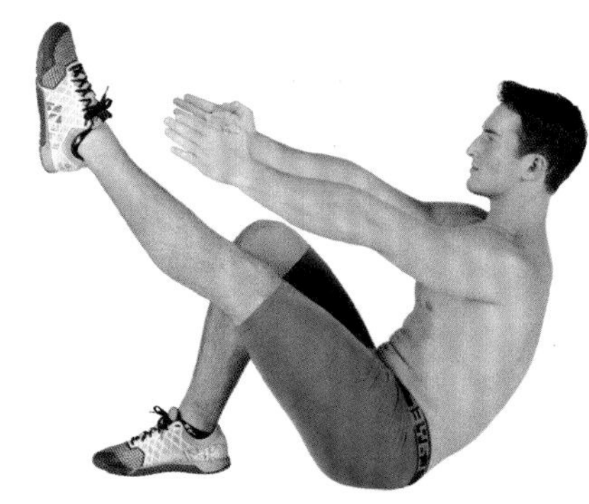

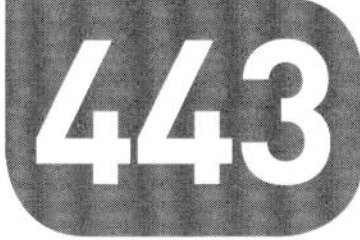

BOSU Jackknife Crunch

Sit on a BOSU trainer placed dome-side up on the floor. Raise your feet off the floor, and bend your knees toward your chest, and extend your arms straight out at shoulder height parallel to the floor. Tighten your abdominals, and straighten your legs until they are parallel to the floor. Bring your knees back toward your chest to return to the starting position, and then continue for the desired repetitions.

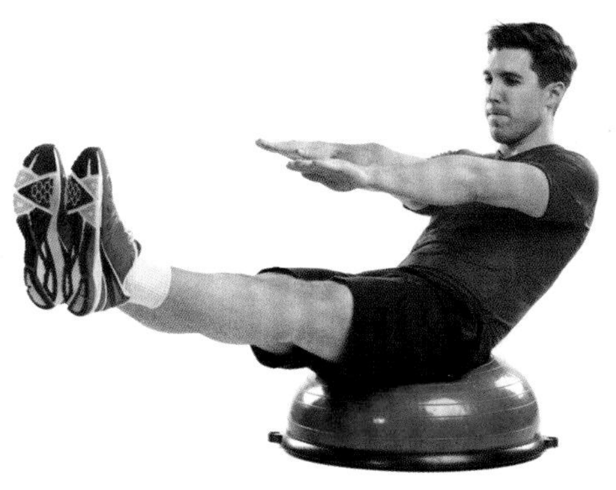

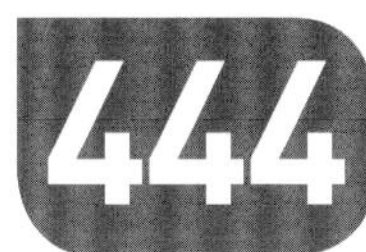

Jackknife Crunch on Aerobic

Sit with your buttock at the edge of an aerobic step or other elevated surface. Lean back slightly with your hands resting on the step, your fingers facing forward. Tighten your abdominals, and straighten your legs until they are parallel to the floor. Bring your knees back toward your chest to return to the starting position, and then continue for the desired repetitions.

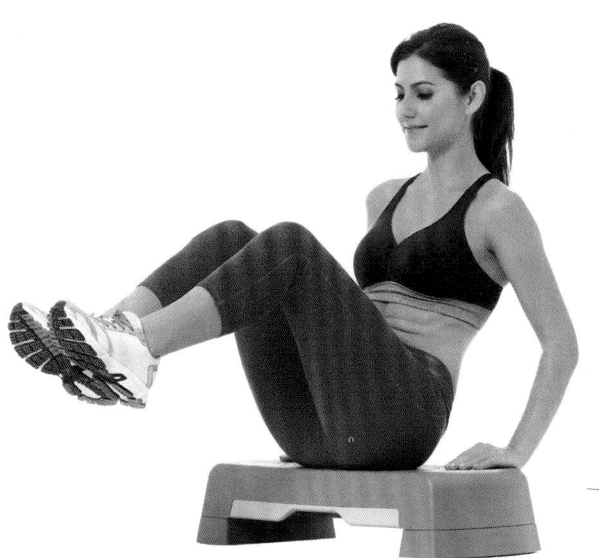

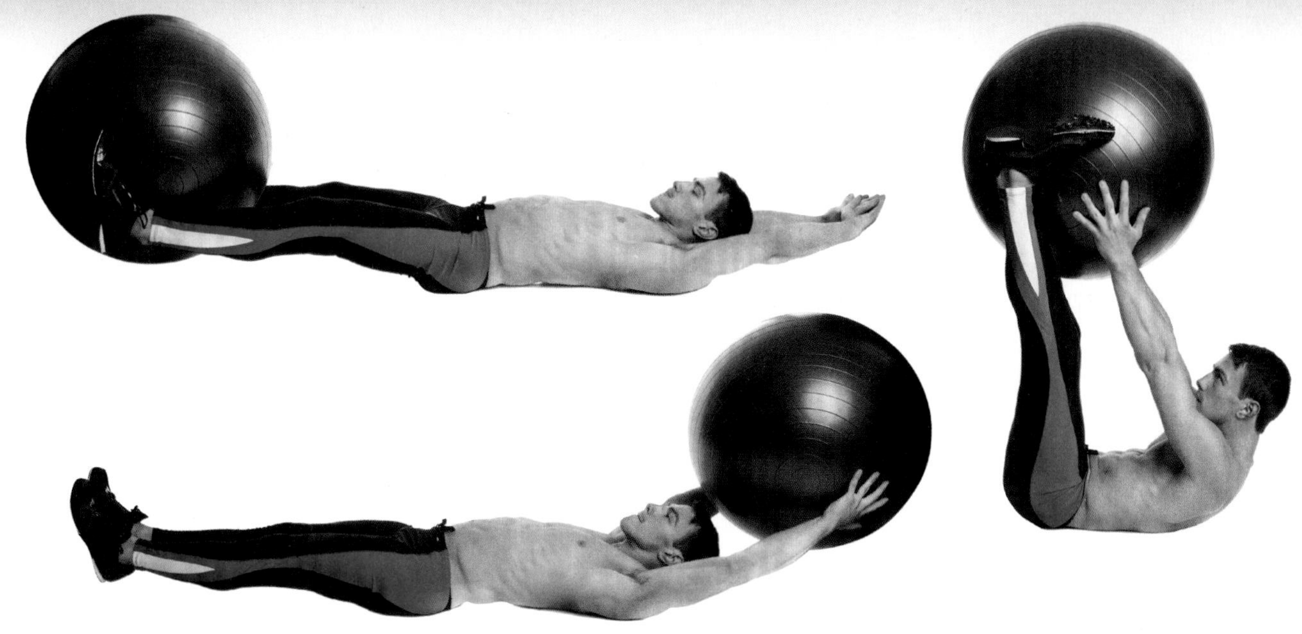

445 V-Up with Swiss Ball Pass

Lie supine on the floor, and extend your arms above your head. Bend your knees so that your feet are slightly off the floor, and then grasp a Swiss ball between your feet. Push your lower back into the floor, keeping your spine long. Contract your abdominals, and lift your upper back off the floor and forward, exhaling as you come up. Simultaneously reach upward with both arms and legs by folding your torso. Transfer the ball from your feet to yours hands, and return to the start positioning. Repeat in the opposite direction to return the ball to your feet. Continue passing the ball from feet to hands for the desired time or repetitions.

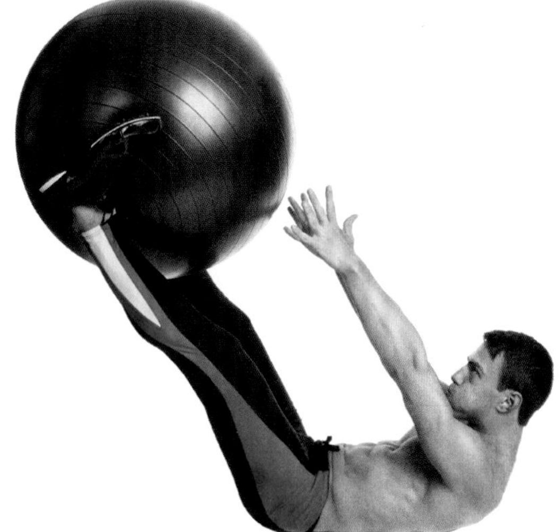

446 The Boat

Sit with your legs extended straight in front of you. Lean back slightly, bending your knees, and support yourself with your hands behind your hips. Your fingers should be pointing forward, and your back should be straight. Exhale, and lift your feet off the floor as you lean back from your shoulders. Find your balance point between your sit bones and your tailbone. Slowly straighten your legs in front of you so that they form a 45-degree angle with your torso. Point your toes. Lift your arms to your sides, parallel to the floor. Pull your abdominals in toward your spine as they work to keep your balance. Stretch your arms forward through your fingertips, and elongate the back of your neck. Hold for up to 30 seconds, and then release. Repeat for the desired repetitions.

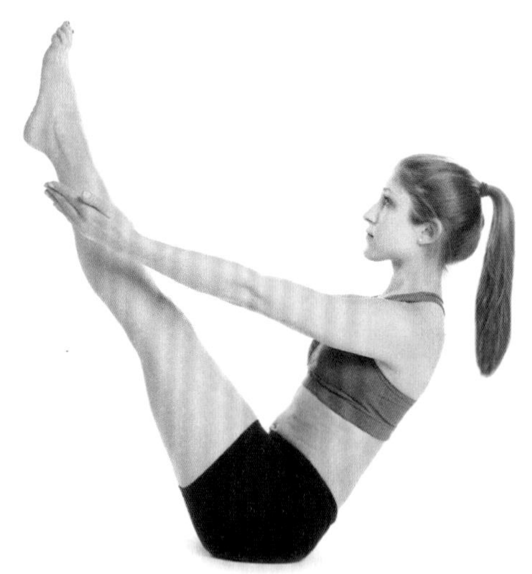

Vertical Leg Crunch

When carrying out Vertical Leg Crunch, you should feel a strong sense that your abs are not just getting stronger but becoming streamlined and defined, too. With your legs up, your abdominals do almost all the work. Keep your movement smooth as you lower yourself to the floor, so that your core stays active throughout all stages of the exercise.

- Lie on your back, with your arms extended behind your head and your legs extended in front of you so that your body forms one straight line.
- Bring your arms over your head so they are reaching straight upward, your hands directly above your shoulders and your arms forming a 90-degree angle with the floor. Raise your legs until they are parallel to your arms.
- Using your abdominals to drive the movement, lift your shoulders off the floor, reaching your extended fingers towards your toes. Lower, and repeat for the desired reps and sets.

FIND YOUR FORM

Keep your arms and legs fully extended, and press your legs together as if they were a single leg. Using your lower-back muscles to drive the movement, making sure to lower your upper back just as slowly as you raised it.

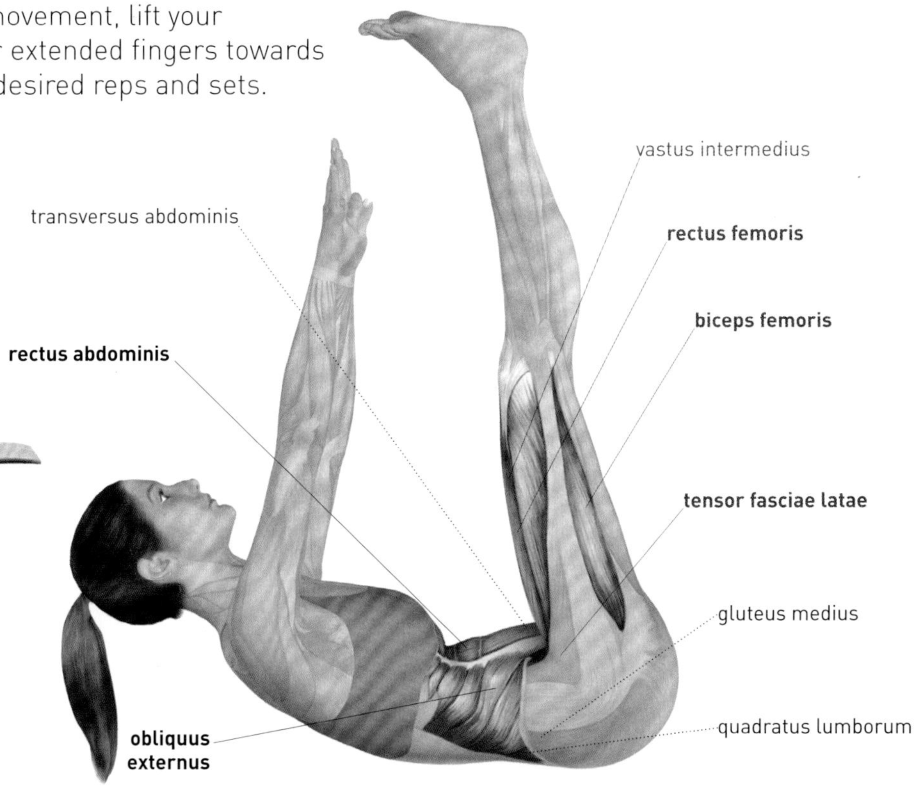

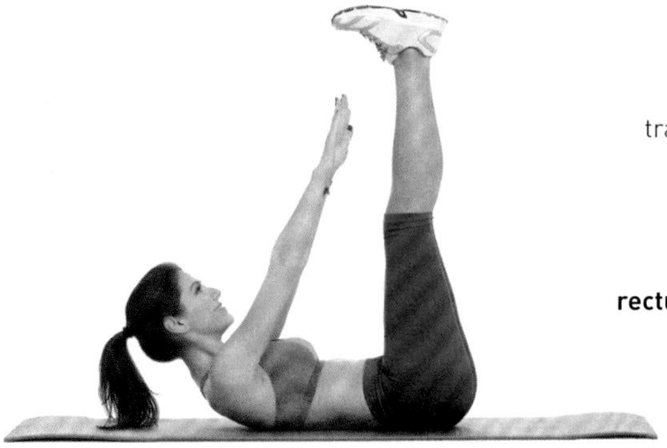

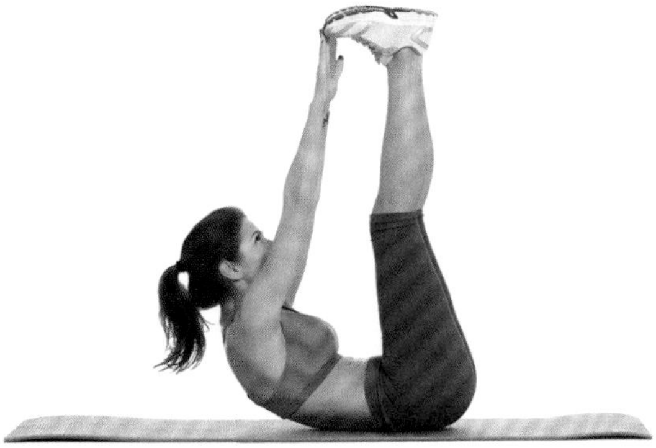

vastus intermedius

rectus femoris

transversus abdominis

biceps femoris

rectus abdominis

tensor fasciae latae

gluteus medius

quadratus lumborum

obliquus externus

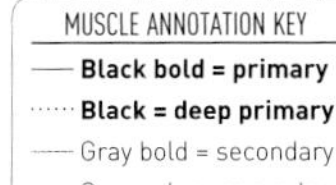

448 Swiss Ball Vertical Leg Crunch

Grasping a Swiss ball between your feet, clasp your hands behind your head, and perform a Vertical Leg Crunch (#447). Repeat for the desired repetitions.

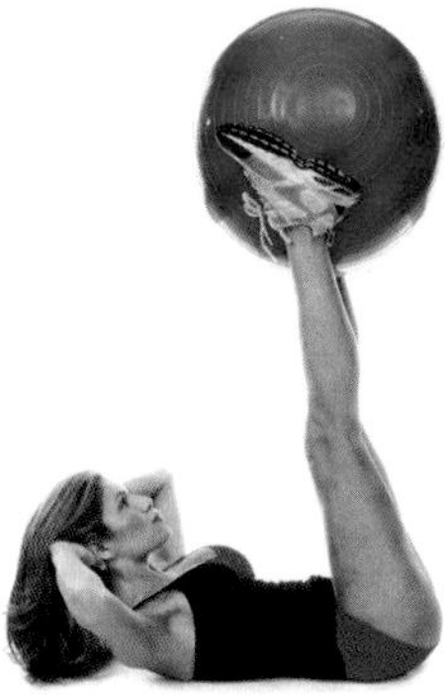

Roll-Up

The Roll-Up is a classical Pilates mat exercise that will challenge your core muscles, flatten your abdominals, and strengthen your back. To execute this move properly, be sure to use the same control rolling down as you do rolling up.

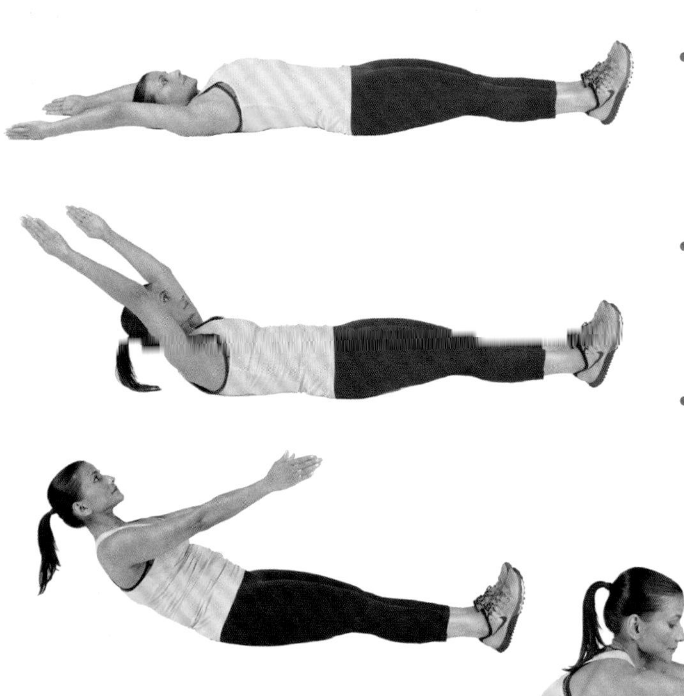

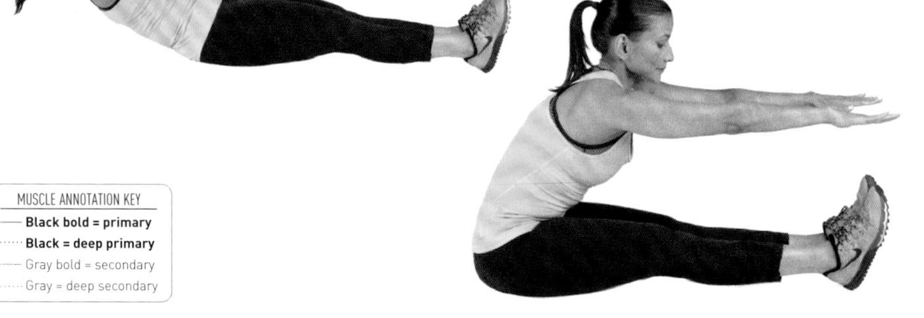

- Lie on your back, with your spine in neutral position and your ankles strongly flexed. Glide your shoulder blades down your back as you lift your arms overhead, extended slightly above the mat behind you. Press your shoulders and your rib cage downward.
- Press your navel to your spine, and, in sequence, roll up each vertebra from the mat, reaching your arms forward into the space above your legs. It helps to really press your heels into the mat.
- Reverse the movement, rolling back down to the mat vertebra by vertebra, resisting the urge to lift your shoulders and collapse your chest. Continue for the desired time or repetitions.

FIND YOUR FORM

Keep your abdominals and rib cage strongly interlaced with your back, and keep pressing your legs and heels into the floor for stabilization. Avoid using shoulder or arm momentum to roll up or down, bouncing, or otherwise compromising the fluid steadiness of the movements.

MUSCLE ANNOTATION KEY
Black bold = primary
Black = deep primary
Gray bold = secondary
Gray = deep secondary

triceps brachii
deltoideus anterior
extensor digitorum
rectus abdominis
transversus abdominis
tibialis anterior
pectoralis major
serratus anterior
obliquus internus
erector spinae
obliquus externus
gluteus maximus
sartorius
rectus femoris

Medicine Ball Roll-Up

Grasp a Pilates ball as you perform as you would the Roll-Up (#449). Keep your arms extended and the ball stable throughout the exercise. Repeat for the desired repetitions.

Roll-Up Triceps Lift

Lie on the floor, with your spine in a neutral position. Hold a body bar in both hands. Bend your elbows so that your arms form a right angle with the body bar above your head. Keeping the rest of your body in place, straighten your arm muscles to smoothly roll up to a sitting position. Keep your arms extended, with the body bar lifted overhead. Slowly roll back to lie in the starting position. Repeat for the desired repetitions.

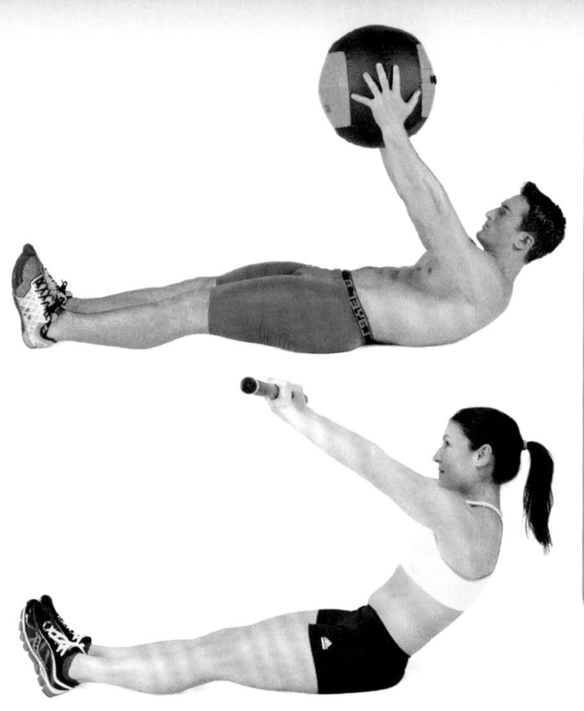

Thread the Needle

Thread the Needle is a multipurpose move that targets your abdominals, while also working your triceps. It also offers your hamstrings a massaging stretch and helps you improve your coordination and agility. Be mindful of how far your roll forward—the roll-back portion of the exercise is more challenging than the roll-out.

- Sit on the floor with your legs outstretched in front of you, with a foam roller placed under your knees. Plant your hands on the floor to support your torso, your fingers pointing toward your buttocks.
- Press into the floor to raise your hips, keeping your legs firm and your abdominals tight.
- Draw your hips backward through your arms, rolling your legs over the roller. Drop your head so that your gaze is directed at your thighs.
- Roll on the roller back to the starting position, keeping your hips lifted off the floor. Continue rolling forward and back for the desired repetitions.

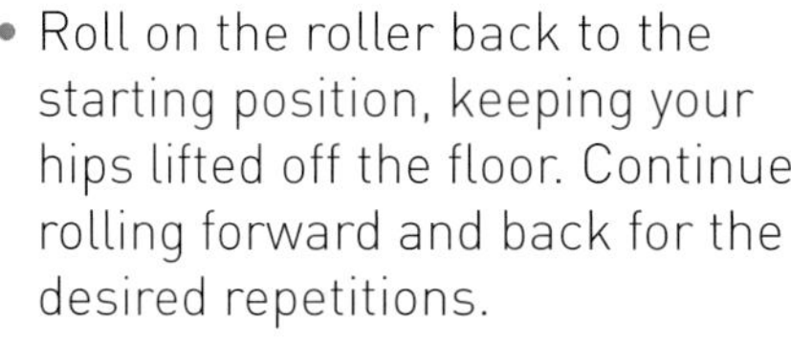

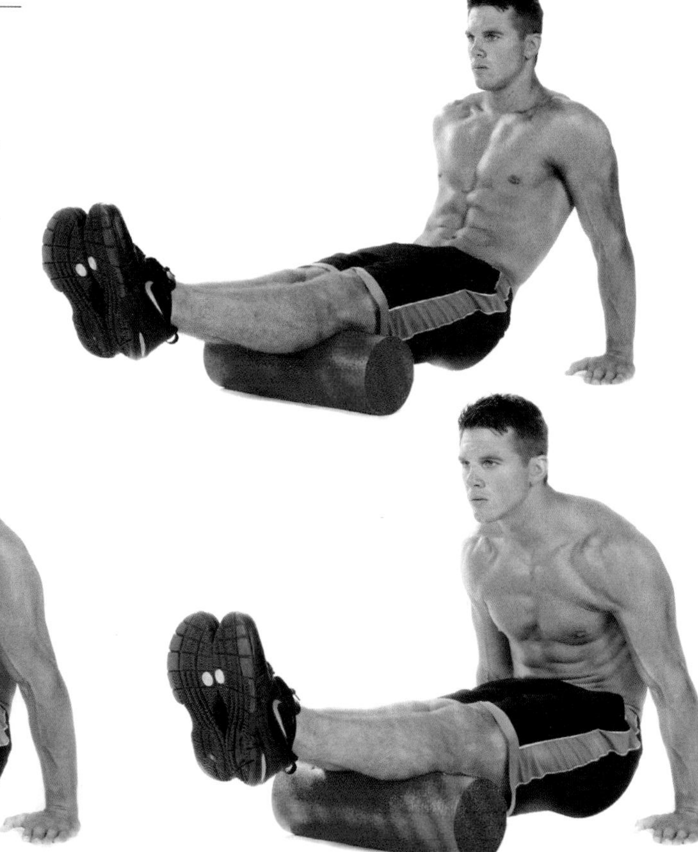

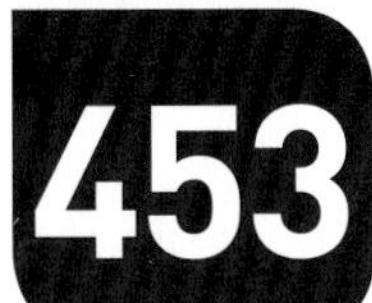

Ab Roll-Out

The Ab Roll-Out is a challenging core-stabilizing exercise from which many movements can build. When you correctly execute a roll-out move, you activate many of the key core muscles. Recent studies have shown that the exercises such as this more efficiently activate the rectus abdominis (the "six-pack muscle") and the obliques than do sit-up or crunch variations.

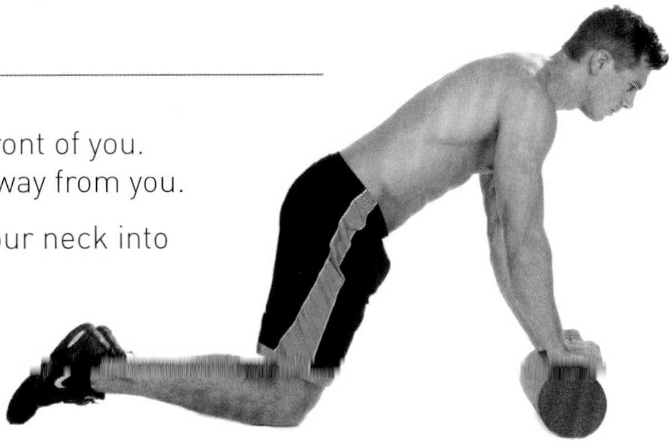

- Kneel on the floor with a foam roller placed crosswise in front of you. Place your wrists on top of the roller, your fingers facing away from you.
- Maintaining a neutral spine and making sure not to sink your neck into your shoulders, roll forward on your forearms.
- Continue to roll forward until the roller reaches your elbows. Press into the roller, keeping your hips aligned, and roll back to the starting position. Continue rolling forward and back for the desired time or repetitions.

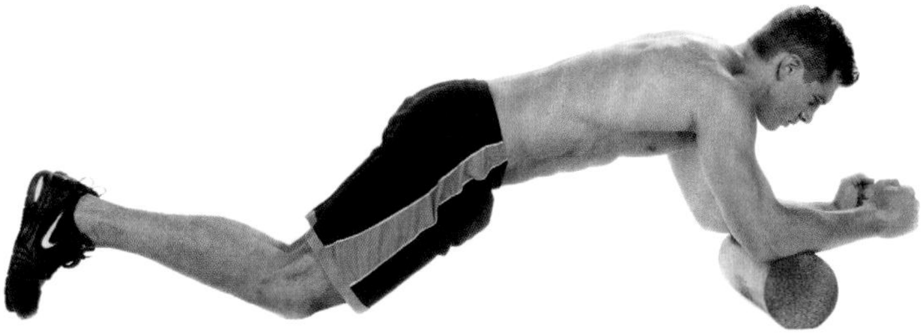

FIND YOUR FORM

Squeeze your abdominals, and concentrate on preventing your back from arching as your roll out.

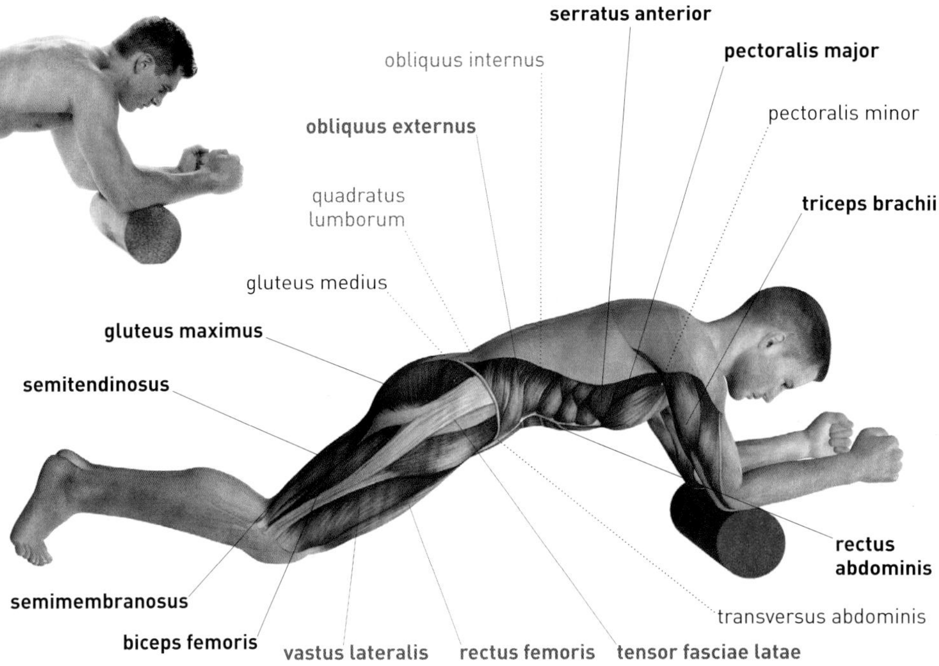

serratus anterior
obliquus internus
pectoralis major
pectoralis minor
obliquus externus
quadratus lumborum
triceps brachii
gluteus medius
gluteus maximus
semitendinosus
rectus abdominis
semimembranosus
transversus abdominis
biceps femoris
vastus lateralis
rectus femoris
tensor fasciae latae

MUSCLE ANNOTATION KEY
Black bold = primary
Black = deep primary
Gray bold = secondary
Gray = deep secondary

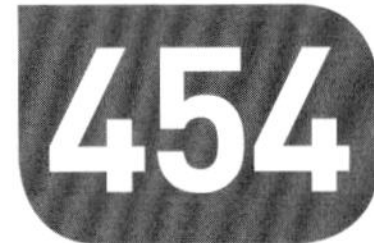

Ab Wheel

Kneel on the floor., and grab the handles of an ab wheel, and then perform as you would the Ab Roll-Out (#453).

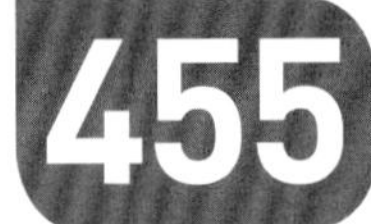

Swiss Ball Roll-Out

Kneel on the floor with your wrists resting on a Swiss ball with your upper back straight and firmly supported, your feet shoulder-width apart, your hips raised, and your arms outstretched to your sides. Perform as you would the Ab Roll-Out (#453).

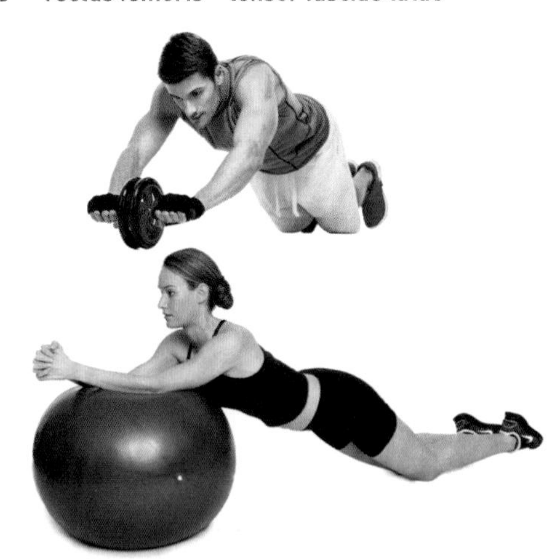

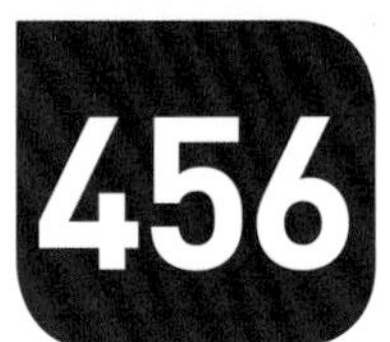

Full-Body Roll

The Full-Body Roll stretches your glutes and tones your core muscles, especially the obliques. It is also a challenging range-of-motion exercise that can help you improve your performance in rotational sports like golf, tennis, baseball, and hockey. This exercise demands impeccable form—you must move with control and precision.

- Lie on your back, with your arms extended at your sides and your legs extended on the floor.
- Raise your right leg so that it is perpendicular to the floor.
- Turn your head to the right, and slowly rotate your lower body to the left, lowering your right leg until your foot is just above the floor.
- Roll your lower body and leg back, and then lower your leg to the starting position. Continue to alternate sides for the desired repetitions.

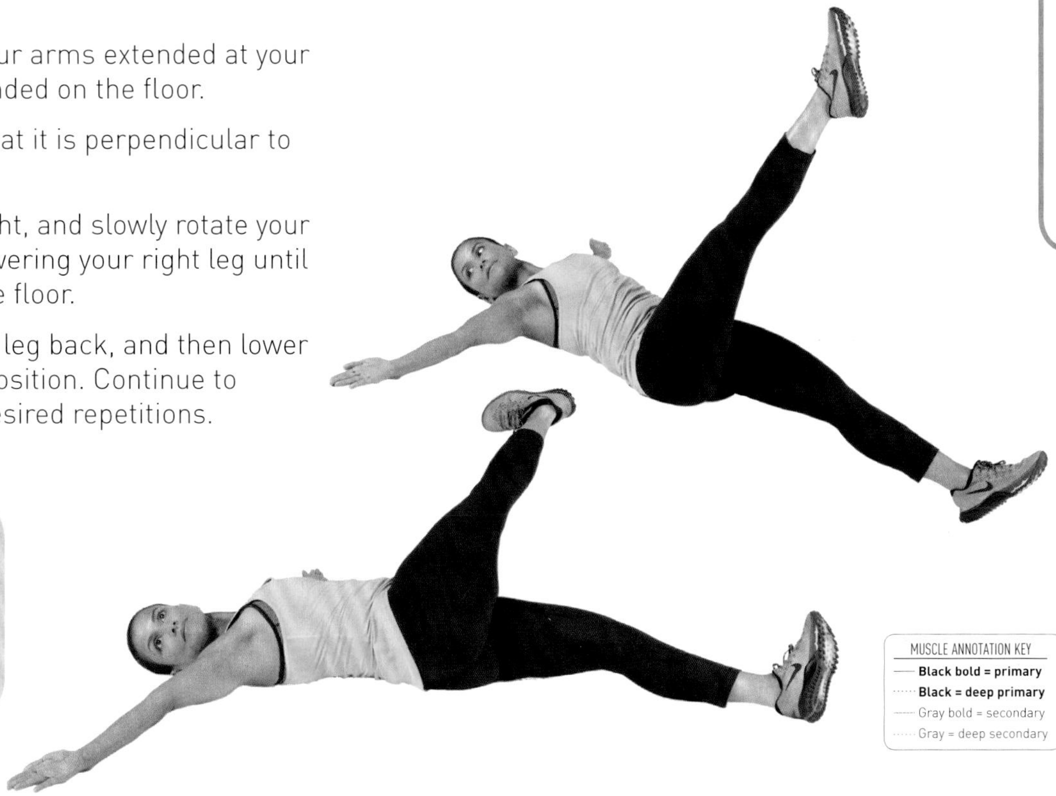

FIND YOUR FORM

Keep your abdominal muscles, especially your obliques, engaged as you roll. Keep your legs straight, and move at a steady pace.

MUSCLE ANNOTATION KEY
- Black bold = primary
- Black = deep primary
- Gray bold = secondary
- Gray = deep secondary

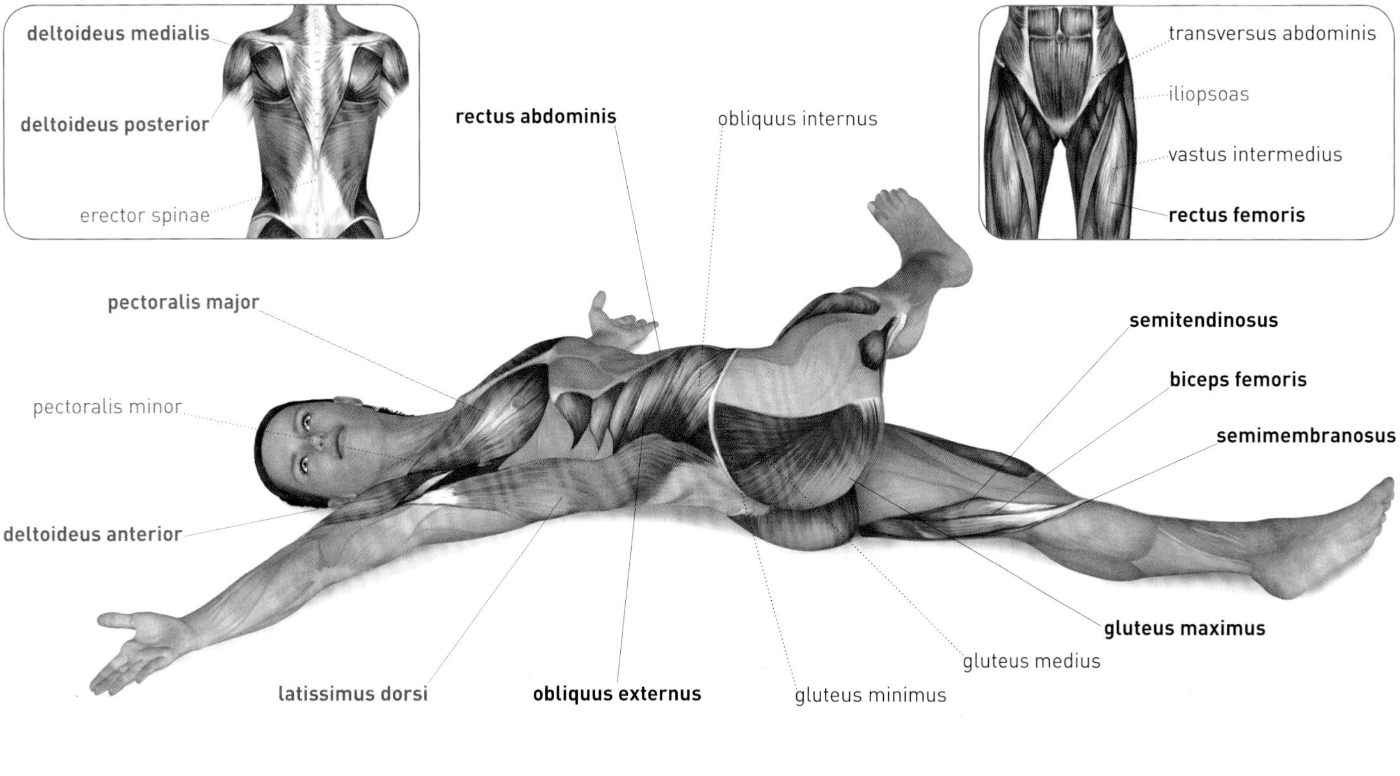

deltoideus medialis
deltoideus posterior
erector spinae

transversus abdominis
iliopsoas
vastus intermedius
rectus femoris

rectus abdominis
obliquus internus
pectoralis major
pectoralis minor
deltoideus anterior
latissimus dorsi
obliquus externus
gluteus minimus
gluteus medius
gluteus maximus
semitendinosus
biceps femoris
semimembranosus

Russian Twist

The Russian Twist works your abdominals and obliques with it torso-rotating motion. Regularly performing this exercise or its variations increases abdominal endurance and builds explosiveness in the upper torso, which may help boost your performance in sports such as swimming, baseball, hockey, golf, lacrosse, and boxing.

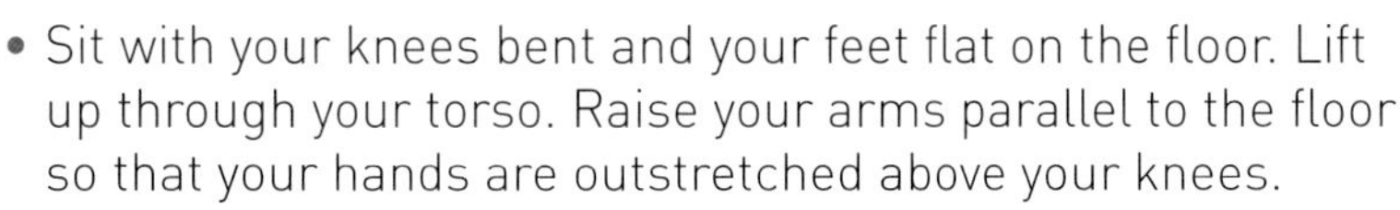

- Sit with your knees bent and your feet flat on the floor. Lift up through your torso. Raise your arms parallel to the floor so that your hands are outstretched above your knees.
- Rotate your upper body to the right, reaching toward the floor with your hands.
- Pass through the center and rotate to the left. Continue moving with control from side to side with [illegible] without stopping for the desired time or repetitions.

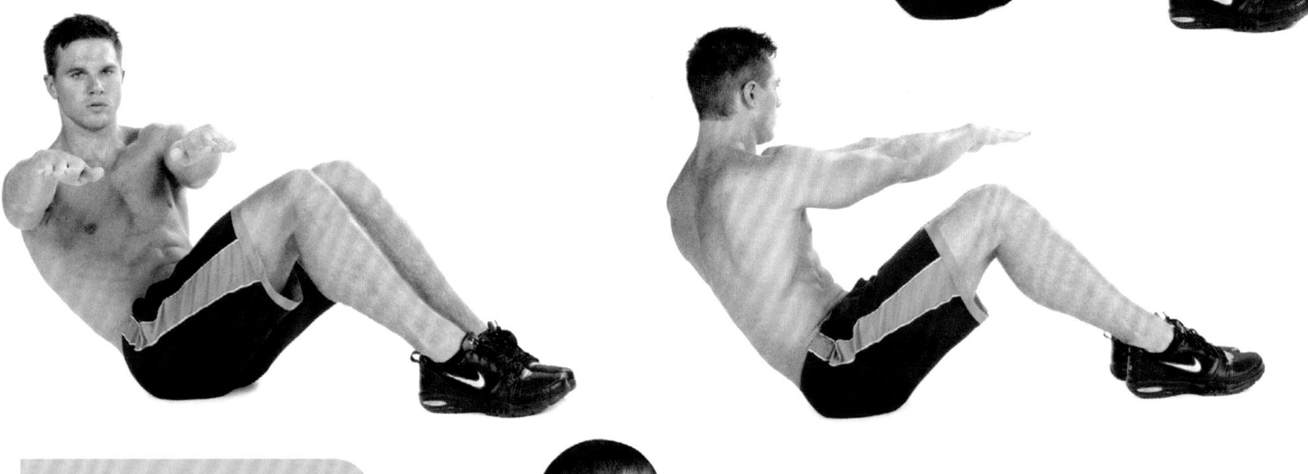

➔ FIND YOUR FORM

To keep your abdominals fully engaged and reaping the benefits of this exercise, be sure to keep moving smoothly with control, without pausing between repetitions, and avoid holding your breath.

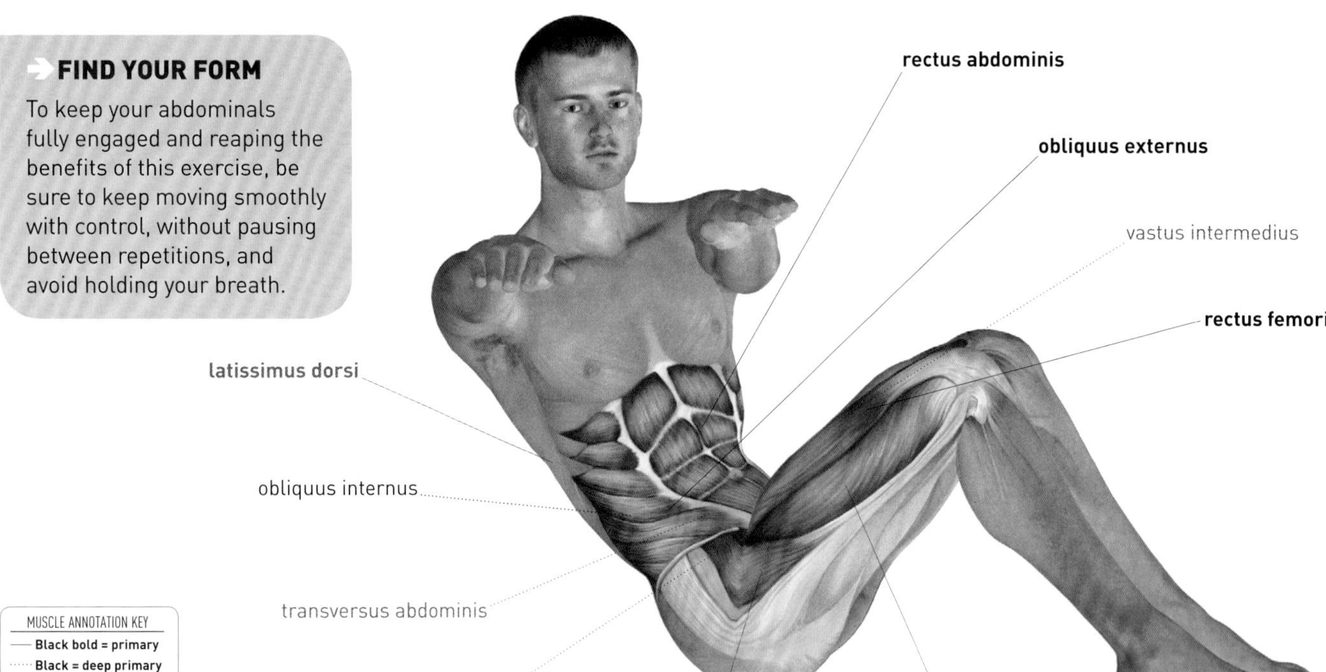

MUSCLE ANNOTATION KEY
- Black bold = primary
- Black = deep primary
- Gray bold = secondary
- Gray = deep secondary

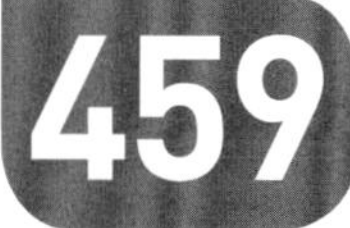

Raised-Leg Russian Twist

Sit with your knees bent and your arms extended at shoulder height. Lift your feet off the floor, and perform as your would a Russian Twist (#457.) Continue moving with control from side to side with a steady pace without stopping for the desired time or repetitions.

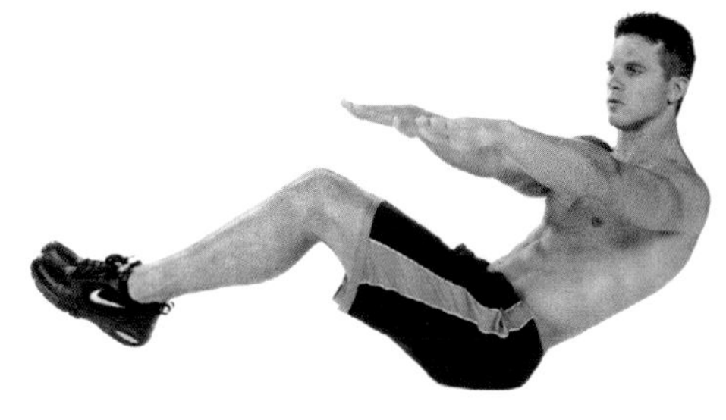

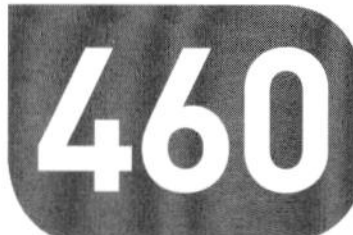

Seated Dumbbell Russian Twist

Holding a dumbbell in both hands, sit with your legs extended in front of you, knees bent and feet about hip-width apart. Lean back slightly, and perform as your would a Russian Twist (#457.) Continue moving with control from side to side with a steady pace without stopping for the desired time or repetitions.

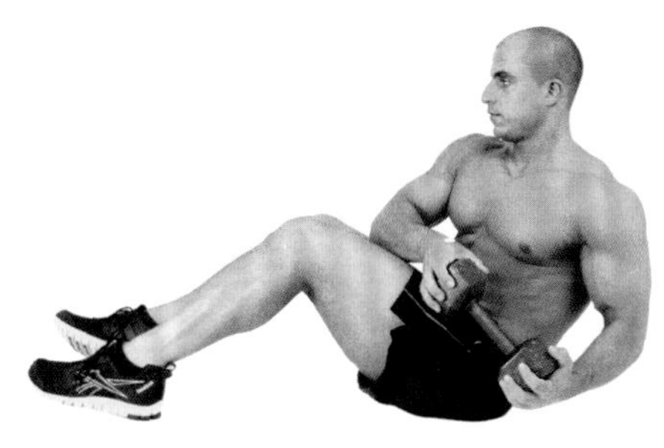

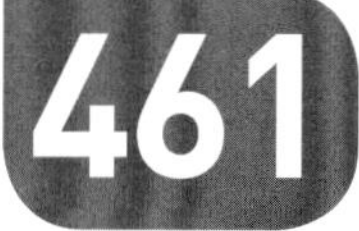

Medicine Ball Twist

Holding a medicine in both hands, sit with your knees bent and feet about hip-width apart. Lean back slightly, and perform as your would a Russian Twist (#457.) Continue moving with control from side to side with a steady pace without stopping for the desired time or repetitions.

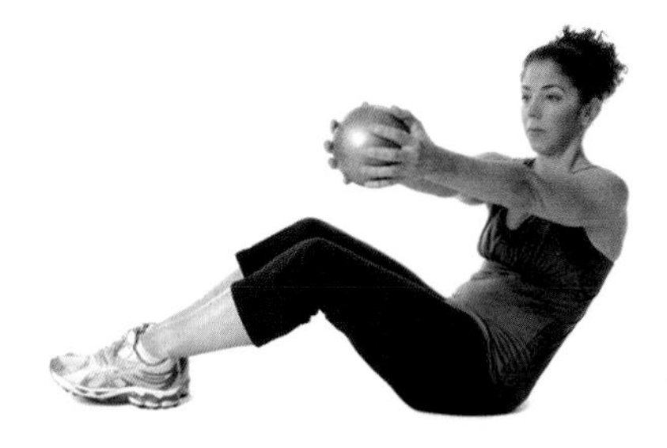

Tabletop Russian Twist

Sit with your legs elevated, your calves parallel to the floor. Lean back slightly, and perform as your would a Russian Twist (#457.) Continue moving with control from side to side with a steady pace without stopping for the desired time or repetitions.

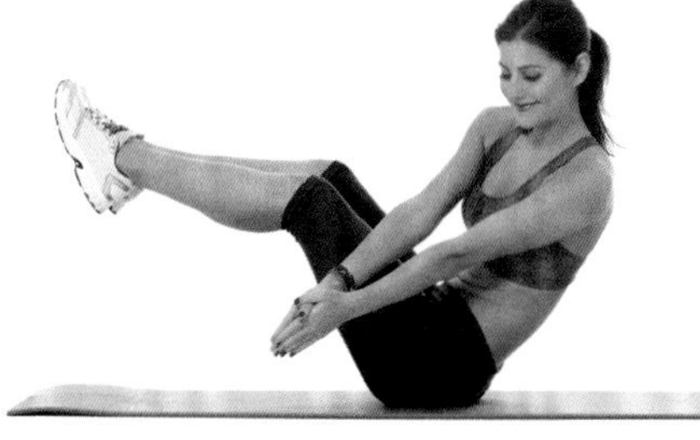

462 Spine Twist

Sit on the floor, with your back straight. Extend your legs in front of you, slightly more than hip-width apart. Lift up and out of your hips as you pull in your lower abdominals. Twist from your waist to the left, and then return to the center. Lift up and out of your hips again, twisting in the other direction. Return to the center, and repeat for desired repetitions.

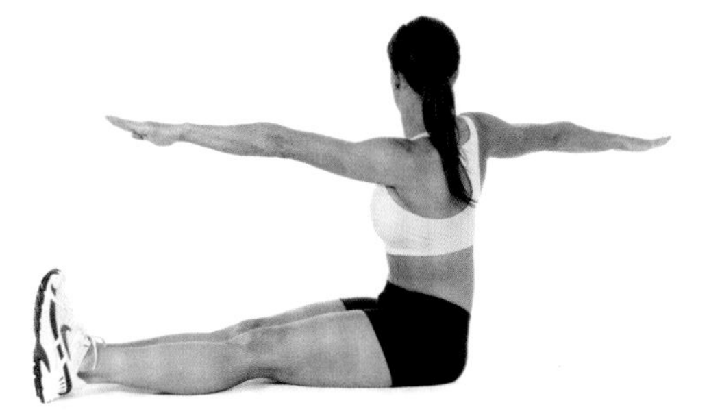

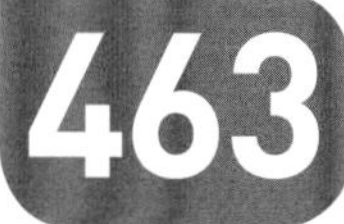

Oblique Roll-Down

Sit with your arms extended to the sides, parallel to the floor. Contract your abdominals, and while simultaneously rotating your torso to one side, roll backward, and then rotate your torso back to the center. Rotate to the other side, return back to the center, and repeat sequence for the desired repetitions.

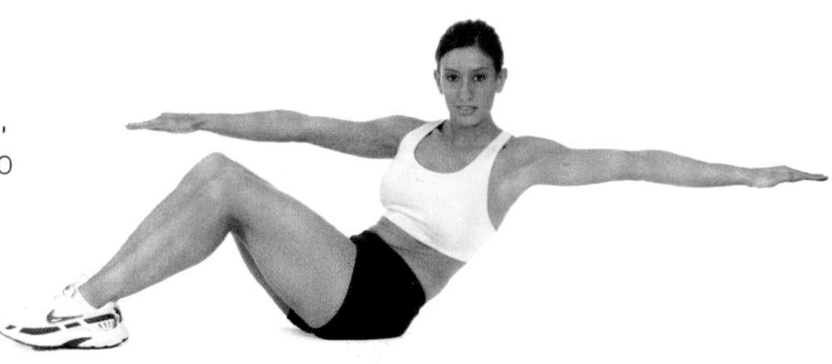

464 Pull-Up

One of the exercises used in numerous fitness qualifying tests, the Pull-Up is a fundamental upper-body-strength compound exercise that works a large number of muscles in your back, shoulders, and arms, with a particular emphasis on the latissimus dorsi. It calls for you to pull your own body weight, using an overhand, or pronated, grip. It is a versatile move that can be combined with other exercises to amp up the intensity—think Burpee with pull-ups, for example. Adjustable pull-up bars that can be installed in a home doorway are readily available.

- Using an overhand grip, place your hands just outside shoulder-width on a bar, and hang until your arms are straight.
- Pull yourself up until your chest touches the bar. Hold yourself in this position for one second, and then lower yourself slowly to the hanging position.
- Repeat, performing the desired repetitions.

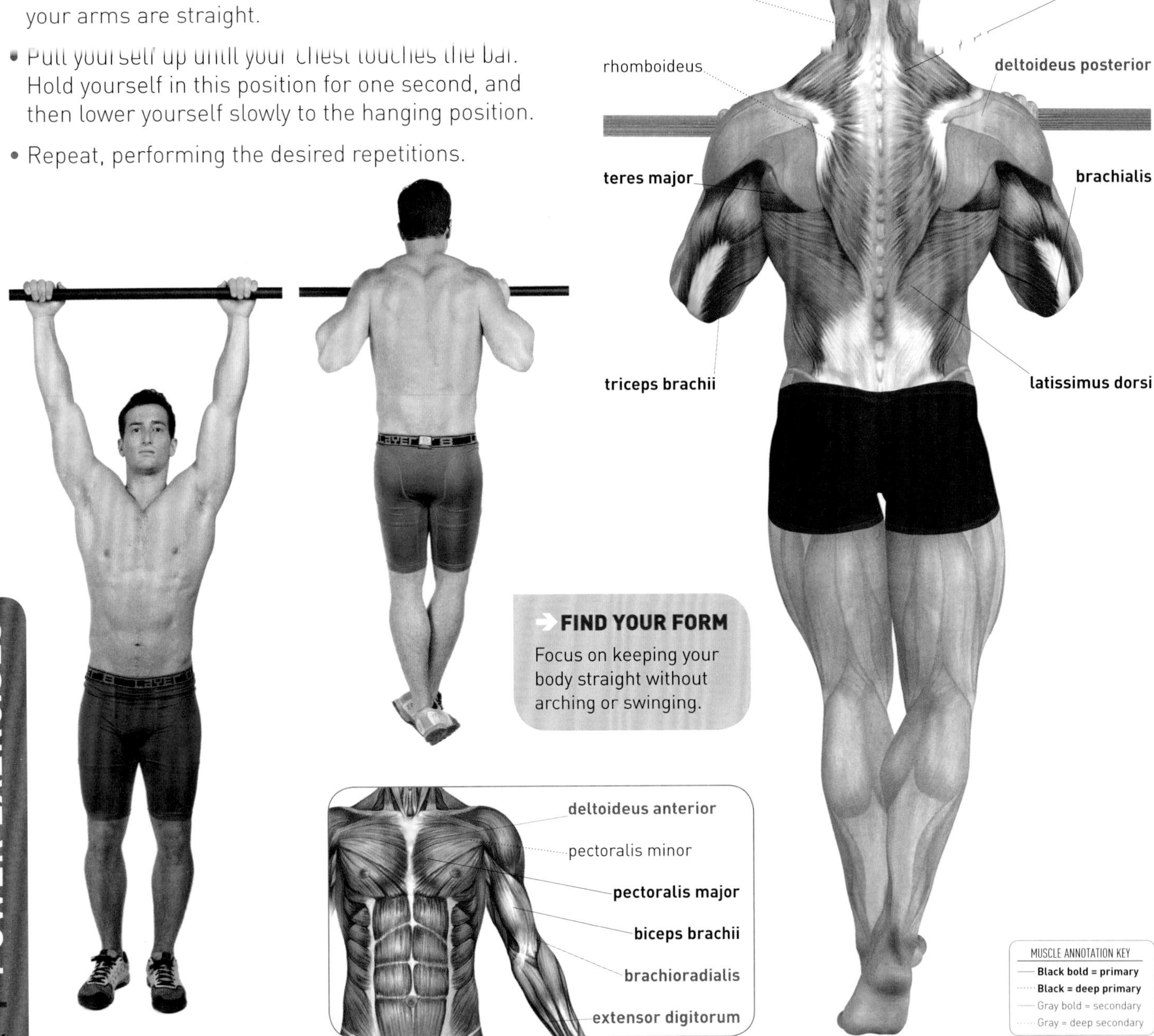

FIND YOUR FORM
Focus on keeping your body straight without arching or swinging.

Chin-Up

A Chin-Up reverses the grip that you use during a Pull-Up, so that you grasp the bar in an underhand, or supinated grip, hands about shoulder-width apart with your palms facing you. This places more focus on the biceps.

- Using an underhand grip, place your hands about shoulder-width on a bar, and hang until your arms are straight. Bend your knees back, and cross your ankles.
- Pull yourself up until your chin touches the bar. Hold yourself in this position for one second, and then lower yourself slowly to the hanging position.
- Repeat for the desired repetitions.

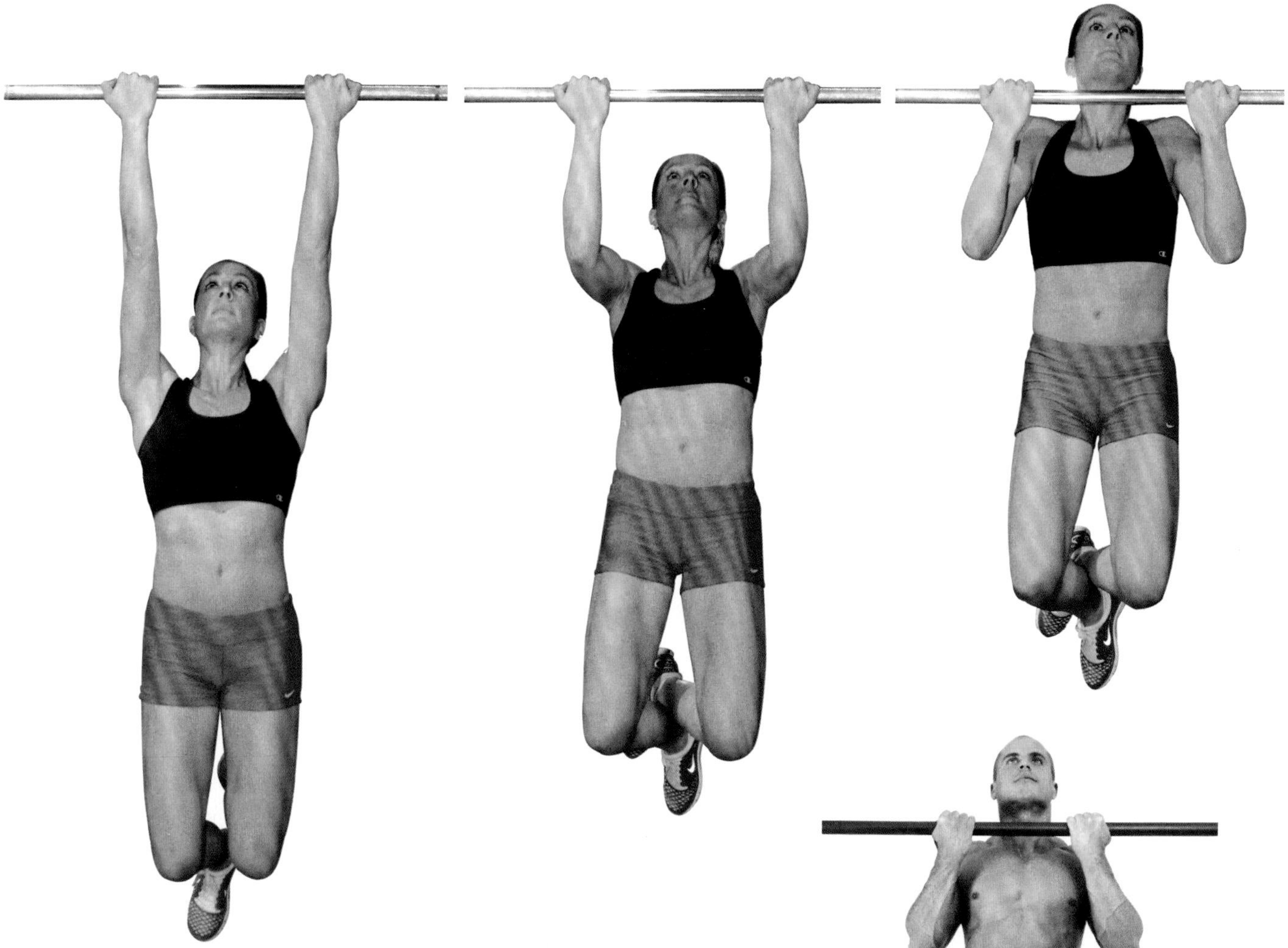

466 Chin-Up with Hanging Leg Raise

Using an underhand grip, place your hands about shoulder-width or slightly wider on a bar, and hang until your arms are straight. Bend your knees and cross your ankles. Perform as you would a Chin-Up (#465), but as you raise your chin to the bar, bend your knees, bring them upward toward your chest. Repeat for the desired repetitions.

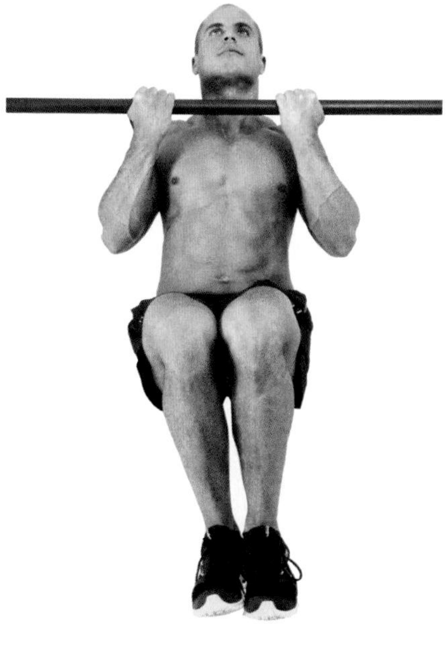

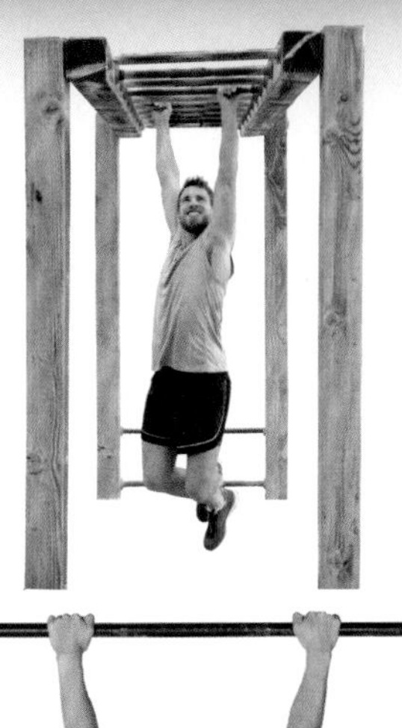

467 Monkey Bar Hand Walk

This is performed on special equipment—known as monkey bars, the jungle gym, or climbing frame—that is like a ladder that is suspended overhead high enough to hang from. To perform, hang from both arms at one end, and "walk" your hands to the other end of the ladder and back.

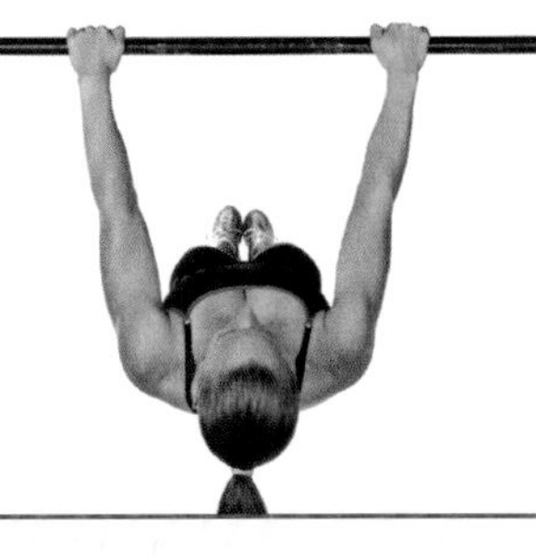

468 Body Row

Hang from a bar with your body in a flat plane. Move your feet away from the bar until your arms are straight, keeping on your heels. Pull your body toward the bar until your chest touches it. Lower yourself slowly, and repeat for the desired repetitions.

PULL-UP GRIPS

There is a wide variety of ways to perform Pull-Ups, especially in how you hold the bar. Here are some of the most common grip variations that you may encounter in your gym.

469 Wide Grip

Place your hands at least five inches wider than shoulder-width. This grip reduces the involvement of the pecs, which calls for you to work your back muscles more, especially the latissimus dorsi (more than the rhomboids).

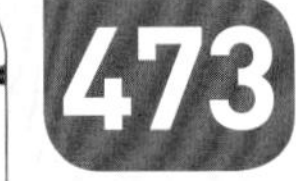

470 Mountain Climber Grip

With the bar at your side, place one hand in front of the other, palms facing each other. Military trainees use this grip to simulate situations like pulling the body into windows or up ropes and climbing.

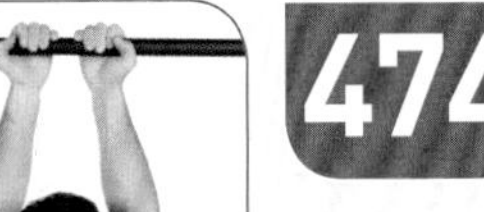

471 Close-Grip Underhand

Place your hands inside shoulder-width. Moving your hands close together leads to greater pectoral activation.

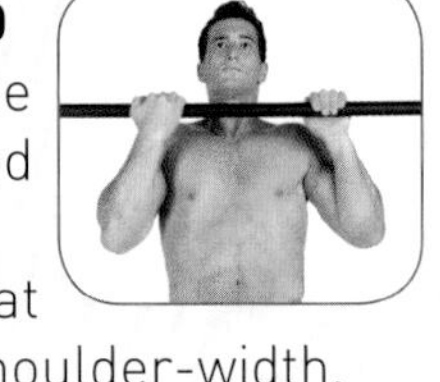

472 Alternating Grip

Place one hand on the bar using an overhand grip and the other using an underhand at slightly wider than shoulder-width. This position improves grip strength, making a great option for heavily weighted Pull-Ups.

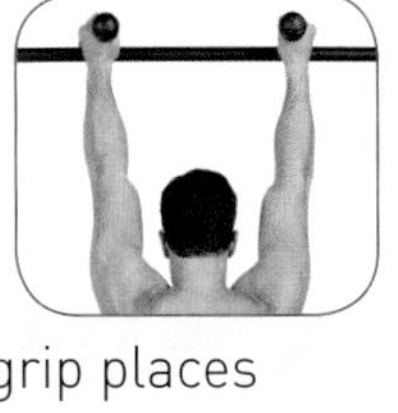

473 Neutral Grip

Place your hands shoulder-width apart, palms facing each other, on a set of parallel handles. This grip places the least amount of stress on your shoulders, and it also emphasizes the brachialis, an upper-arm muscle.

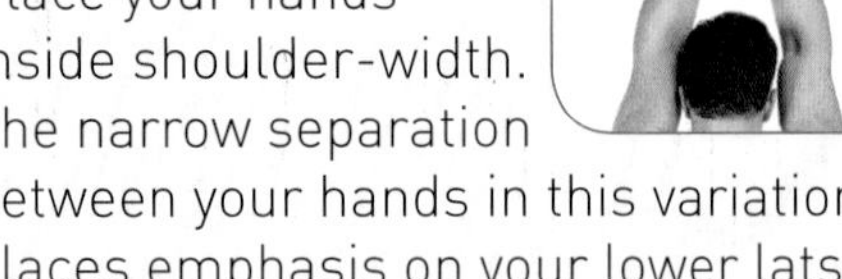

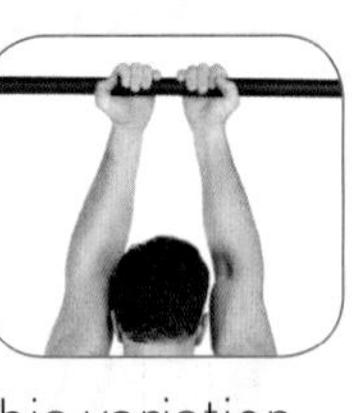

474 Close-Grip Overhand

Place your hands inside shoulder-width. The narrow separation between your hands in this variation places emphasis on your lower lats.

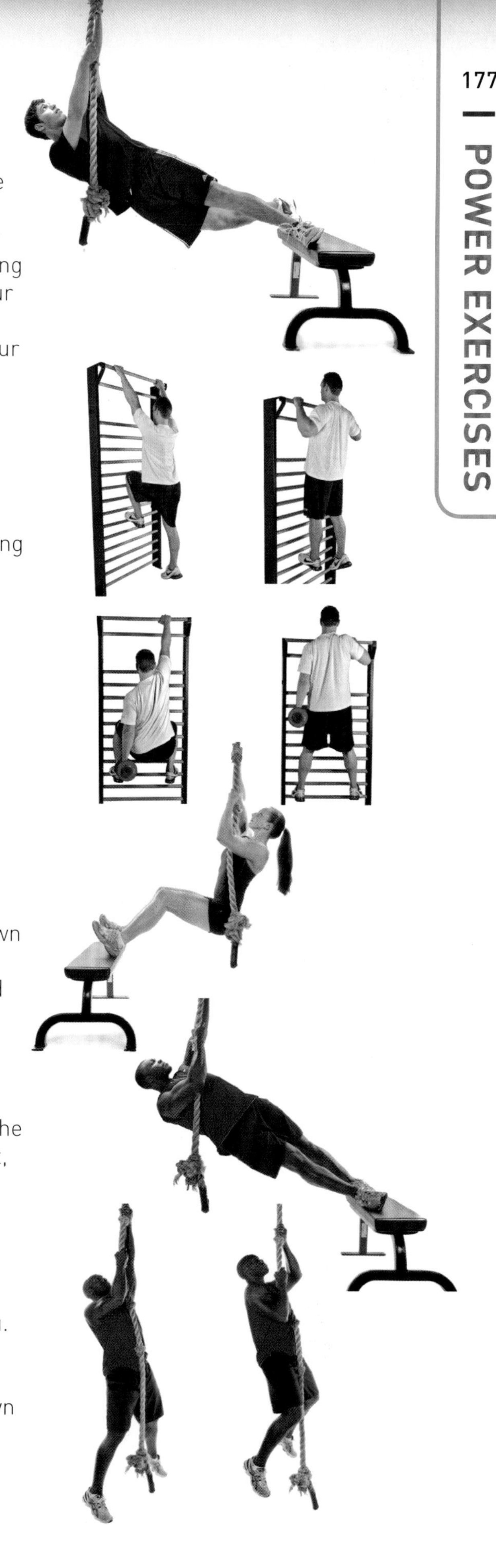

475 Drop and Pull

Stand on a bench, and grasp a rope with an alternating grip. Drop your body, and rotate to one side of the rope, moving yourself toward the floor until your arms are completely extended and your feet, hips, and torso are turned 45 degrees. Keeping your body rigid, pull on the rope while rotating your lower body and pushing into the floor with your toes until your body is adjacent to rope. Extend your arms, pushing rope away and body up, and out to return to the starting position.

476 Step Chin

On one foot, stand on a wall bar, grasping the top bar with an overhand grip. Extend your arms completely and bend the knee of the weight-bearing leg. Return by pulling your elbows down and pushing through the weight-bearing foot.

477 Dumbbell Step Chin

On one foot, stand on a lower bar of a wall bar, grasping the top pull-up bar with an overhand grip with one hand, and holding a dumbbell in the other. Perform as you would a Step Chin (#477).

478 Vertical Rope with Alternate Grip

Grasp the rope with an alternating grip, one hand in front of your chin, and the other slightly above your head. Step forward so that the rope hangs to one hip, and place your heels on a bench. Pull down on the rope while simultaneously pushing down on your heels. Be sure to keep the knees bent and torso upright throughout the movement.

479 Lateral Rope Pull

Stand on a bench, and lean at a 30-degree angle from the floor, with your feet rigid and weight on the edges of your shoes. With the rope at chest height, grasp it across your body with an alternating grip. Pull down and across your body, keeping the rope adjacent to your chest throughout movement.

480 Rope Chin

Stand on tiptoes with a rope directly in front of you. Grasp the rope with an alternating grip, one arm completely extended, and the other slightly above your head. Step forward so that the rope runs down the middle of your body. Bend your knees slightly, and then hang onto to the rope with only your hands. Pull down on the rope until your chin rises above your bottom hand.

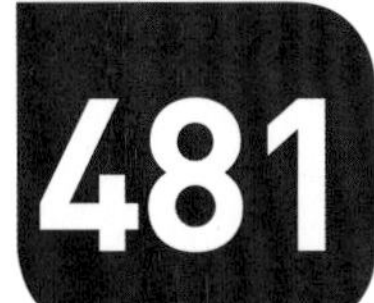

Deadlift

The Deadlift is a class bodybuilding power lift that is based on everyday movement. Just think of lifting a heavy object from the floor, hefting a laundry basket, or even picking up your toddler, and you know the mechanics of a Deadlift. You can perform it with just about any weight, form barbells to dumbbells to kettlebells to your own body weight. Its primary benefits are hip, leg, and lower-back strength, as well as improved position (posture) and range of motion (flexibility). Once you've master the basic version, try one of its many variations.

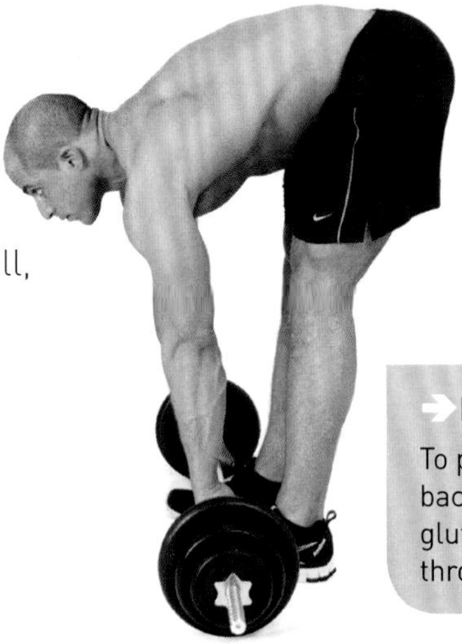

- Stand with your feet shoulder-width apart, with a barbell at your feet. Lean over to grasp the weight with both hands.
- Using your core muscles as well as your arms, raise the barbell, hinging at the hips as you slowly rise to a standing position.
- Smoothly return the barbell to the floor, again hinging at the hips. Repeat for the desired repetitions.

FIND YOUR FORM

To protect your lower back, contract your glutes and abdominals throughout the exercise.

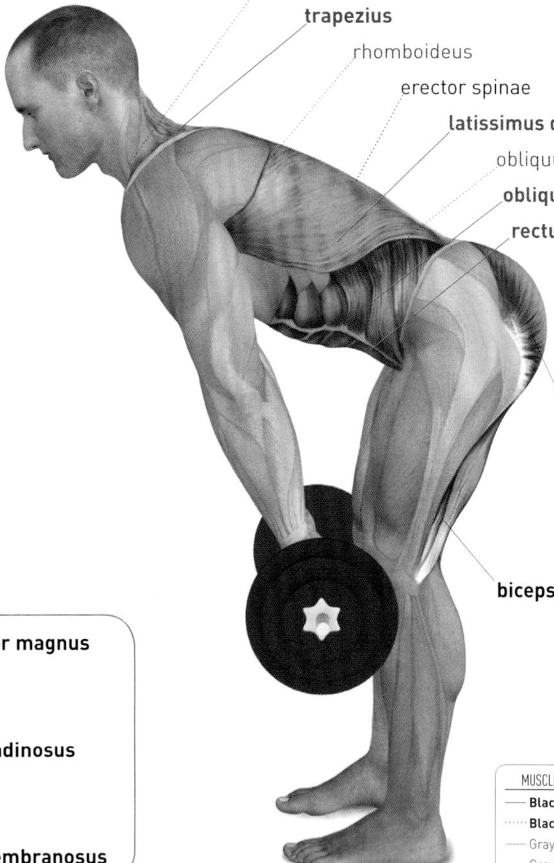

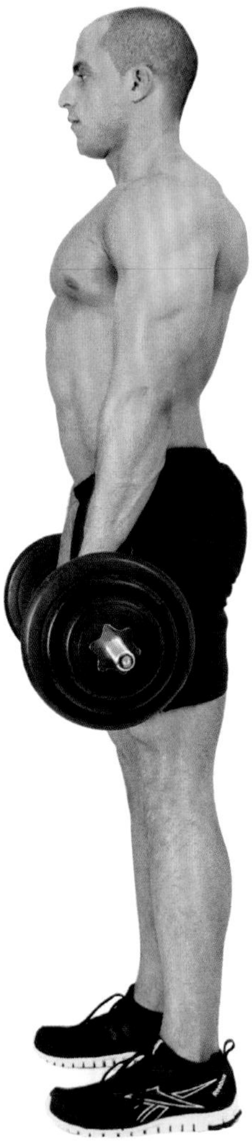

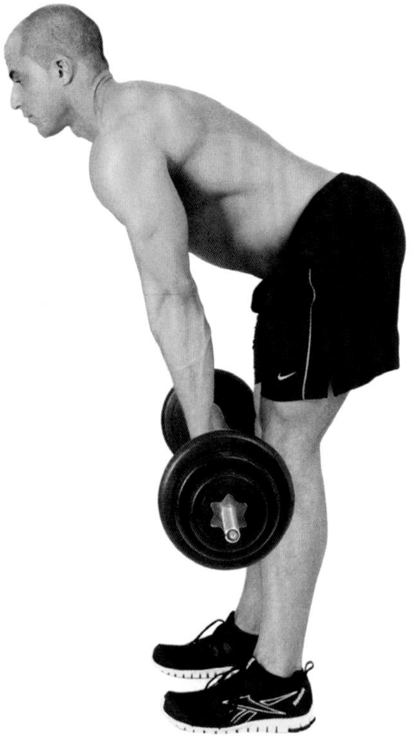

levator scapulae
trapezius
rhomboideus
erector spinae
latissimus dorsi
obliquus internus
obliquus externus
rectus abdominis
gluteus maximus
biceps femoris

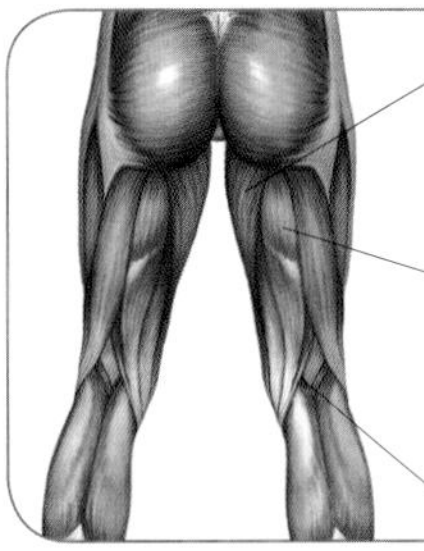

adductor magnus
semitendinosus
semimembranosus

MUSCLE ANNOTATION KEY
Black bold = primary
Black = deep primary
Gray bold = secondary
Gray = deep secondary

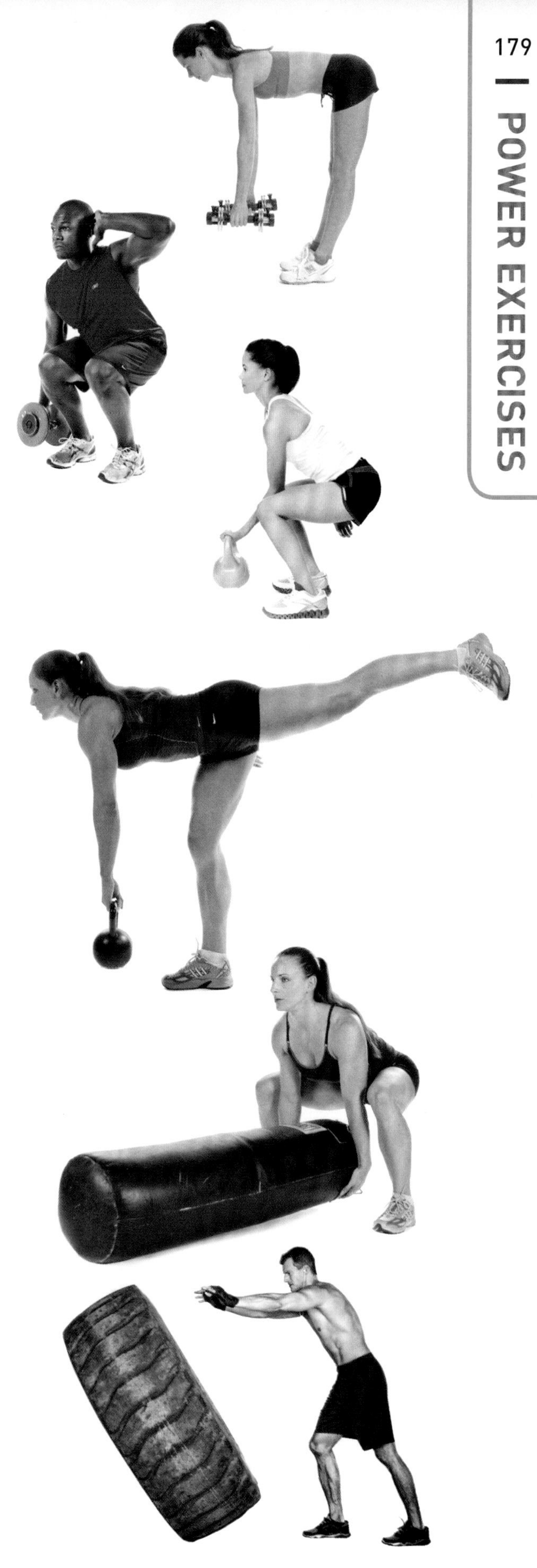

482 Dumbbell Deadlift

Stand with your feet shoulder-width apart, with a set of dumbbells at your feet. Lean over to grasp the weights with both hands, and perform as your would a Deadlift (#481).

483 Single-Arm Dumbbell Deadlift

Stand with your feet shoulder-width apart, with a dumbbell next to one foot. Lean over to grasp the weight, and perform as your would a Deadlift (#481).

484 Kettlebell Single-Arm Lift

Stand with your feet shoulder-width apart, with a kettlebell between your feet. Lean over to grasp the weight with one hand, and perform as your would a Deadlift (#481).

485 Single-Leg Straight-Leg Kettlebell Deadlift

Stand on your right leg, and keep your left slightly behind your right heel, bearing little to no weight. Hold the kettlebell in your left hand. Bend your right leg very slightly as you bend over from your hip, and reach the kettlebell toward the floor. Make sure that you keep your chest up and your back slightly arched. Your left leg remains in line with your spine throughout the exercise. Once you've touched the floor or gone as deep as you can, squeeze your glutes, hamstrings, and shoulder blades as you stand up on your right leg, while your left leg returns to starting position.

486 Sandbag Flip

Stand with your feet shoulder-width apart with a sandbag in front of you. Grasp the bag with your palms facing each another, and squat deeply. Exhale, and drive your torso upward and your hips up and forward. Push your feet into the floor, extending your knees and pulling upward on the bag, forcefully and quickly, with your upper back, shoulders, and elbows. Elevate onto your toes and follow through with your hands upward and forward away from your body, releasing the bag all in one fluid movement.

487 Tire Flip

Stand with your feet shoulder-width apart with a tractor tire in front of you, and perform as you would a Sandbag Flip (#486).

Bottoms-Up Kettlebell Clean

The Bottoms-Up Kettlebell Clean might look easy, but it really is a complicated move that takes your upper body through a range of movement that will help you burn fat and build muscle. It also helps you to develop hand strength and coordination.

- Stand upright, with your feet shoulder-width apart, holding a kettlebell in your left hand. Swing the kettlebell backward, then bring it forward and above your head forcefully, squeezing the handle as you do so.
- Once your upper arm is parallel to the floor, hold the position, and then lower your arm again. Complete the desired repetitions, and then repeat with the other arm.

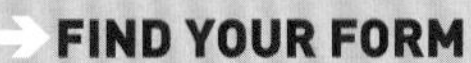

FIND YOUR FORM

Keep your upper arm close to your body as if you were tucking a purse or newspaper under your arm.

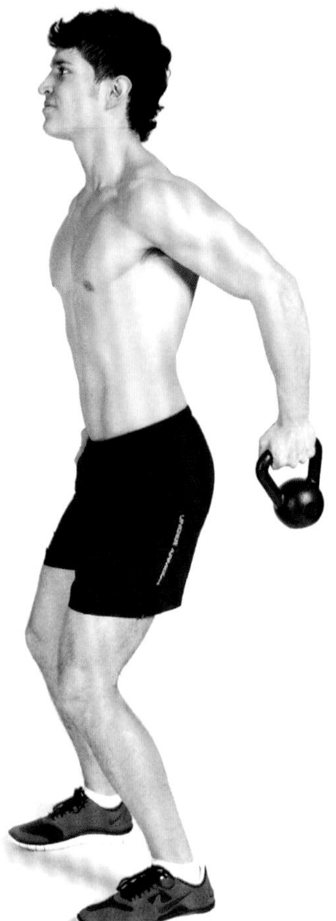

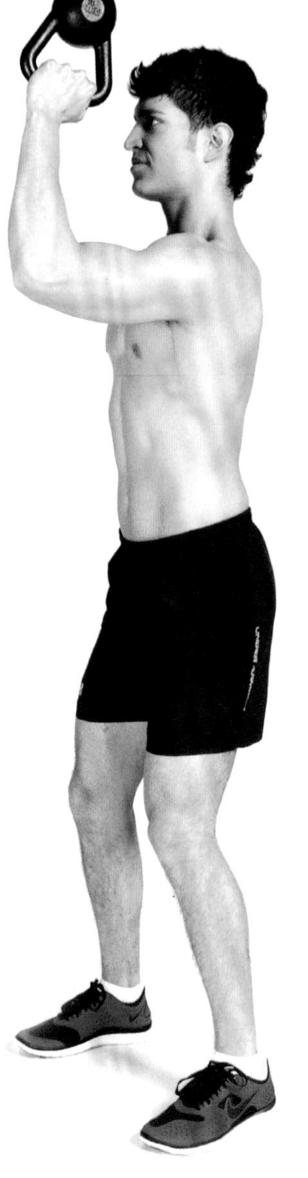

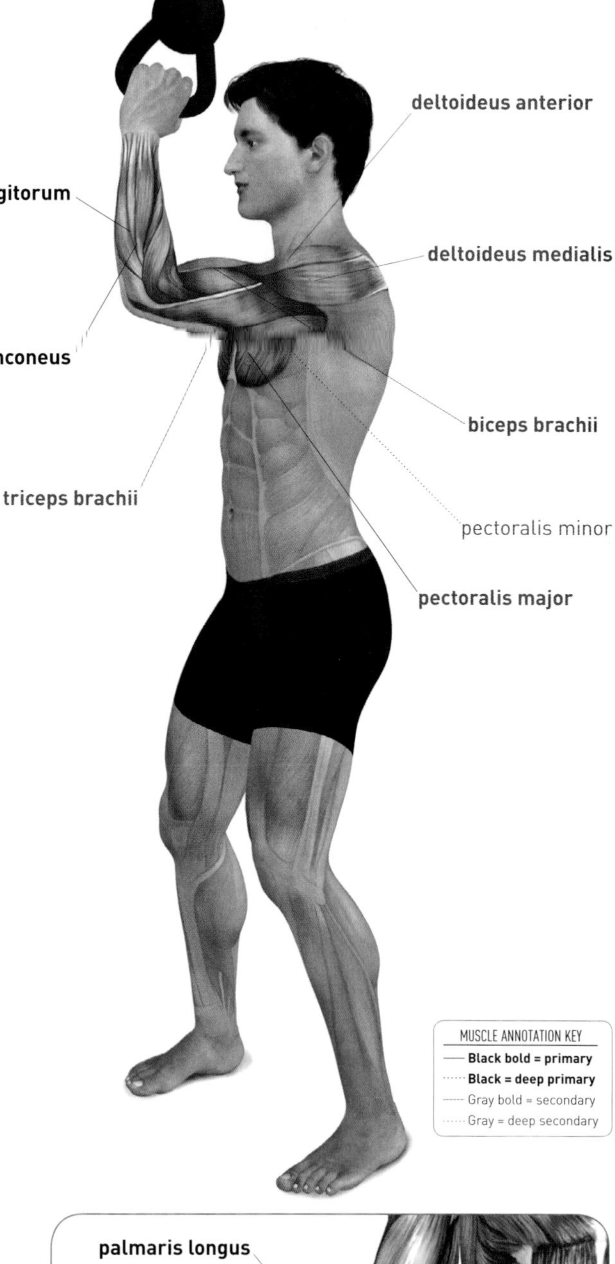

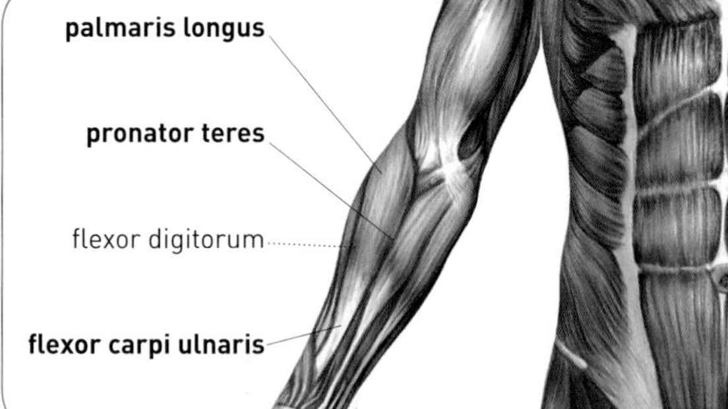

489

Body-Weight Clean

Perform as you would the Bottoms-Up Kettlebell Clean (#488) without a kettlebell,making a fist instead, being sure to contract your arm muscles throughout.

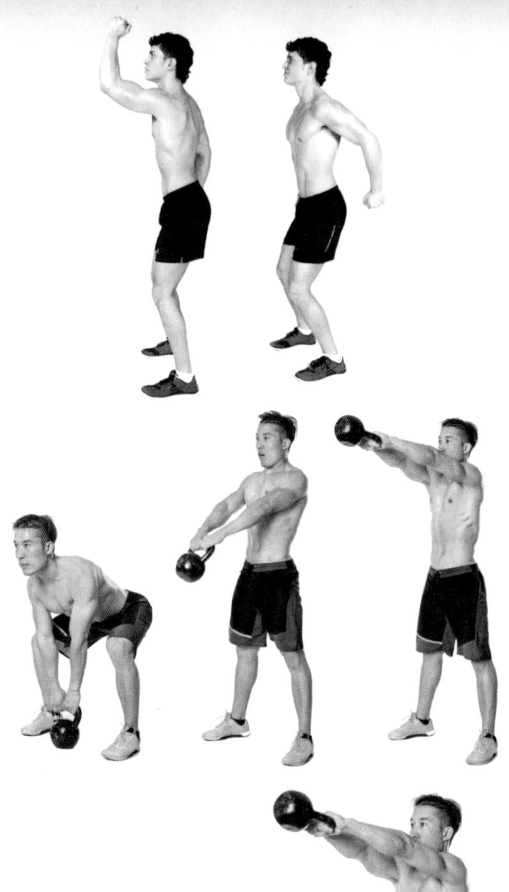

490

Kettlebell Swing

Stand over the kettlebell with your feet hip-width apart, chest up, and shoulders back and down. Squat down and grip the kettlebell with your palms facing you and your thumbs wrapped loosely around the handle. Stand tall, and then driving through your heels, explode through the hips to send the weight swinging upward from your quads, aiming to reach chest height with your arms extended. As the kettlebell begins to descend, shift your weight back into your heels while hinging at the hips and loading both the hamstrings and glutes. Receive the weight, allowing the kettlebell to ride back between your legs. As the weight makes the transition from backward to forward, drive through the heel to move into the next rep.

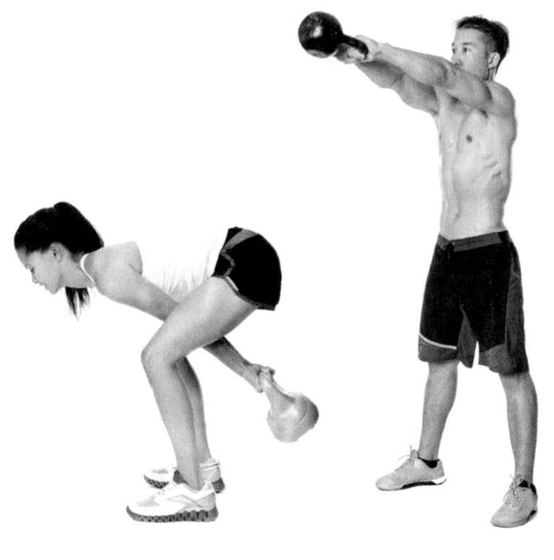

491

Kettlebell Overhead Arc

Being sure to use a weight you can safely control, perform a Kettlebell Swing (#485) bringing the weight above your head.

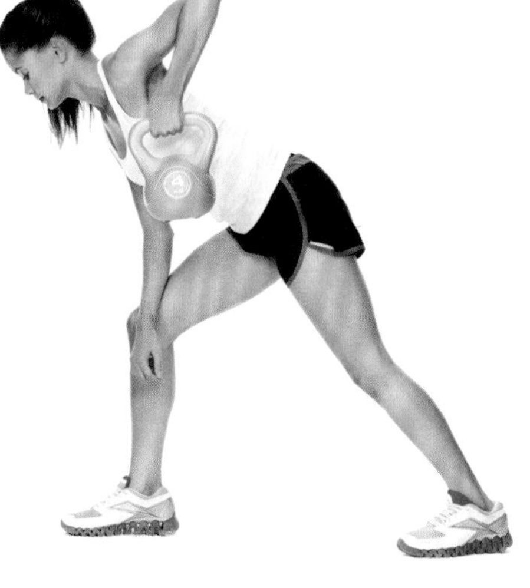

492

Kettlebell Row

Stand with your right leg extended several feet in front your, with your right leg bent, holding a kettlebell in your. Rest your right hand above your knee, and lean forward slightly. Bend your arm as you pull the weight up toward your chest. Lower, and repeat for the desired repetitions, and then repeat on the other side.

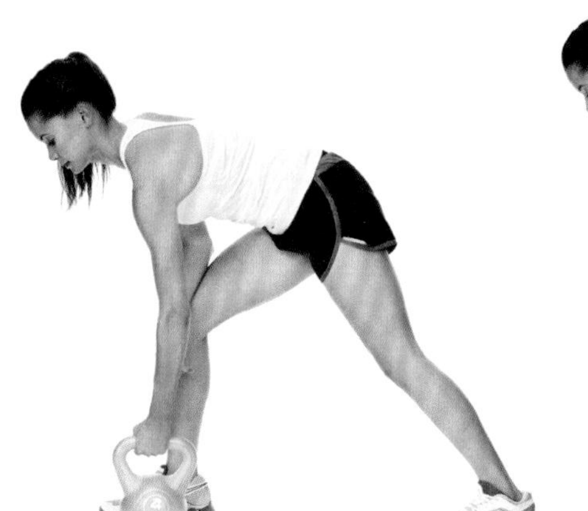

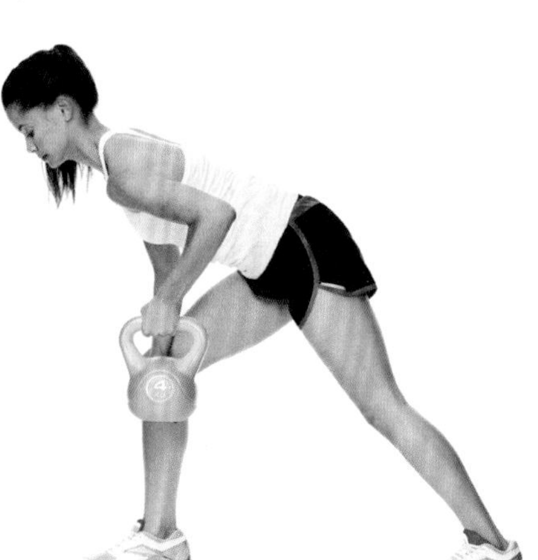

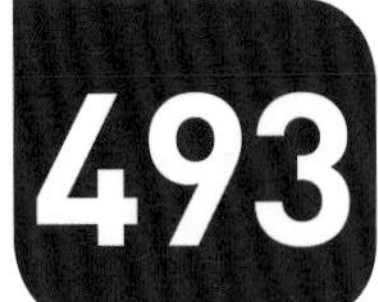

Double Kettlebell Snatch

The Kettlebell Snatch is an advanced bodybuilding move with multiple benefits: it builds strength, elevates heart rate, and increases mobility. Work with a trainer for the best results, so that you learn proper lockout form and how to execute it for your goals—performing it quickly with lighter weights reaps maximum volume of oxygen benefits, while using heavier weights at low speeds results in full-body strength.

- Stand with your feet a little more than shoulder-width apart, holding a pair of kettlebells at your sides.
- Squat down, leaning forward slightly and sticking out your buttocks. Bring your arms between your legs, so that the kettlebells are next to your inner thighs.
- In one swift and determined movement, drive through your hips and swing the kettlebells overhead. Lower and repeat for the desired repetitions.

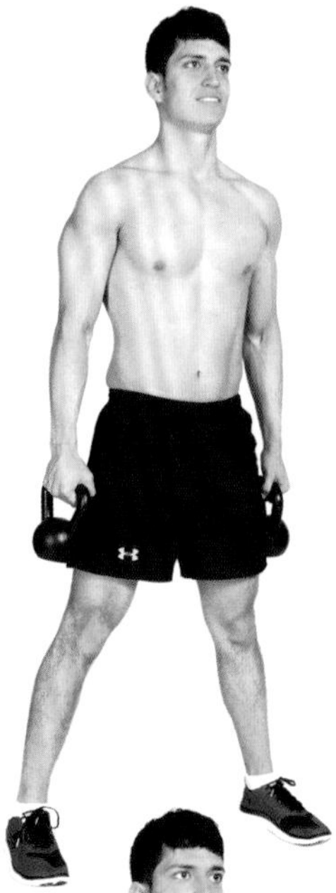

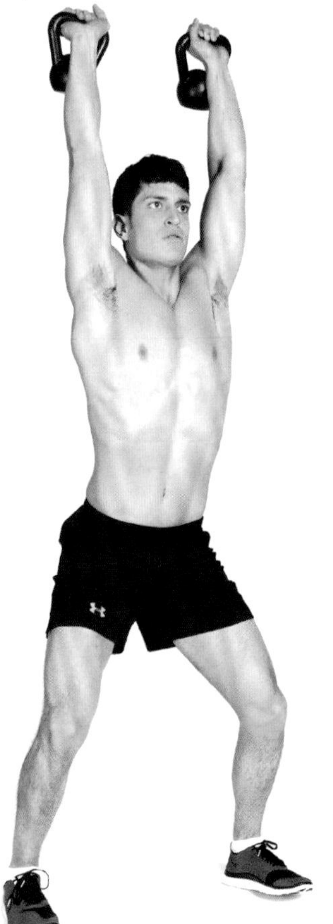

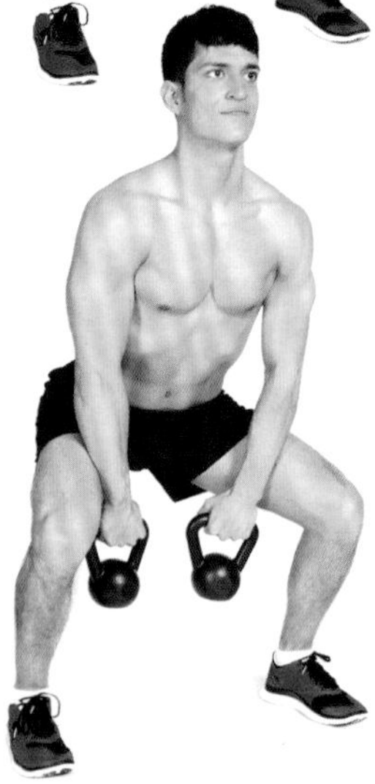

➔ FIND YOUR FORM

As you swing the bell upward, shrug your shoulders backward, which will pull the weights closer to your body, making then feel lighter when they reach the apex.

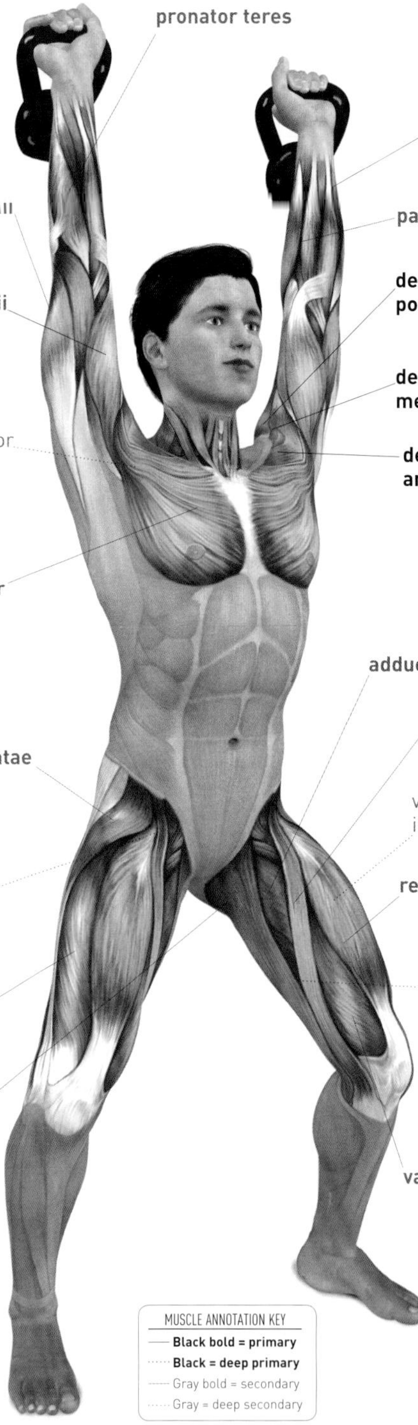

Clean and Press

Another classic bodybuilding power lift, the Clean and Press focuses on your shoulder muscles, but also works your trapezius, triceps, middle and lower back, abdominals, glutes, quadriceps, hamstrings, and calves—making it a highly effective full-body exercise. As well as building lean muscle, the challenging lift will also help you increase your endurance.

- Assume a high squatting position so that your upper legs are parallel with the floor. Hold a body bar in front of you, arms straight.
- Using the muscles in your legs as well as your abdominals, rise to stand as you bend your arms to bring the bar to shoulder height. If you choose, extend one foot in front of the other.
- Move your feet to parallel position, hip-width or wider apart, and bring the body bar above your head. Hold for several seconds.
- Focus on breath and alignment as you bring the bar down to shoulder height in a controlled manner.
- Repeat the lift overhead and the controlled lowering for the desired repetitions.

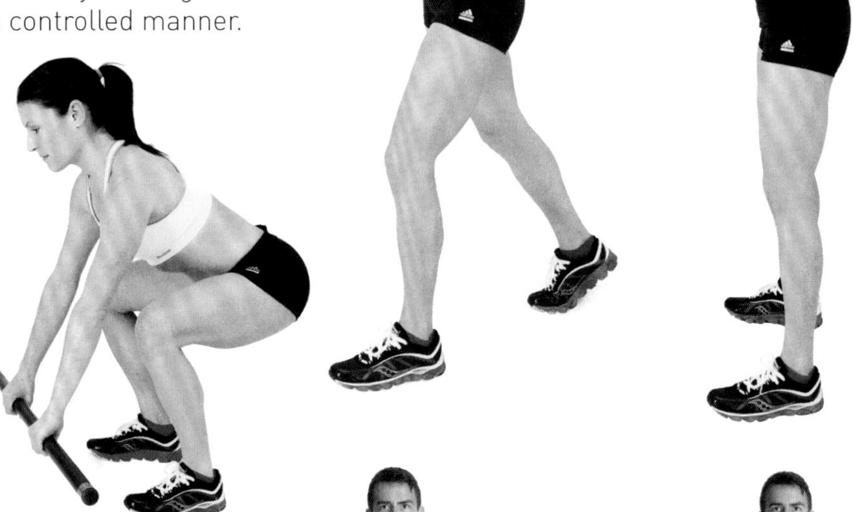

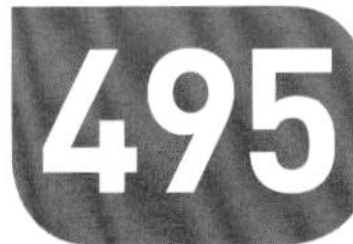

Lateral Raise

Standing with your feet together, holding a dumbbell in each hand with your arms extended at your sides. Keeping your elbows and knees slightly bent, raise your arms out to your sides in wide arcs to about shoulder level. Slowly return to the starting position. Repeat for the desired repetitions. Lifting laterally activates your posterior deltoids and upper-back muscles.

496 4-Count Overhead

The 4-Count Overhead draws its inspiration from special forces stamina/endurance training exercises that call for teams to work in convert under a log to perform a variety of moves, including overhead presses, while instructors call the steps. The 4-Count Overhead. Performed to a steady four-count beat, simulates this kind of training while it works the muscles of your shoulders.

- Stand with your feet hip-width apart. With both hands, grasp a dumbbell of any weight you can press overhead, and bring it to your right shoulder. This is your starting position.
- Press the weight overhead with your arms straight for count 1.
- Lower the weight to your left shoulder for count 2.
- Press the weight overhead with your arms straight for 3.
- Lower the weight to your right shoulder for count 4. Each time the weight touches your right shoulder equals one repetition.

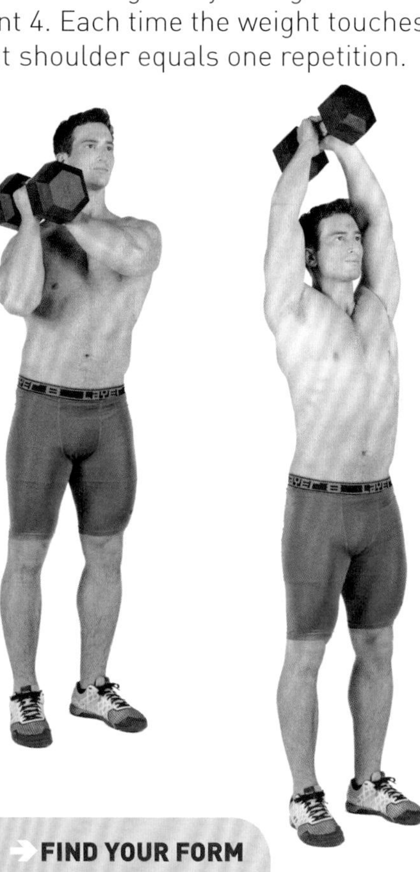

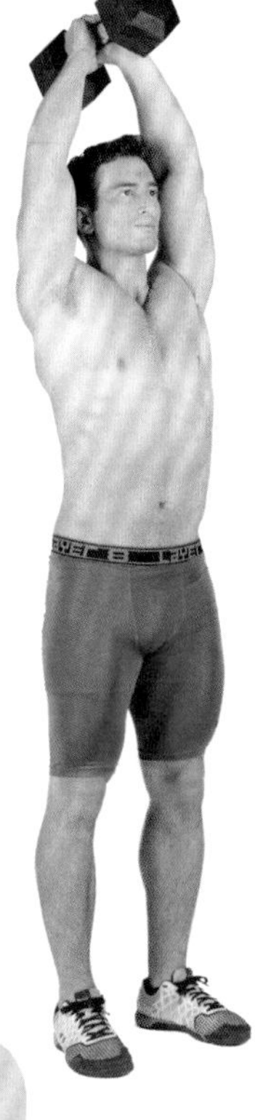

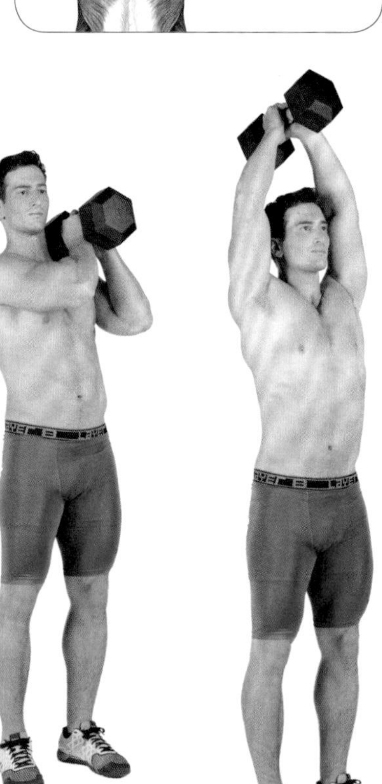

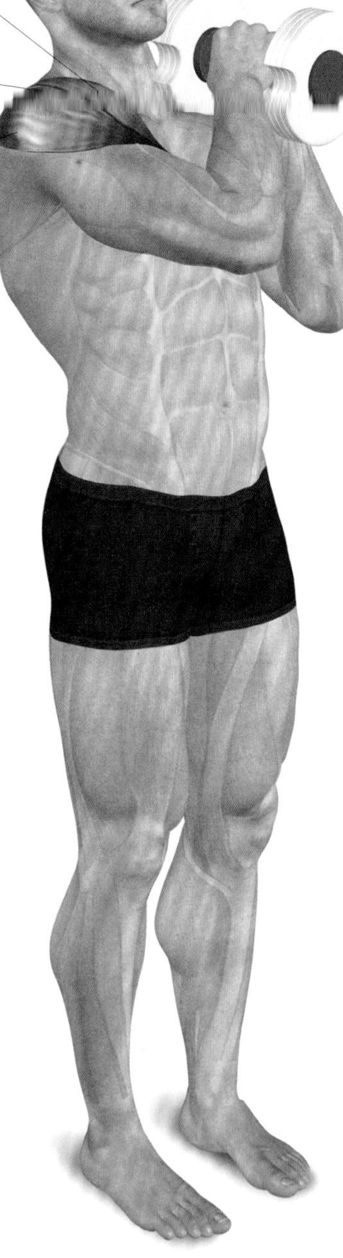

FIND YOUR FORM
Maintain and steady beat, moving quickly but with control.

497 Barbell Row

Stand with your toes pointing slightly outward, holding a barbell with both hands using an underhand grip. Keeping your lower back straight, bend your knees slightly, and hinge forward at the hips. Lead with your elbows, pulling them toward the ceiling until the bar reaches the level of your upper waist. Return the bar to the floor, so that your arms are fully extended and your shoulders are stretched downward. Repeat for the desired repetitions.

498 Upright Barbell Row

The upright row moves the target upward to the trapezius muscles of your upper back, neck, and shoulders and also works the deltoids and biceps. The narrower the grip, the greater the emphasis on the traps. Stand upright grasping a barbell with a shoulder-width or slightly narrower overhand grip. With your elbows leading, pull the bar upward to neck height, allowing your wrists to flex as the bar rises. Lower the bar to the starting position. Repeat for the desired repetitions.

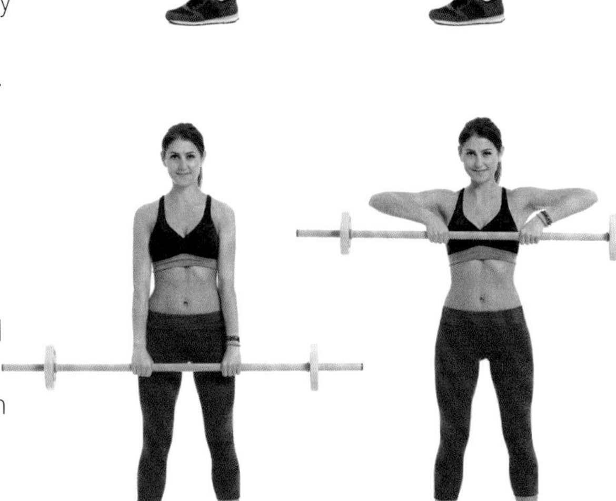

499 Sledgehammers

Stand in front of a tractor tire with your feet in a staggered stance about shoulder-width apart. Hold a sledgehammer, with one hand on the top of the handle and the other near the bottom. Rotate the hammer until it gets aligned directly over your head. At the point when the hammer feels weightless overhead, drop your hips downward as your top hand slides toward the bottom of the hammer. Catch the hammer up high on the rebound, and then repeat for the desired alternating your hand position to work each side.

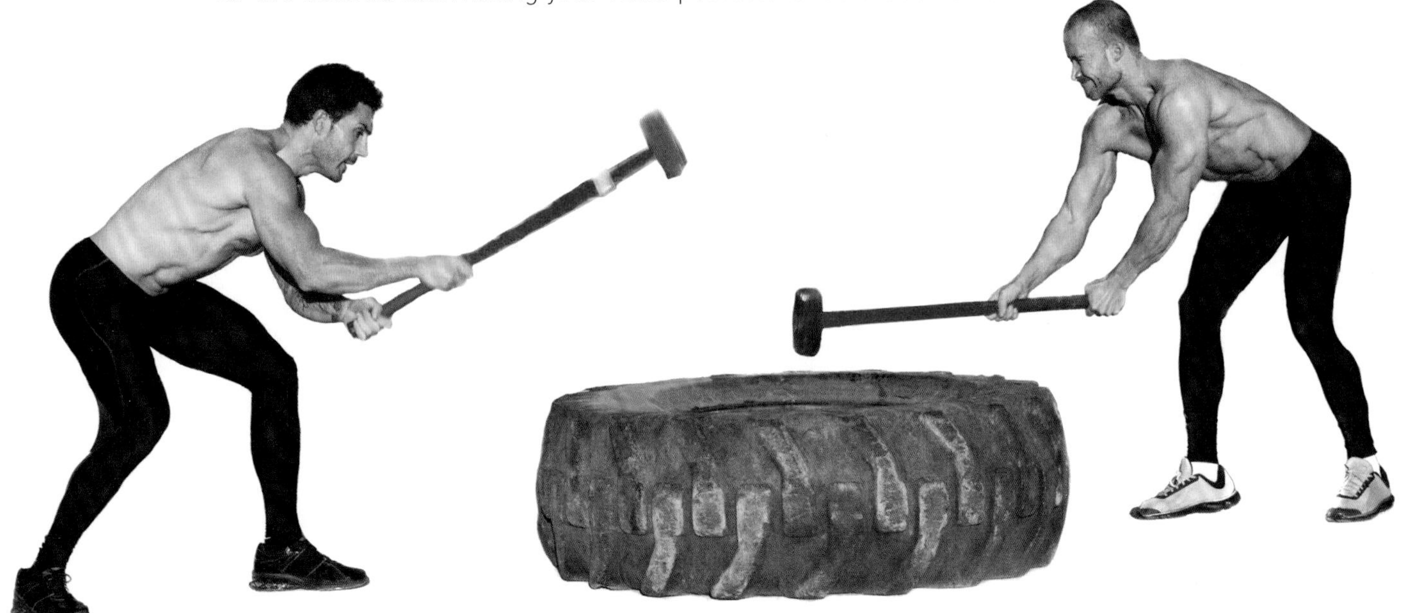

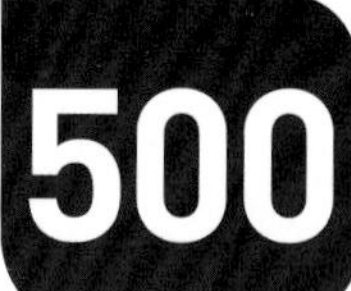

Shoulder Crusher

As its name implies, the Shoulder Crusher zeros in on your deltoids to give your shoulders an grueling, intense workout. Like many boot camp training exercises, it calls for you to perform a series of positions in rapid succession to the beat of a count. Each position of the counts can be called as a command in any sequence, or you can perform the counts in the order listed below.

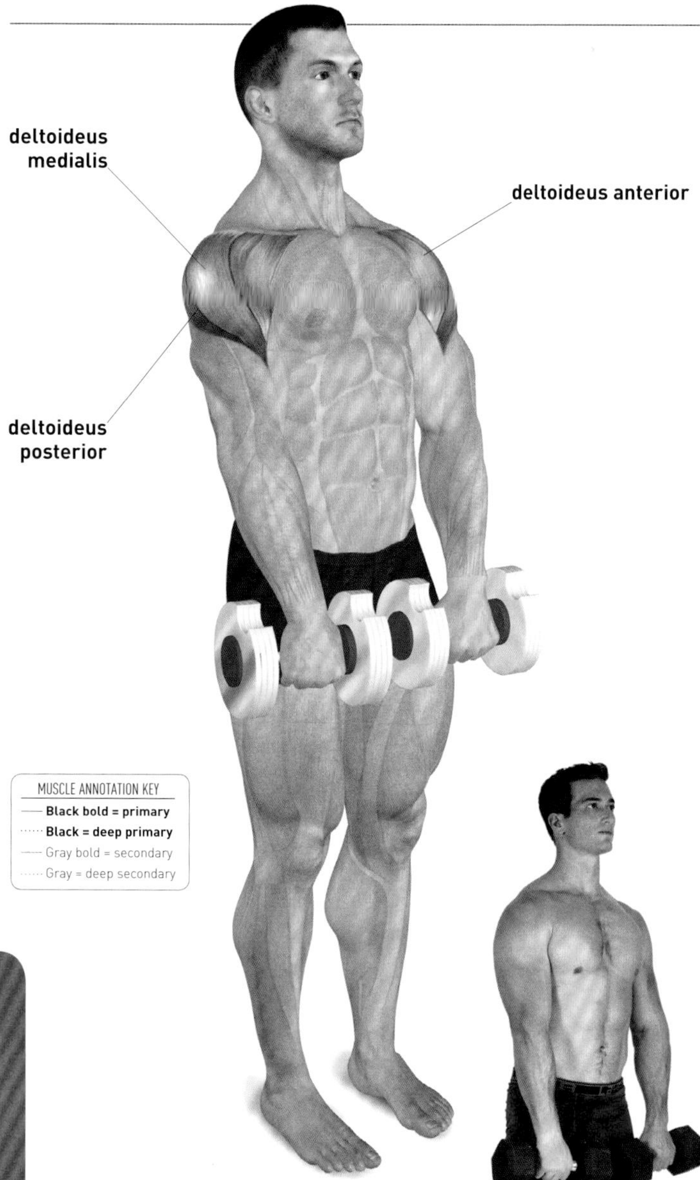

deltoideus medialis

deltoideus anterior

deltoideus posterior

MUSCLE ANNOTATION KEY
Black bold = primary
Black = deep primary
Gray bold = secondary
Gray = deep secondary

- Start with a dumbbell in each hand resting at the front of your thighs.
- Bring your hands to your chest for count 1.
- Move your arms straight out in front of your body at chest level for count 2.
- Keeping your arms straight, bring your hands overhead, and hold for count 3.
- Lower the weight to your shoulders, and hold for count 4.
- Press your arms overhead, and hold for count 5.
- Keeping your arms straight, bring them back in front of your chest for count 6.
- Pull your hands into the chest for count 7.
- Drop your arms to the front of each thigh for count 8. Each time your hands hit your thighs equals one rep. Perform all steps for the desired repetitions.

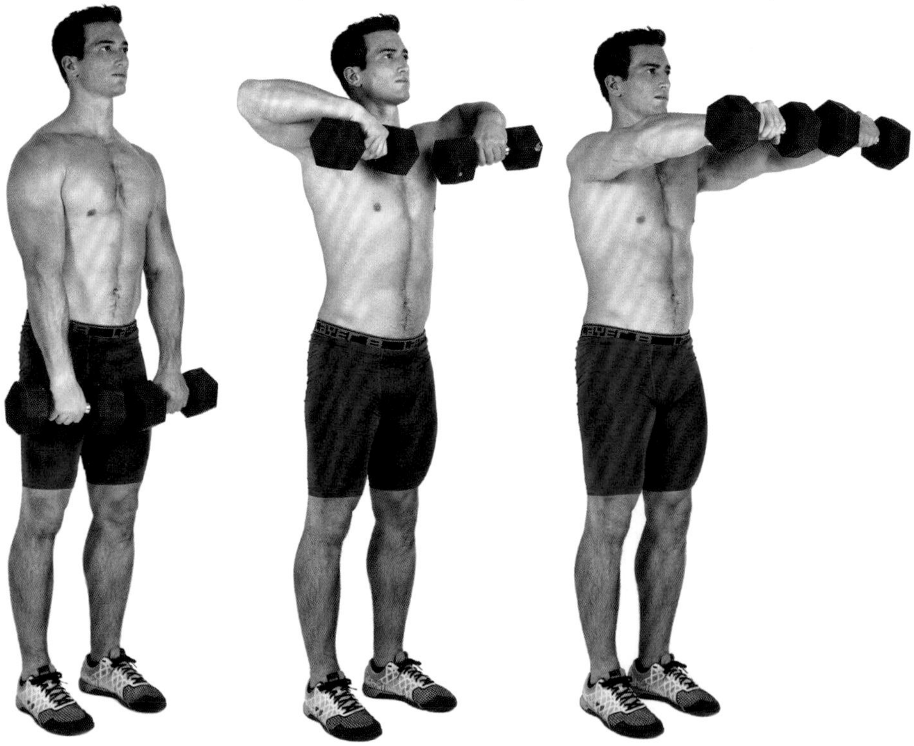

➔ FIND YOUR FORM

When bringing the dumbbells overhead, make sure that your hands are directly overhead and not in front of your center of gravity. Be sure to work with a weight that is not too heavy for your strength level.

Military Press

Stand holding a dumbbell in each hand, and raise them to shoulder level with palms facing out and elbows bent. Press the weights up and toward each other as you straighten your arms, keeping a slight bend in your elbows at the top. Slowly bring down the weights, and return to the starting position.

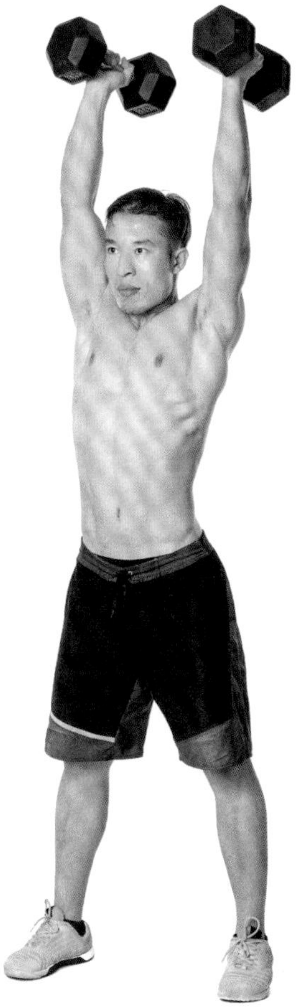

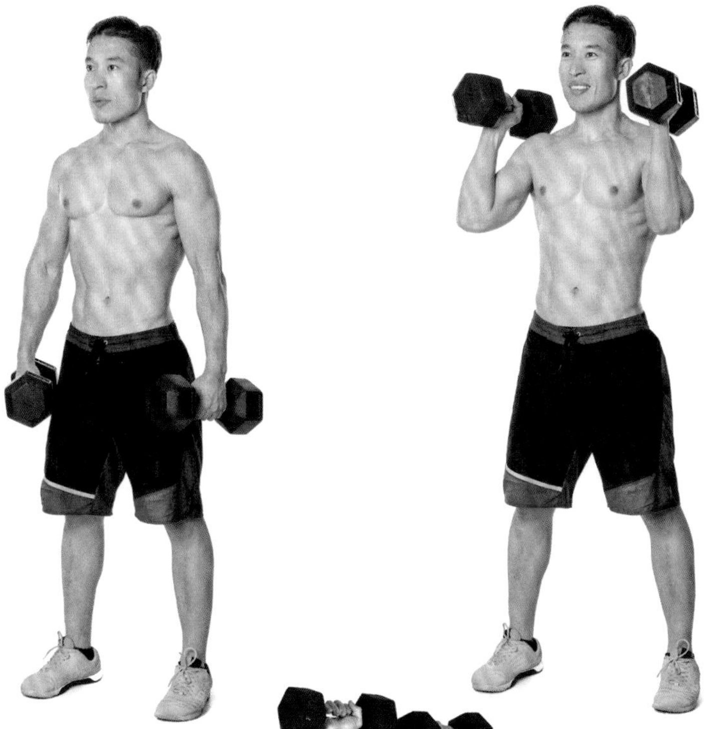

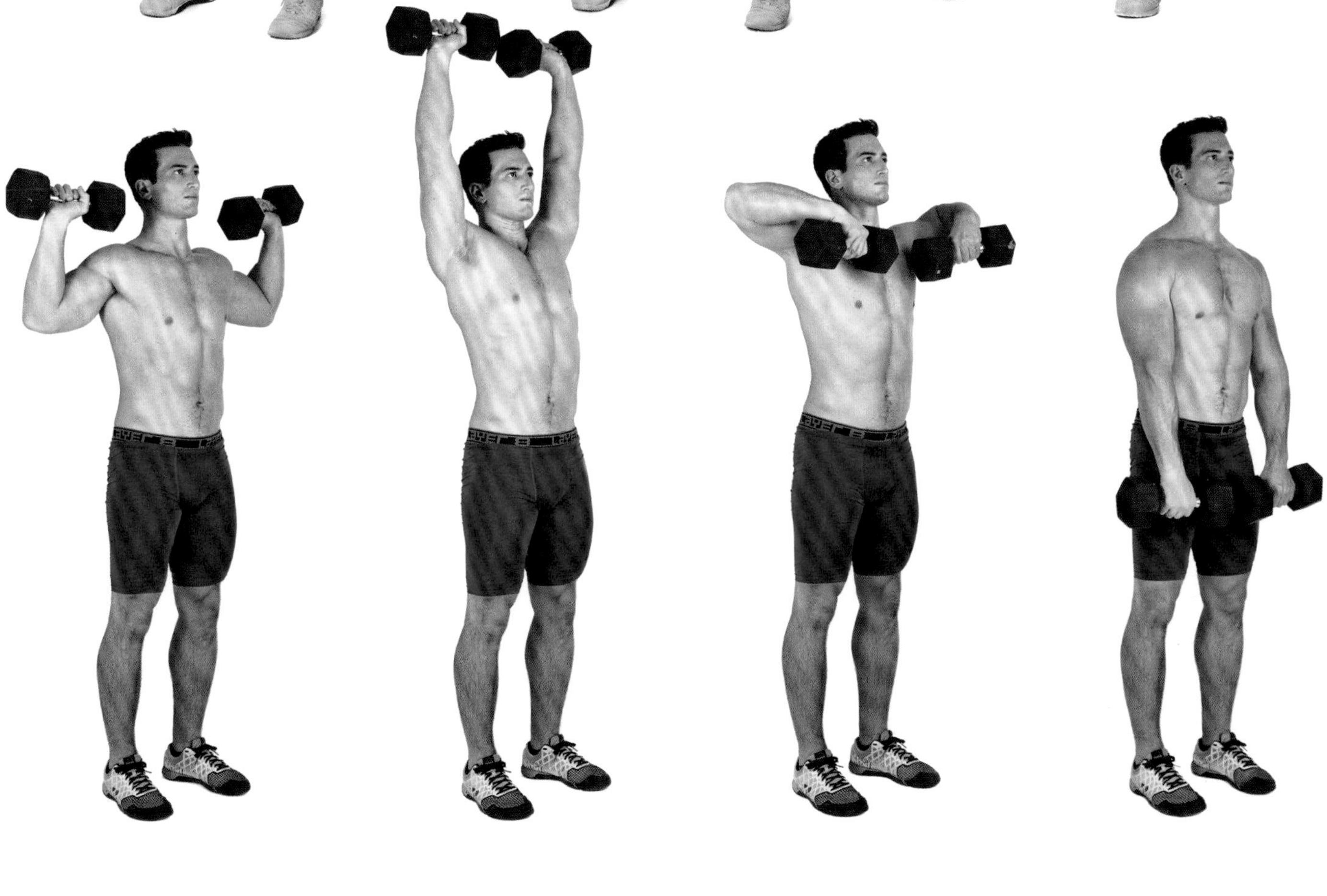

ALPHABETICAL INDEX

N–O–P

R

S

CREDITS & ACKNOWLEDGMENTS

Illustration Credits

All anatomical illustrations by Hector Diaz/3DLabz Animation Limited

Insets by Linda Bucklin/Shutterstock.com

Photography Credits

NAILA RUECHEL

Title page, 022, 024, 031, 037, 038, 043, 047, 048, 049, 050, 051, 055, 059, 066, 067, 072, 074, 075, 077, 078, 079, 082, 092, 097, 098, 101, 102, 105, 110, 112, 115, 116, 119, 124, 125, 134, 137, 138, 140, 146, 149, 162, 167, 168, 170, 171, 173, 174, 175, 176, 179, 180, 181, 182, 184, 185, 187, 188, 190, 192, 196, 212, 213, 215, 217, 218, 219, 220, 221, 222, 223, 224, 225, 253, 254, 263, 264, 268, 274, 278, 279, 283, 304, 307, 334, 338, 340, 341, 342, 344, 362, 379, 381, 382, 383, 384, 385, 386, 387, 388, 389, 390, 398, 400, 418, 430, 441, 442, 449, 450, 456, 464, 469, 470, 471, 472, 473, 474, 496, 500

JONATHAN CONKLIN PHOTOGRAPHY

004, 011, 016, 032, 039, 040, 041, 045, 046, 076, 091, 099, 100, 113, 169, 177, 183, 204, 206, 207, 209, 231, 232, 236, 237, 238, 247, 252, 257, 258, 260, 269, 270, 273, 275, 276, 277, 290, 293, 299, 303, 311, 313, 317, 318, 319, 320, 322, 324, 329, 336, 337, 339, 343, 347, 350, 359, 360, 361, 363, 364, 366, 371, 372, 373, 374, 377, 391, 392, 393, 394, 395, 396, 397, 399, 401, 402, 403, 404, 405, 406, 407, 408, 409, 413, 414, 416, 417, 420, 424, 427, 429, 431, 432, 434, 435, 437, 438, 446, 446, 451, 452, 453, 455, 457, 458, 460, 462, 463, 468, 475, 476, 477, 478, 479, 480, 482, 483, 485, 486

FINE ARTS PHOTOGRAPHY GROUP

005, 006, 017, 018, 023, 042, 057, 063, 064, 065, 085, 086, 096, 097, 106, 107, 108, 118, 123, 130, 131, 132, 133, 144, 150, 151, 155, 178, 198, 199, 200, 201, 202, 203, 205, 227, 233, 267, 280, 281, 294, 308, 321, 330, 331, 345, 346, 365, 368, 369, 378, 436, 439, 459, 465, 466, 481, 488, 489, 493, 494

ROBERT WRIGHT

104, 114, 250, 292, 433

The following photos courtesy Shutterstock.com

1759443 Ontario Incorporated 239; 2xSamara.com page 129 box; Ahturner 156; Alan Poulson Photography 234, 255, 261, 312; Andrew Rafalsky 243, 244; Angela Aladro mella page 83 box; Apollofoto 121, 287, 288; baranq 159; Billion Photos 356; Catalin Petolea 230; Claire McAdams 164; Comaniciu Dan 087; Creativa Images 354; cristovao 002; Dana Heinemann 422; Daniel_Dash 411, 412, 421, 428; Daxiao Productions 484, 492; Dean Drobot page 10–11 introduction, 012, 161, 228, 265, 302, 454; Dmytro Zinkovych 251, 262, Egor Tetiushev page 139 box; Elnur 053, 089,152; Eviled 289; FeyginFotolSS page 91 box; fizkes 080, 083, 084, 090, 285, 298, 305, 367, 425; GG Pro Photo139; Halfpoint 241; holbox page 10 introduction, 189, 240, 426, 499, 423; Julenochek 248; Kinga 410; Kzenon Chapter One opener, page 8 introduction, 015; LifetimeStock 165, 166; lipik 014, 271, 272, 306, 349, 358; Ljupco Smokovski 147; Lucky Business page 11 instroduction, 103, 127,136; Luis Molinero 044; Maksim Shmeljov 069, 088; Maridav 467; Mihai Blanaru page 9 introduction, 003, 008, 013, 019, 020, 021, 025, 026, 027, 028, 033, 034, 035, 052, 054, 058, 060, 061, 062, 068, 073, 081, 093, 094, 095, 126, 128, 129, 135, 141, 143, 145, 148, 158, 160, 172, 191, 194, 195, 210, 229, 259, 295, 296, 297, 300, 301, 309, 310, 315, 316, 323, 325, 326, 327, 328, 332, 333, 351, 353, 357, 370, 375, 376, 380, 440, 444, 447, 461, 498; mtphoto19 Chapter Two inset; nanka 284; Nicholas Piccillo 348, 445, 495; ostill 036; PanicAttack 286; Petar Djordjevic 007, 111, 153, 214, 443; Piotr Marcinski 109, 355,142; Producer 314; Real Deal Photo 211, 448; Rommel Canlas 163; Ronald Sumners page 85 box; ruigsantos 010, 030; Serghei Starus 235; Skydive Erick 415; spwidoff page 37 box; Stanislaw Tokarski page 109 box; Stefano Cavoretto 242; studioloco 001, 009, 029, 249, 497; Syda Productions Chapter Two opener, 120, 122; Tom Kuest - Fotograf 282, 487; Vaclav Volrab 056; Vadim Martynenko 157; Vereshchagin Dmitry Chapter One inset; Ververidis Vasilis page 18 box; Viktor

Acknowledgments

Moseley Road and photographer Naila Ruechel would like to thank models Yesenia Linares, Roya Carreras, Fahmida Molla, Philip Chan, and Alex Geissbuhler for giving this project their all.